Perception, Cognition, and Decision Training

The Quiet Eye in Action

Joan N. Vickers, PhD

University of Calgary

Human Kinetics

Library of Congress Cataloging-in-Publication Data

Vickers, Joan N., 1945-
  Perception, cognition, and decision training : the quiet eye in action / Joan N. Vickers.
    p. cm.
  Includes bibliographical references and index.
  ISBN-13: 978-0-7360-4256-7 (hard cover)
  ISBN-10: 0-7360-4256-3 (hard cover)
  1. Sports--Physiological aspects. 2. Sports--Psychological aspects. 3. Visual perception. I. Title.
  RC1236.E38V53 2007
  613.7'11--dc22

                                2006103463

ISBN-10: 0-7360-4256-3
ISBN-13: 978-0-7360-4256-7

The Web addresses cited in this text were current as of 3/7/07 unless otherwise noted.

Acquisitions Editor: Judy Patterson Wright, PhD; **Developmental Editor:** Amanda S. Ewing; **Assistant Editors:** Melissa McCasky and Heather M. Tanner; **Copyeditor:** Alisha Jeddeloh; **Proofreader:** Pamela Johnson; **Indexer:** Michael Ferreira; **Permission Manager:** Carly Breeding; **Graphic Designer:** Nancy Rasmus; **Cover Designer:** Robert Reuther; **Photographer (cover):** Frank Fife/AFP/Getty; **Photographer (interior):** Joan N. Vickers, unless otherwise noted; **Photo Asset Manager:** Laura Fitch; **Visual Production Assistant:** Joyce Brumfield; **Photo Office Assistant:** Jason Allen; **Art Manager:** Kelly Hendren; **Illustrator:** Mic Greenberg; **Printer:** Sheridan Books

Printed in the United States of America   10 9 8 7 6 5 4 3

The paper in this book is certified under a sustainable forestry program.

Human Kinetics
Web site: www.HumanKinetics.com

United States: Human Kinetics
P.O. Box 5076
Champaign, IL 61825-5076
800-747-4457
e-mail: humank@hkusa.com

Canada: Human Kinetics
475 Devonshire Road, Unit 100
Windsor, ON N8Y 2L5
800-465-7301 (in Canada only)
e-mail: info@hkcanada.com

Europe: Human Kinetics
107 Bradford Road
Stanningley
Leeds LS28 6AT, United Kingdom
+44 (0)113 255 5665
e-mail: hk@hkeurope.com

Australia: Human Kinetics
57A Price Avenue
Lower Mitcham, South Australia 5062
08 8372 0999
e-mail: info@hkaustralia.com

New Zealand: Human Kinetics
P.O. Box 80
Torrens Park, South Australia 5062
0800 222 062
e-mail: info@hknewzealand.com

CONTENTS

For the past 25 years I have focused my research on the visual system and the role of gaze and attention in sport performance. I had a good start, taking courses and seminars from some of the world's greatest cognitive psychologists: Anne Treisman, discoverer of feature integration theory; Daniel Kahneman, whose research in decision making won the Nobel Prize in 2002; and Stan Coren, a superb perception psychologist who taught me about doing research on eye movements.

Despite these wonderful beginnings, I left my doctoral program a committed follower of James Gibson, founder of ecological psychology. From the start I was determined to study the gaze of athletes as Gibson advised—in real-action worlds where the invariants, affordances, and other optic clues underlying elite performance lay. I fully expected to find support for Gibson's ideas, but in my first experiments with elite actors (athletes), I did not find eye movements that occurred quickly and without apparent thought. Instead, in both slow- and fast-paced tests, they fixated the critical cues in their sport environments both earlier and longer than did those with lower skill levels. There was also an elegance and efficiency in their gaze (even amidst the hustle and bustle of their sport worlds) that I called the "quiet eye." The quiet eye has since been identified in a range of motor tasks, and in *Perception, Cognition, and Decision Training*, I share that information with you. Once a hidden world, the gaze of the performing athlete is now known. It is an exciting world, one where old mysteries are set aside and new insights gained.

At the same time as I was carrying out my gaze research in sport, I worked extensively with coaches and sport leaders in applying what I was learning to the sport setting. I have had the opportunity to work with those who have trained many Olympic and world champions, and they often comment that at the highest level, everyone is fit, strong, and able. Instead, what matters most during those final high-pressure contests is the ability to focus on what is most important and make the right decisions at the right time while physically performing at the maximum level. Successful athletes are able to focus and make the best decisions under all the conditions they encounter in their sports.

I have therefore structured *Perception, Cognition, and Decision Training: The Quiet Eye in Action* to focus on the following questions that are often asked by those involved in research and preparation of elite athletes:

➤ What are the dominant theories that explain the neural and psychological aspects of motor performance?

➤ What is the role of the visual system in motor performance? In particular, how does the control of the gaze affect attention (or vice versa), and what does this mean in terms of sport outcomes?

➤ How is the brain organized to process visual information, and how is this used to control physical movements?

➤ How is the gaze of the performing athlete recorded and analyzed?

➤ Does the gaze of an elite athlete differ from a nonelite athlete?

➤ How is the gaze controlled in targeting tasks, in interceptive timing tasks, and in tactical tasks, and how does this affect sport outcomes?

➤ What is the quiet eye and why has it emerged as an important predictor of sport performance?

➤ What do we know about decision making in sport settings? How does the control of the gaze affect decision making in sport?

➤ What is meant by the paradox in modern motor learning research? Why does this paradox provide guidance in terms of how to provide instruction, design practices, and give feedback to athletes?

➤ Is there a systematic way that all this new literature (from perception, cognition, neuroscience, vision, gaze control, dynamic systems, and motor learning) can be incorporated into a comprehensive model that is effective in improving athletes' decision making?

As is evident from this list of questions, *Perception, Cognition, and Decision Training: The Quiet Eye in Action* concentrates on motor performance, which in this book is narrowly defined according to the outcome of the motor task (success or failure). This approach differs from the expertise approach, which describes how experts in sport differ from novices, but does not describe the specific gaze, attention, and motor characteristics that define success and failure in sport. An attempt has been made to bring together in one book as many perception–action and vision-in-action studies where the gaze and motor behavior of sport performers have been studied during successful and unsuccessful performance. The compilation of this information is designed to help students understand how humans optimally control their focus and attention and make decisions not only in sport but also in all areas where there is a need to perform physical skills at a high level.

Organization

Perception, Cognition, and Decision Training is a unique mixture of cognitive science, ecological psychology, dynamic systems, and the constraints-led approach to perception and action. What athletes see when they perform is influenced by three factors: the inherent limits of their visuomotor system, factors imposed by specific task constraints, and factors they impose as a result of their understanding (or misunderstanding) of the task at hand. Understanding how these constraints function in real-world sport environments opens a new level of understanding of what underlies optimal decision making in human performance. The general characteristics of the quiet eye are identified, along with a selection of tasks where they have been found.

Part I is Visual Perception, Cognition, and Action. Chapter 1 focuses on the visual system and the parts of the brain used in the processing of visual information. Two information-processing systems are emphasized, one best suited for processing information for short durations and the other for long durations. Each perspective is characterized by several emerging dichotomies: focal and ambient vision; top-down and bottom-up processing; ventral and dorsal processing; and closed- and

open-loop motor control. The focal, top-down, ventral, closed system is tailored for situations where the movement times are longer and there is adequate time for cognitive processing to occur. The ambient, bottom-up, dorsal, and open-loop control system is specialized for tasks performed when movement times are shorter and therefore affected by time constraints. It is important to stress at the outset that the two systems work together and permit the great range of actions humans perform. Chapter 1 concludes with two neural processes, called synaptogenesis (or the growth and refinement of existing neurons), and neurogenesis (or the birth of new neurons), that lead to continual change in the brain, or plasticity. Although these concepts are controversial in humans, a weight of evidence from animal studies shows that extensive participation in physical activities, especially those that occur in enriched and challenging environments, contributes to higher levels of both synaptogenesis and neurogenesis.

Chapter 2 describes how the gaze of the athlete is recorded using the visual-search and vision-in-action paradigms. The visual-search paradigm records the gaze of novice and expert athletes as they view videotaped stimuli from a sport but does not require that they physically perform the skills found in that sport. In contrast, the vision-in-action paradigm (also called perception–action studies) records the athletes' gaze as they physically perform specific tasks under conditions similar to those found in the sport. This book concentrates on the vision-in-action paradigm.

Chapter 3 describes the relationship between gaze control and attention and stresses a newfound relationship between the control of the gaze and attention. Emerging research from cognitive science shows a strong relationship between shifts of gaze and shifts of attention, thus opening a window that objectively explains how focus and concentration, or lack thereof, contribute to various levels of motor performance.

Part II, Gaze Control and the Quiet Eye in Sport, is covered in chapters 4 through 8. Chapter 4 presents a unique framework of gaze control that has been derived from the available perception–action and vision-in-action studies completed to date. Three major categories of gaze control are identified: targeting tasks, interceptive timing tasks, and tactical tasks. Within each category, control of the gaze is affected by the number of visuomotor workspaces found in the task, the number and type of locations and objects that exist within the visuomotor workspace, the spotlight of attention, and gaze–action coupling.

Chapter 5 presents gaze control in fixed targeting tasks. Gaze control in basketball shooting (free throw and jump shot) and rifle shooting (standing shots and biathlon) are presented as exemplars. The quiet eye is described in detail in each of these tasks, and two training studies are presented. The final part of chapter 5 concentrates on biathlon shooting and the interactive effects of physical arousal, high pressure, cognitive anxiety on the quiet eye, and focus of attention on shooting accuracy.

Chapter 6 describes gaze control and quiet eye in abstract targeting tasks as well as those involving moving targets. Abstract targeting tasks require the gaze to be directed to locations that are not as obvious as those found in fixed targeting tasks. Examples are golf putting on a sloped surface and billiards. The quiet eye is explained in each of these tasks, along with a study of quiet-eye training in golf. At the conclusion, four underlying interpretations for the quiet-eye phenomenon are presented: cognitive neuroscience, ecological or dynamic systems theory, sport psychology, and the Setchenov phenomenon, which links optimal levels of external attention to higher capacities for physical work.

Chapter 7 describes gaze control in interceptive timing tasks where an object is propelled toward the athlete and must be controlled in some way. Interceptive timing tasks are defined by both predictable and unpredictable object flights; each requires a unique type of gaze control. Examples include catching a ball, hitting a baseball or cricket ball, receiving a serve in volleyball, hitting a table tennis ball, and goaltending.

Chapter 8 concentrates on gaze control in tactical tasks. Tactical tasks often subsume the gaze control found in targeting and interceptive timing tasks but require another capacity, which is pattern recognition, or the ability to read complex patterns of moving players and objects. Tactical tasks require ongoing decision making and an ability to extract meaning from only fleeting glimpses of critical tactical cues. Examples include locomotion over and around obstacles, speed skating, shooting on a goaltender, soccer, and ice hockey tactics.

Part III, Decision Training in Sport, is covered in chapters 9 through 12. These chapters describe how the information on perception, cognition, and gaze control presented in parts I and II can be used for enhancing teaching and coaching in any sport or activity and at any age or skill level. Decision training incorporates high levels of cognitive effort into the practice environment while preserving or increasing the amount of physiological, technical, and tactical training that normally occurs. Decision training is designed to improve the performer's attention, anticipation, concentration, memory, and problem-solving skills through the design of practices where cognitive training is integrated with physical and technical training. The overall goal is to lead to the development of an athlete who is able to make effective decisions under the pressures of competition.

Chapter 9 presents the four scientific foundations of the decision-training model. The first two foundations are presented in parts I and II. These chapters provide insight into the nature of the visuomotor workspaces that athletes use, the critical object and location cues that are present, the spotlight of attention (or quiet eye) employed by athletes, and optimal perception–action coupling. The third foundation of decision training comes from its extensive use in the field. Decision training has been used for more than 15 years in a range of sports. Research has been conducted on its effectiveness and is presented in chapter 9. In addition, the fourth foundation is introduced, which comes from recent research on motor learning. Research findings in this field have revealed a curious paradox showing that our traditional approaches to sport training, with their high levels of repetition, feedback, and direct instruction, lead to impressive gains in the short term, but athletes trained exclusively under these conditions often falter in the long term. Motor learning research now advocates the use of new methods that incorporate high levels of athlete decision making into the training environment. These motor learning methods, which are called decision-training tools, provide practice environments in which long-term decision-making skills can be trained and acquired in a systematic way. Chapter 9 concludes with an overview of the three-step decision-training model, with its seven cognitive skills, seven cognitive triggers, and seven decision-training tools. The seven decision-training tools can be used alone or in combination.

Chapter 10 concentrates on designing practices with a decision-training focus. Two of the decision-training tools are featured: variable practice (or smart variations) and random practice (or smart combinations). Research underlying the use of variable practice and random practice is explained. Variable and random practice methods are more apt to be effective than blocked training in leading to permanent changes in the neural structures underlying motor performance. Three examples of the three-step decision-training model are presented (from badminton, freestyle skiing, and golf putting) followed by a number of case studies and decision-training exercises.

Chapter 11 presents the three-step decision-training model within the context of bandwidth feedback, questioning, and video feedback. The chapter begins with an overview of the many types of feedback found in sport teaching, coaching, and therapy. The way a sport practitioner provides corrective feedback has a profound effect on how well athletes learn and perform in the long term. The three-step decision-training model is applied in biathlon skiing and counseling. The chapter concludes with case studies and decision-training exercises.

Chapter 12 covers the last two decision-training tools: hard-first instruction and modeling and external focus of instruction. Several converging lines of research support a change in how instruction is provided to athletes, including the use of hard-first rather than easy-first instruction, the extensive use of modeling, and the use of instruction where an external rather than internal focus of attention is emphasized. The chapter concludes with examples of the three-step decision-training model in cycling and speed skating, along with a number of case studies and decision-training exercises.

Learning Tools

Perception, Cognition, and Decision Training: The Quiet Eye in Action explores the principles of cognition, neuroscience, gaze research, dynamic systems, and motor learning. To help students learn the concepts as well as apply the activities of interest to them, the text presents several learning aids.

➤ *Where Have We Been? Where Are We Going?* Each chapter starts with Where Have We Been? and Where Are We Going? sections. The Where Have We Been? sections help students review the important concepts that were covered in the previous chapter, and the Where Are We Going? sections explain what the text explores next.

➤ *Glossary terms.* Many terms are shown in bold throughout the book. These terms are central to understanding the theories, principles, and methods presented. Each of the boldfaced terms is defined in the body of the chapter and again in the glossary. Each scientific discipline involves precise definitions for the critical ideas, concepts, and principles of the field. It is only through the process of definition that a science becomes both understandable and easier to use.

➤ *Vision-in-action data.* Throughout the book are several photos of vision-in-action data that were captured directly from the videotapes when an eye tracker was used. These frames show the gaze of the athlete and motor behavior at critical moments in the tasks performed. This type of gaze data has never been presented in a textbook before; therefore, students are provided with unique insight into what athletes see when they perform many of the sport tasks presented in this book.

➤ *Gaze control, quiet eye, and decision-training exercises.* Many of the chapters include gaze control and quiet-eye exercises that are designed to broaden the experience of students as well as provide applied exercises of a personal and professional nature. For example, in part I, Web sites are listed that students are encouraged to view. In part II, students are asked to complete quiet-eye training exercises in one or all of the targeting tasks, interceptive timing tasks, and tactical tasks. In part III, students are shown how to use the three-step decision-training model in creating coaching practices in their area of interest. Students are also asked to select a task of their choice and develop a decision-training drill using the three-step decision-training model.

➤ *Case studies.* Both quiet-eye training and decision training have been used in the field for several years, and case studies are presented from coaches and athletes who have experienced one or both of these methods. Their stories give readers a firsthand account of using quiet-eye training or decision training (or in some cases failing to use either). Seeing how others have fared using many of the concepts within the book provides a valuable aid for students who want to experiment with quiet-eye training and decision training.

➤ *References.* Every effort has been made to include the latest research studies in each of the areas highlighted. An extensive reference list brings together in one place all the research in these areas, making it a great resource for those who want to further study gaze control and decision training.

ACKNOWLEDGMENTS

I dedicate this book to the memory of Aftab E. Patla.

I have been fortunate to take part in many aspects of sport, as an athlete, a physical education teacher, a coach, a parent, an athletic director, a university professor, and a researcher of eye movements and decision making in sport. I have been privileged to know and work with many marvelous people along the way. First I must thank many in my family and my friends and loved ones for their tireless devotion for so many years. To my mother Pauline, who raised the six of us to persevere and make the most of what we had, I say thanks first of all. I remember her words often and her quiet way of bringing out the best in everyone she knew. To my sons, Robert and James, who are the light of my life and also my best friends—I am very proud of you and delighted to vicariously enjoy the adventurous lives you lead. To Hannah and Lillian, my granddaughters, whose purity of gaze is the gift of the young, and to their fabulous mother, Janette, who takes such good care of everyone in the family. To my brother John, who being two years younger than I, always indulged my penchant for playing any sport on earth and to his family: Judy, Nick, Todd, and Joanne, who all inspire and then inspire some more. To Michael Coster, the principal of my high school and coach, who was an inspiration at a time when this was most crucial in my life; to Ross Eddy for his twinkle and enthusiasm in all aspects of life; to Nancy Webster for being stalwart and regal; to Sally Ross and Jen and Noel Villard for their enduring approach to life and sport. To Bob Morford for his inspiration and academic guidance a la Thomas Kuhn (1970) and to the marvelous years we had together; to Pat Klinck, Shirley Murray, Claudia Emes, Keith Kendall, and Fleurette Collins for their wonderful insights into what underlies a successful life and education system and for being such great friends; to Nancy Buzzell—psychologist, decision trainer and friend par excellence.

Second I want to thank those in academia that I have had the pleasure to work with as both friends and colleagues. To Stan Coren for his insights into perception and eye movements which are reflected in this book; to Gary Sinclair for his wisdom and the gift of his applied sports methods; to Brian Gaines for his quick intelligence and charm in all things at all times; to Barry Morton for his solid work over so many years as head technician in my lab; to Mark Williams and Chris Janelle for their vision and rigor in the areas of research presented within, as well as their encyclopedic knowledge of the many diverse areas that make up this fascinating multi-disciplinary field. Both reviewed this book for me and provided many valuable suggestions. To Aftab Patla, who I had the pleasure to collaborate with on a number of gaze in human locomotion studies. Aftab is gone now, but I will always remember his wonderful way of working together. To Sue McPherson for her humor and insights into the role of knowledge in sport; to Janet Ronsky, Barb Ramage, Geoffrey Edwards, and everyone in the MIME project for thinking way outside the box; to Warren Veale, past Dean of Kinesiology, who could see the sense of my work when many could not and helped at a crucial time in a crucial way.

Next I want to thank my students who have made so many contributions to the development of either my quiet eye or decision training work, many of whom are referenced in the chapters to follow. I especially want to thank Raissa Adolphe, Kristine Chambers, Dan Holden, Shawnee Harle, Flora Hillis, Lori Livingston, Tania Marshall, Steve Martell, Joshua Nugent, Derek Panchuk, Dan Ota, Dan Pittman, Sergio Rodrigues, Ruth-Morey Sorrentino, and Sheri Umeris for your hard work as students and scholars. You were often the reason the ideas in this book kept marching forward.

I also want to thank a number of sport leaders, who were instrumental in putting the quiet eye and/or decision training into their sport and professional worlds—to Mary Ann Reeves, Director of National Coaching Institute (Turin) for her unique ability to help coaches reach levels they would never achieve without her; to Jacques Thibault, Director of Olympic Oval (Turin), Calgary; to Gord May, Director of the Coaches Association of BC; to Andre Fournier, Director of the National Coaching Institute Montreal; to John Bales, President of the Coaching Association of Canada; to Jean-Pierre Brunnelle of Sherbrooke University, who has led the way in decision training in Quebec; to Bernard Petoit of Cirque d'Soleil; to Gail Donahue, past Director of the National Coaching Institute in Vancouver; to Gene Edworthy of the Edworthy Vision Clinic; to Mark Sharp of Alpine Canada; to Dave Wood of Cross Country Canada; to Rainer Martens and Judy Wright of Human Kinetics; to Scott Smith, who as Instructional Editor of Golf Digest put the quiet eye on the front cover; to Allan Chadd of Chadd-Angiers and Alan Alda of Scientific American Frontiers and their marvelous work on the quiet eye; to Julie Clothier of CNN for the opportunity to show the world a bit of what the quiet eye is all about; to Alix McDonald of the Discovery Channel, Canada; to Allison Toms of Continuing Education at the University of Calgary for taking the decision training certification forward, and to all at Applied Sciences Laboratories in Boston.

To the many athletes and their coaches who have volunteered to be my subjects in gaze experiments; I especially want to thank the men's and women's basketball teams at the University of Calgary; Team Canada Volleyball; National and Alberta Speed skating teams; Team Canada Men's and Women's Ice Hockey; the National Biathlon Team of Canada; members of the table tennis clubs in Calgary; Alberta Ballet and Alberta School of Ballet; the Alberta Professional Golfers Association and so many golfers of all skill levels from Calgary, Arizona, and elsewhere; Team Canada Women's Ice Hockey Team and many other ice hockey players from Calgary; the Calgary Baseball Association; the Andrews Hockey Growth School of PEI and the many students from the Human Performance Laboratory, University of Calgary, and City of Calgary who have taken part in our experiments. Thank you all for your tireless support over the many years I have been carrying out gaze and decision training research in sport.

And finally, to the many coaches who I have had a chance to work with throughout Canada and the world in applying decision training. I especially want to recognize Todd Allison, Melody Davidson, Janos Engelbert, Dave Hill, Martin Jensen, Ron Pike, Murray Cluff, Marcel Lacroix, Lisa Woodcock, Neil Gondek, Mike Marshall, Dave McMaster, Jean Pichette, Julie Stegall, Jeff White, Debbie Fisher, Kurt Innis, Sean Ireland, Dave Matthews, Kathy Berg, Kristine Chambers, Moira D'Andrea Marshall, Shawn Holman, Karl Taylor, Xiuli Wang, Derrick Campbell, Neal Marshall, Dan Proulx, Jason Smith, Walter Corey, John Jacques, Bernie Ontkean, Ozzie Sawicki, Ayako Tsubaki-Francis, Gail Niinimaa, Christian Hrab, Derrick Schoof, and Sonya Seyfort. To all of you I salute your wonderful work over the years in the development of the quiet eye and decision training. You are a very special group.

Finally, I claim any errors within as strictly my own.

Introduction to the Theoretical Foundations

➤➤ *Where Are We Going?*

The theoretical orientation of this book is a unique mixture of cognitive psychology (Kahneman, 1973; Solso, 1995; Sternberg, 2003; Treisman & Gelade, 1980), ecological psychology (Gibson, 1966, 1979), dynamic systems (Bernstein, 1967; Kelso, 1982), and the constraints-led perspective (Newell, 1986; Newell & McDonald, 1994; Williams, Janelle, & Davids, 2004). Over the past 20 y these four theoretical approaches have increased our understanding of how people learn and control motor skills.

In truth, no theory today is able to do this on its own. Instead, each theory provides insight into how movements are controlled within certain constraints. In the sections to follow, visuomotor coordination, motor learning, and motor performance are first defined. The four theories are then explained given the state of research today and the overall purpose of this book, which is to explain how athletes control their gaze in the environments in which they perform and how this affects their performance. The quiet eye is defined, within a unique gaze control framework that has been derived from the available eye movement and gaze studies in sport. At the conclusion of the chapter, selected aspects of each theory are incorporated into an adaptation of the constraints-led model, which provides the theoretical scaffolding for this volume.

Visuomotor Coordination

Humans use information from the perceptual systems (vision, audition, touch, taste, smell) to produce goal-directed movements. Although inputs from all the perceptual systems are important, this book concentrates on the visual system and its integration with the motor system. The term **visuomotor coordination** refers to the ability to use visual information to generate appropriate motor commands (McLeod, 1994). Visual information is acquired through shifts of gaze that bring information onto the retina, where neural processing begins. One of the goals of this book is to show that the processing of visual information is critical to understanding how people both learn and control motor skills.

Visual information is essential for both **motor learning** and **motor performance** to occur. People engage in motor learning when they go through a number of phases, stages, steps, or transitions on their way to becoming proficient in a motor skill. Motor learning requires physical practice and is affected by age, maturation, amount of time devoted to practice, plus a host of other factors. In contrast, a person is engaged in motor performance when most of the learning of the skill has been done and the challenge is now one of **motor control,** or the ability to plan and produce a movement that successfully achieves a particular goal. The outcome of the skill is important, as is determining the reasons why one is successful or unsuccessful. There is no single point where motor learning ends and motor performance begins. This is because a person may be an elite performer in one aspect of a sport and still be a novice learning a particular skill in another. For example, it is not unusual for a golfer to be good at putting and poor with the driver, or vice versa.

Cognitive Psychology

Cognitive psychology offers a formal way to study how the brain functions in terms of information processing. Sternberg (2003, p. 527) defines cognitive psychology as "the study of how people perceive, learn, remember, and think about information." Solso (1995, p. 2) explains that "cognitive psychology is the scientific study of the thinking mind and is concerned with how we attend to and gain information about the world, how that information is stored in memory by the brain and how that knowledge is used to solve problems, to think and to formulate language." Summers (2004, p. 7) explains that when a cognitive approach is used, "the processing of information occurs through discrete stages that can be isolated and studied thorough appropriate chronometric methods. Using flow-diagram techniques borrowed from computer programming, the flow of information is typically traced through three primary stages involving perceptual processes, decision making and response selection, and response programming and execution."

Note that the critical word in these definitions is *information*. To this day we do not have a concrete way of measuring information used in cognitive processing in the same way that we can measure the oxygen levels in the blood, the strength of a muscle, or the pressure under our feet. It is perhaps for this reason that cognitive psychologists have developed a number of cognitive psychology sub-areas that together define how information is acquired and processed within specific domains or areas of interest and the effect this processing has on human behavior. Some of the major sub-areas are as follows:

➤ *Cognitive neuroscience.* Describes the structure and function of the brain. Recent brain imaging techniques, such as fMRI (functional magnetic resonance) and PET (positron emission tomography), permit scanning of the brain when different types of information are processed under different conditions. These studies allow for the identification of the areas of the brain involved in processing different types of information and the effect this has on behavior.

➤ *Sensation and perception.* Explains how we process sensory information in very short periods of time, usually less than 100 ms (note there are 1000 ms in one s).

➤ *Attention.* Explains how we select information for more extensive processing in thresholds that minimally range from 120 to 200 ms depending on the sensory modality—vision, hearing, touch, smell, or taste.

➤ *Consciousness.* Explains why we are aware of some things but not others and the effect this has on learning and performance. This "is both the most obvious and the most mysterious feature of our mind" (Dennet, 1987, p. 160).

➤ *Memory.* Describes how information is stored in the brain, how we access it and represent it as knowledge, and how we use it to guide our actions.

➤ *Language.* Explains the nature of speech, audition, comprehension, writing, and other forms of literary expressions.

➤ *Problem solving.* Explains how we use perception, attention, and other cognitive abilities to arrive at solutions in both old and new situations.

➤ *Decision making and reasoning.* Explains how we choose from the alternatives that are available.

➤ *Creativity.* Explains how the human mind generates original thought.

➤ *Cognitive development.* Describes what happens in the brain from birth to old age.

➤ *Intelligence and expertise.* Attempts to explain why individuals have different abilities in art, sport, science, and other domains.

➤ *Artificial intelligence, robotics, human factors, and ergonomics.* Explores how humans interact with the world and how to build machines that act like humans or animals in thought and action.

There is no attempt in this book to include all the areas in this list, but instead the seven areas shown in figure 1 are emphasized. Sport performers must be able to anticipate what is most important in the environments in which they play. They must be able to attend to critical cues and concentrate at appropriate moments. They must be able

to retrieve from memory the information that is needed at the right time, solve problems when they arise, and ultimately make the right decision under time constraints. One of the most comprehensive models that incorporates many of these cognitive areas with the motor system available today is that of Richard Schmidt (Schmidt, 1991; Schmidt & Lee, 2005; Schmidt & Wrisberg, 2004). This model is composed of various information-processing stages used in the control of both short- and long-duration movements. This model is presented in more detail in chapter 3.

It is through cognitive psychology that the following types of questions can be answered. What part of the brain is activated when we plan a movement and make the movement? How long does it take to anticipate and respond to different types of information (for example, how long does it takes to perceive a simple signal versus a complex one, what part of the brain is activated by that information, what is the effect of skill level on the processing of information)? How long does it take to perceive a cue and make a movement with one hand, or two hands, or with the hands and feet? How are movements organized in the brain? What information do athletes see when they are successful and unsuccessful? What visual information underlies the ability to make effective decisions under all conditions? What is the relationship between verbal responses to an action and the actual action? What changes occur within the cognitive system when a person moves from learning a skill to performing it at a high level?

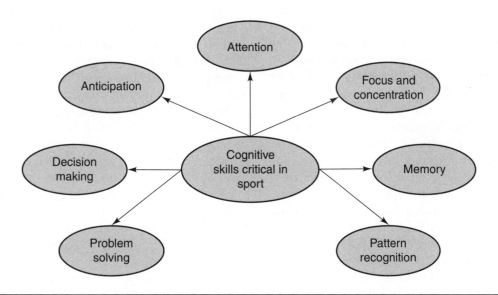

➤ **Figure 1** The seven areas of cognitive psychology that are emphasized in this book.

Sport is an excellent place to find an answer to these questions since highly skilled athletes have discovered the specific information that leads to performing at a high level. They have also discovered how to control the acquisition of information as they perform in terms of perception–action cycles. And they have discovered how to perform even when opponents make it difficult to acquire the best information. In this book you will learn that with the advent of mobile eye trackers and new methods of research, we are able to discover the types of visual information that underlie athlete success and then use this knowledge in teaching, coaching, therapy, and a host of other areas.

Ecological Psychology

Ecological psychology was founded by James Gibson (1966, 1979). Ecological psychology is also called **direct perception** and is identified as *direct* because it is believed that people perceive the environments in which they perform unaided by inference, memories, or other neural representations as suggested by cognitive psychology (Michaels & Carello, 1981). Cognitive psychology involves **indirect perception,** meaning the act of perceiving involves the intervention of memories and knowledge representations stored in the brain. Gibson (1979) stated that movement through the world is dependent on the establishment of direct optical relationships that develop without any apparent need for the many processing stages described in cognitive psychology. Central to Gibson's theory is the idea that visual information exists as invariances in the environment that are naturally perceived (or picked up) through the act of direct perception. An invariant is any aspect of the environment (or people or events) that does not change but retains the same qualities in all situations.

One of Gibson's greatest contributions is the discovery of the optic array and optic flow. The **optic array** includes the projections of the surrounding visible environment. **Optic flow** includes changes in the optic array created by observer movement, for example, how visual information is perceived as it moves toward or by us as a consequence of our own movements. Gibson realized that "permitting the observer or the observed scene to move made certain supposed problems of spatial perception appear to

vanish" (Warren & Shaw, 1985, p. 2). For example, figure 2 shows a pilot's orientation and heading with respect to the earth's surface when flying across an airfield and the patterns of optical flow that occur as the pilot flies over and perceives the airfield. The length of the lines reveals how fast the information is approaching. Note that at the farthest extreme on the horizon the lines are very short, and indeed at their convergent point they cease to move. This location is an invariant called the focus of expansion, which is the point in space toward which the person is moving. Michaels and Carello (1981) define an **invariant** "as a constant pattern, usually amid change in other variables of stimulation" (p. 31). Invariances are "those high-order patterns of stimulation that underlie perceptual constancies, or more generally, the persistent properties of the environment that an animal is said to know. Invariant structures in light and sound not only specify objects, places, and events in the environment, but also the activities of the organism… Thus invariants are, by virtue of the laws that support them, information about the environment and the animal's relation to it" (p. 40).

Another type of optic flow occurs when information expands or contracts in size on the retina as a consequence of movement in the environment (Cutting, 1996; Lee, 1976; Lee & Aronson, 1974; Savelsberg, Whiting, & Bootsma, 1991). Lee & Aronson (1974) created a swinging room with walls that moved toward and away from a person standing in the room. If the wall moved toward the person, then the person swayed backward to compensate; if it moved away, then the person leaned forward. Other experiments showed that when an object travels toward a person (such as a ball approaching [Lee et al., 1983]) or the person moves toward the object (such as toward the take off point in long jumping [Lee, Lishman, & Thomson, 1982]) or when stepping over irregular ground (Warren, Young, & Lee, 1986), the change in size of the image on the retina is enough to trigger a change in action. Clearly, humans do not always process information through all the elaborate stages as described in cognitive psychology; instead we directly perceive what is in the environment and organize the appropriate behavior without any apparent need for conscious thought.

This subconscious aspect of ecological psychology is appealing to many because the acquisition

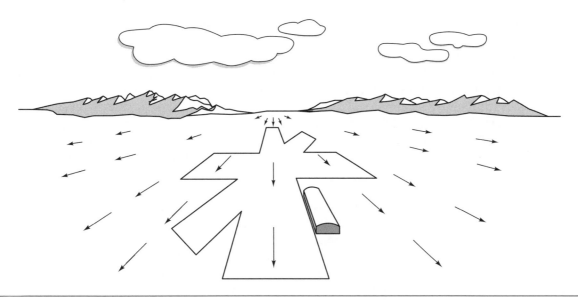

➤ **Figure 2** Retinal motion perspective looking ahead.

Reprinted, by permission, from E. Reed and R. Jones, 1982, The ability to judge distance and space in terms of the retinal motion queue. In *Reasons for realism: Selected essays of James Gibson*, edited by E. Reed and R. Jones (Hillsdale, NJ: Lawrence Erlbaum), 140.

of motor skills often occurs without an awareness of what is happening. Most people cannot explain exactly how they move, let alone elaborate on the underlying processes involved. Usually it takes a period of formal study to gain insight into the many subconscious aspects of a movement, whether it involves participating in a sport, using a computer, making tea, or engaging in a conversation. We move through the world and perform many actions with little conscious thought.

Gibson (1979, p. 12) also introduced another term called **affordances.** He explained that "the affordances of an environment are what it offers the animal" (p. 127). For example, a hard, flat pathway affords walking that is easy, while a steep slope covered with small stones affords a more difficult walking situation. Gibson (1979) also stressed that people do not perceive the affordances of an environment in the same way. For example, ice is frozen water that is hard and is often slippery. It has some properties that are invariant (hard) and others that are perceived in different ways (slipperiness). For example, if you come from a country such as Canada, where ice is common, then you learn over time whether ice on the walkway is slippery just by looking at it. If you come from a tropical country where ice on walkways does not exist, however, then you do not know how to perceive its properties, or affordances. This example shows that although affordances exist naturally in the environment,

the degree to which they are perceived is also affected by the experiences of the perceiver.

Sport is an ideal place to apply Gibson's theory since it is defined by continual motion, both in terms of athlete movement and the movement of objects. Patterns of optical change define playing in sport and are captured when a mobile eye tracker is placed upon the head of an athlete who is performing *in situ*, which is a Latin term that means in its original place. It is a term that is important in this book as many studies are presented in which the athlete's gaze is recorded in task environments that are very similar to those found in real-world settings. Sport environments are often structured the same way around the world and thus present similar conditions within which the perceptual-motor system evolves. Within a particular sport, the rules also dictate that athletes must often play within the same kinds of spaces, use the same kinds of equipment, and play by the same rules. In addition, athletes are often trained technically and physically in ways that are more similar than different, given a specific period of time. All sports also require many years of training, and it is not unusual for an elite athlete to spend more than 10,000 hours practicing in their sport (Ericsson, Krampe, & Tesch-Romer, 1993; Helsen, Starkes, & Hodges, 1998; Howe, Davidson, & Sloboda, 1998). To replicate this amount of training within a laboratory context is very difficult yet readily available for investigation when studies are carried out *in situ*. However, even though the environment and training conditions may be similar, some athletes emerge as more elite than others. The pickup of affordances within these highly structured environments occurs differently for athletes of differing skill levels. One of the goals of this book is to provide new insight into why this occurs.

Finally, there was one area where Gibson (1979) was incorrect, and this was his explanation of how eye movements occur in dynamic action environments. He stated that "the prolonged fixing of the eyes on an object or part of an object, the bringing of its image to the fovea and keeping it there, does not occur in life. It is a laboratory artifice, brought about when an experimenter tells an observer to stare at a fixation point that is usually of no interest to her. No one stares at a fixed point in the world for long unless she is so preoccupied that she is actually not seeing what she looks at. Seeming exceptions arise in the aiming of a rifle or the threading of a needle, but these are actually cases where different objects are aligned, not where a single object is fixated. The eyes normally search, explore or scan, and there are seldom fewer than several saccadic jumps per second. They look at but do not fixate" (p. 211).

Studies presented in the following chapters show that elite athletes, even in dynamic tasks such as ice hockey goaltending, do fixate specific locations or objects in space for extended periods, often approaching a full second (Panchuk & Vickers, 2006). The rapid and continual shifts in gaze that Gibson thought underlie all actions are not borne out by existing gaze research in sport. Overall, the gaze control of the elite athlete is not only directed to specific information in the task environment, but their fixations and tracking eye movements tend to be both earlier and longer in duration when performance is at its highest level.

There are two reasons why Gibson may have held the view that fixations and tracking gaze were not a part of skilled behavior. First, accurate mobile eye trackers had not been developed during his lifetime and so the gaze data presented throughout this book did not yet exist. Second, his belief in optic flow was so strong that he may have assumed that information continually washed over the eyes due to the movements of the eyes, body, and objects in the environment. He may have assumed that it was impossible for the same information to be processed for a long duration by the moving person. But athletes bring the critical information required to perform well onto the part of the eye that sees with clear acuity (the fovea) and do so for prolonged durations, even as they move dynamically in cluttered and difficult environments. Evidence supporting this ability is found throughout this book, especially in chapters 4 through 9, where the gaze of elite athletes is presented in a number of well-known sport tasks.

Dynamic Systems

At the same time that the cognitive and ecological approaches were emerging, the **dynamic systems** perspective grew out of the work of Bernstein (1967) and later that of Turvey (1977a, 1977b), Kelso (1982), and others. In a dynamic systems approach, "movement patterns arise from the synergistic organization of the neuromuscular system based on morphological factors (i.e., biological constructs), biomechanical factors (i.e., Newtonian Laws), environmental factors (i.e., spatial and temporal configuration of events), and task constraints (e.g., walking at slow or fast speeds)" (Kurz & Stergiou, 2004, p. 93). In a manner similar to Gibson (1979), researchers of dynamic systems attach little importance to higher-level cognitive processes, but instead study the behavior of the joints and muscles using biomechanics, quantum physics, and other approaches.

Central to the dynamic systems theory is the notion that skill emerges when the individual exerts control over the degrees of freedom of a movement. Bernstein (1967) explained that "the coordination of a movement is the process of mastering redundant degrees of freedom of the moving organ, in other words, its conversion to a controllable system" (p. 127). The **degrees of freedom** of a movement is the number of separate independent elements that must be controlled in the body to produce a coordinated action. Turvey, Fitch, and Tuller (1982) in Kelso (1982, p. 242) depicted the basic idea of the degrees of freedom using the diagram of the arm shown in figure 3. This diagram shows the degrees of freedom that occur in the arm. The arm has four joints: the shoulder, the elbow, the radioulnar joint, and the wrist. Turvey at al. explain that the shoulder joint has 3 degrees of freedom (horizontal, vertical, longitudinal), the elbow has 1 degree (flexion–

extension), the radioulnar joint has 1 degree (rotation about its length), and the wrist has 2 degrees (horizontal, vertical), making the total degrees of freedom equal to 7 degrees. But the degrees of freedom can also be expressed in terms of the number of muscles operating at each joint, and when these are also considered, Kelso states there are 26 degrees of freedom in the arm. When a person is unable to move the arm effectively, such as when learning a skill or as a consequence of injury or disease, then the number of degrees of freedom remains large and uncontrollable. However, when the person becomes skilled, then the number of degrees of freedom decreases as a coordinated dynamic system emerges.

Bernstein (1967) and Vereijken, van Emmerick, Whiting, and Newell (1992) further explained that when we first learn a skill, we tend to freeze the degrees of freedom in a way that limits coordination and control. Then as skill is acquired, we free some of the degrees of freedom, thus allowing the movement to be performed more efficiently and accurately. Finally, we learn to exploit the degrees of freedom, an evolution in skill development that is needed to perform at a high level in any context. **Freezing, freeing, and exploiting the degrees of freedom** therefore can be viewed as stages the performer goes through in the attainment of higher levels of skill.

Another major idea emanating from the dynamic systems approach is that of **self-organization**, which Kelso (1995, p. 1-2) describes as existing in all forms of life "without any agent-like entity ordering the elements, telling them what to do and where to go." Self-organization is often used to describe the process of development, where humans grow from infants to crawlers to toddlers to children to adolescents to adults and finally to elderly adults without any external agent appearing to exert control. Kelso (1995,

p. 8) explains that self-organization is defined by "spontaneous pattern formation" where the system organizes itself without any input from the "self, or other agent within the system doing the organizing."

Proponents of the dynamic systems perspective give little weight to representations in the brain, such as schemas, motor programs, and neural networks, or to processes involving the processing of information or other higher-level cognitive constructs. Kelso (1995, p. 257) explains that the "brain is fundamentally a pattern forming self-organized system governed by potentially discoverable, non-linear dynamical laws. More specifically, behaviors such as perceiving, intending, acting, learning, and remembering arise as meta-stable spatiotemporal patterns of brain activity that are themselves produced by cooperative interactions among neural clusters. Self-organization is the key principle." A dynamic systems perspective does not seek to identify any brain-based, higher-level agents (e.g., neural networks, motor programs) that control motor behavior. A notable exception to this is the work of Newell (1986) and Newell and McDonald (1992, 1994) who incorporate many of the concepts from dynamic systems into what is called a constraints-led perspective, which is presented in the following section.

The dynamic systems perspective provides a theoretical basis for describing how the motor system is reorganized as motor skills are learned and controlled. The development of skill in sport is a process of mastering the degrees of freedom found in the many skills and tactics. Freezing, freeing, and exploiting degrees of freedom is something most sport performers can remember doing as they moved from being a tentative to a confident performer able to handle all the nuances of their sport environments. In the past,

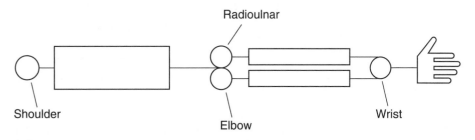

➤ **Figure 3** Degrees of freedom in the arm as illustrated by Kelso.

Reprinted, by permission, from J.A. Kelso, 1982, *Human motor behavior* (Hillsdale, NJ: Lawrence Erlbaum).

we used to believe that changes in motor control occurred with little overt cognitive processing, but now it is known that all the changes that occur in motor behavior must be accompanied by changes in the brain. A model of motor learning and control that presents this view, while being supportive of the cognitive, ecological, and dynamic systems models, is the constraints-led perspective, as proposed by Newell (Newell, 1986; Newell & McDonald, 1994).

Constraints-Led Perspective

Thus far we have reviewed the cognitive psychology, ecological psychology and dynamic systems theories of motor learning and control. Each provides a unique contribution to our understanding of human movement, but none alone is adequate in itself in explaining how humans learn all types of motor skills. A theoretical approach that attempts to incorporate many aspects of the cognitive psychology, ecological psychology, and dynamic systems models is provided by the **constraints-led perspective** (Newell, 1986; Newell & McDonald, 1994; Newell & Vaillancourt, 2001; Williams et al., 2004; Williams, Davids, & Williams, 1999). Newell and McDonald's (1994) model is shown in figure 4 and illustrates how three categories of constraints (organism, task, and environment) "interact to determine for a given organism, the optimal pattern of coordination and control for any activity" (Newell, 1986, p. 348). The model also shows the importance of a perception–action cycle that actively seeks information from the perceptual-motor workspace, resulting in motor coordination. Following is a description of each component of the constraints-led model as defined by Newell and colleagues,

as well as an application of each category of constraints as used in this book.

Organismic Constraints

Organismic constraints include various biological and functional aspects of a person, such as body weight, height, and shape, as well as synaptic connections that control cognitive and body functions. Organismic constraints are inherent in the person and are affected by genetics, nutrition, development, and training experiences.

Organismic constraints are recognized in this book as those that reside within the athlete—physiology, height, weight, maturation, and acquired skill level. Elite athlete and near-elite athlete comparisons are made whenever possible, where **elite athletes** are defined as those who consistently achieve the highest statistics in a specific task in their sport, as documented by external authorities such as statisticians, league officials, and so on, as well as by testing in the experimental environment. In contrast, **near-elite athletes** compete in the same task environment and therefore possess similar height, weight, and other biological attributes needed to compete at the same level, but they differ significantly from elite athletes in how well they perform the tasks selected for investigation.

By using the elite–near-elite comparison, there is an attempt to hold the organismic contributions to performance constant while isolating the contribution of the gaze and attention to performance outcomes. For example, Vickers and Adolphe (1997) recruited elite Team Canada volleyball players from the same team. The elite receivers had pass-reception statistics in competition that were similar to those of the world's best receivers

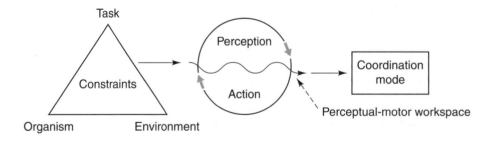

➤ **Figure 4**   Schematic representing the different frames of reference for considering the constraints that influence a task, the perception–action cycle, and the perceptual-motor workspace.

(62%), while the near-elite athletes had statistics under 50%. Furthermore, analysis of the athletes' organismic constraints (height, weight, jump height, $\dot{V}O_2$max, strength, flexibility) found no significant differences in the two groups on any of these measures, yet the two groups differed significantly in their ability to read the server as the ball was delivered and to track the ball before reception. This study is explained in depth in chapter 7.

Environmental Constraints

Environmental constraints are external to the body and include "gravity, natural ambient temperature, natural light and other environmental features that are not usually simply adaptations of the task" (Newell & McDonald, 1994, p. 350). Environmental constraints are often manipulated by the athlete in ways that allow skillful performance to occur. For example, skiers learn to use the bumps (or moguls) in the hill as aids to turning and therefore exploit a naturally occurring environmental constraint.

Environmental constraints are defined in this book as those not only imposed by the sport within which performance occurs, but also by how researchers carry out their research. Newell and McDonald (1994) and Williams et al. (2004) stress the importance of carrying out research in natural environments where the normal constraints on behavior can be studied within tasks where perception–action coupling can be realistically observed. Two research methods, called the *visual search* and *vision-in-action paradigms,* have been developed to study the contributions of vision and gaze to motor performance.

When the **visual-search paradigm** is used, videotapes or other pictorial stimuli are shown to athletes as their eye movements are recorded. These studies have the advantage of showing the same stimuli to all participants, but the major limitation is that the motor behavior is rarely performed at the same time. Motor responses are limited to pressing a key, moving a joystick, stepping on a mat, or similar movements. The visual-search paradigm is an observer paradigm, and it does not explain the relationship between control of the gaze and motor success and failure within realistic sport contexts. In contrast, researchers who use the perception–action paradigm (Bard & Fleury, 1976; Bahill & LaRitz, 1984; Ripoll & Fleurance, 1988) record the per-

formers' gaze as they perform within contexts that are similar to those encountered in the real world. More recently, the **vision-in-action paradigm** (Vickers, 1992; Vickers, 1996a; Williams, Singer, & Frehlich, 2002) has evolved to the point where the gaze and motor behavior are recorded simultaneously as sport tasks are performed *in situ*, making it possible to objectively determine which gaze and attention characteristics are associated with successful and unsuccessful performance.

Task Constraints

As Newell (1986) explains, **task constraints** include "a) the goal of the task; b) the rules specifying or constraining response dynamics; and c) implements or machines specifying or constraining response dynamics" (p. 352). In addition, "all goals relate to the outcome of the product or outcome of the action" (p. 352). This perspective is also emphasized in this book. Whenever possible, gaze differences are described not only in terms of skill level, but also in terms of the outcome of the task. Rules and equipment constrain how a task is performed and affect the response dynamics. For example, the development of the klap skate in speed skating increased speed and quickly changed how the sport was performed.

Task constraints are recognized in three ways in this book. First, the goal of the task is preserved. Therefore, if the goal of a task is normally to hit a target consistently, then assessment of accuracy is the outcome reported (Vickers, 1996a; Janelle et al., 2000; Williams, Singer, & Frehlich, 2002). If the goal of the task is to receive an object and pass to a target (Vickers & Adolphe, 1997; Rodrigues, Vickers, & Williams, 2002), then this focus is maintained. Or, if the goal of the task is to stop a shot on net, then how this is accomplished is reported (Martell & Vickers, 2004; Panchuk & Vickers, 2006). The second task constraint is abeyance of the rules of the sport. The rules of the sport are preserved in the research protocols so that the task is performed under the constraints normally found in the sport. Finally, the implements used to perform the task are preserved in that athletes are tested within environments that are exactly the same or very similar to those within which they actually play. Athletes are also required to use the equipment they normally use, and when relevant, compete against individuals similar to those found *in situ*.

Perception–Action Cycle and the Perceptual-Motor Workspace

The constraints-led perspective also includes perception–action cycles and perceptual-motor workspaces (see figure 4). **Perception–action cycles** link information perceived in the environment to specific physical behaviors in time-dependent ways. In this book, we concentrate on how the gaze of the athlete is coupled with his or her actions both in terms of absolute and relative time. Absolute measures of time are normally expressed as seconds (s) or milliseconds (ms), while relative time is expressed as a percentage of the total time taken. Perception–action cycles function within **perceptual-motor workspaces**, which are "nonstationary, that is, the nature of the workspace changes over time because of a variety of influences, including ongoing interactions of the performer with the environment" (Newell & McDonald, 1994, p. 527). It is within perceptual-motor workspaces that visual information is acquired and critical decisions are made that affect sport performance.

Three Categories of Gaze Control

Newell & McDonald (1994) originally described the perception–action cycle as an abstract concept, one where it was not yet possible to specify the relationship between a performer's gaze and his or her physical actions as they occur in real-world tasks. However, with the advent of mobile eye trackers, coupled with motor analysis systems, it is now possible for researchers to objectively determine the relationship between an athlete's gaze and his or her motor behavior within specific sport-task environments. In addition, this research shows that, instead of one generic perception–action cycle existing for all motor tasks, the gaze behaviors of performers may be grouped into the three large gaze control categories as found in targeting tasks, interceptive timing tasks, and tactical tasks as shown in figure 5. Each of these perception-action cycles has been derived from the existing gaze control research in sport, which shows that the gaze control found in targeting tasks is distinct from that found in interceptive tasks, which in turn is distinct from that found in tactical tasks. While some sport tasks require only one type of gaze control, others require all three. For example, in basketball, gaze control when shooting (a targeting task) differs from gaze control when receiving a pass (an interceptive timing task), which in turn differs from the gaze control when reading a zone defense or executing a fast break (a tactical task). These three large categories are part of a unique gaze control framework that will be explained in detail in chapter 4.

The Quiet Eye

In a typical gaze study in sport, all gaze (fixations, pursuit trackings, saccades, blinks) found in the task to all locations are analyzed in an effort to

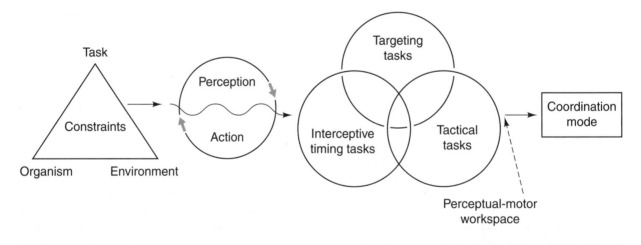

> **Figure 5**   Constraints-led model, adapted to show three categories of gaze control (targeting, interceptive timing, tactical) that have been derived from recent gaze research in sport.

determine which ones contribute to higher levels of performance. One gaze has emerged, called the **quiet eye** (Vickers, 1996a), that has been shown to underlie higher levels of skill and performance in a wide range of sport tasks. The quiet eye is a final fixation or tracking gaze that is located on a specific location or object in the visuomotor workspace within 3° of visual angle (or less) for a minimum of 100 ms. The onset of the quiet eye occurs prior to the final movement of the task, and the offset occurs naturally when the gaze deviates off the location or object by more than 3° of visual angle for a minimum of 100 ms. Since elite performers exhibit an optimal control of the quiet eye relative to the final movement, the quiet eye may be viewed as an objective measure of optimal perceptual-motor coordination. Some studies where the quiet eye has been shown to be a characteristic of higher levels of sport performance are as follows:

- ➤ Golf (Vickers, 1992; Vickers, 2004)
- ➤ Basketball (Harle & Vickers, 2001; Oudejans, Koedijker, Bleijendaal, & Bakker, 2005; Oudejans, van de Langenberg, & Hutter, 2002; Vickers, 1996a, b, c)
- ➤ Volleyball (Adolphe, Vickers, & LaPlante, 1997; Vickers & Adolphe, 1997; McPherson & Vickers, 2004)
- ➤ Darts (Vickers, Rodrigues, & Edworthy, 2000)
- ➤ Rifle shooting (Janelle et al., 2000; Vickers & Williams, in press)
- ➤ Billiards (Williams, Singer, & Frehlich, 2002)
- ➤ Table tennis (Rodrigues et al., 2002; Williams, Vickers, & Rodrigues, 2002)
- ➤ Ice hockey tactics (Martell & Vickers, 2004)
- ➤ Ice hockey goaltending (Panchuk & Vickers, 2006)

The quiet eye of elite athletes is both earlier and longer than that of athletes with lower skill levels. It is also trainable, and in a number of studies such training has been shown to contribute to unusually large increases in performance (Harle & Vickers, 2001; Oudejans, Koedijker, Bleijendaal, & Bakker, 2005; Vickers, Morton, & Panchuk, in progress). Information on the quiet eye will be elaborated upon in chapters 4 through 8, where the quiet eye is described as found in targeting tasks, interceptive timing tasks, and tactical tasks.

Summary of Theoretical Orientation

Thus far the four major theories that contribute to our understanding of visuomotor coordination have been introduced and the major concepts defined in terms of understanding motor learning, motor control, and visuomotor coordination. From cognitive psychology comes the concept of information processing and the cognitive processes of sensation, perception, anticipation, attention, pattern recognition, memory, problem solving, and decision making. From ecological psychology come the concepts of direct perception, invariances, optic array, optic flow, and affordances. From dynamic systems come the notion of degrees of freedom and their freezing, freeing, and exploitation and self-organization.

The constraints-led perspective attempts to pull together many of the competing views contained in the cognitive, ecological, and dynamic systems theories and explains that organismic constraints, environmental constraints, and task constraints all influence the perception–action cycle as found in specific perceptual-motor workspaces. Each constraint was elaborated upon in terms of how it is used in this book. Organismic constraints were defined through elite–near-elite comparison, and environmental and task constraints were incorporated through the use of research methods situated within realistic performance environments, thus increasing the **ecological validity** of the findings. A study is considered to be ecologically valid when its methods, materials, and the setting of experiments approximate the real-life situation that underlies the study. Gaze control studies situated within realistic sport environments have identified three major categories of gaze control as found in targeting, interceptive timing, and tactical sport tasks. Finally the quiet eye was described. These concepts were only briefly explained since they make up the bulk of the information presented in chapters 4 through 8.

It is clear from the many concepts outlined here that there are a number of distinct, and in some cases competing, ways of understanding visuomotor coordination. In this final section, the ability of each of the four theories to explain both fast and slow movements is explained. To be successful, a theoretical framework must account for how humans are able to perform rapid dynamic tasks (such as ice hockey goaltending, cricket batting) as well as those that are slower (as found when walking or shooting a free throw). Slow and fast movements are normally defined by the duration of their movement times (see chapter 3) since this dictates the extent to which feedback (and additional cognitive processing) can be used to modify or change the movement. An overview of the theoretical concepts is presented in two columns below. Those concepts in the first column are best at explaining how tasks with slow movement times are controlled, while those in the second column are best at explaining tasks with fast movement times. Note that some concepts are effective in explaining how both slow and fast actions are performed. At the end

of the overview, a number of new concepts are listed that will be covered in the next chapters, the main ones being focal and ambient vision, top-down and bottom-up processing, ventral and dorsal processing, and closed- and open-loop motor control. It will be shown in the next chapters that the combination of **focal vision**, top-down processing, ventral stream, and closed-loop control is tailored for situations where there is ample time for cognitive processing to occur, while the combination of the ambient vision, bottom-up processing, dorsal stream, and open-loop control is specialized for tasks performed under time constraints. The two systems work together to permit the great range of human actions we find in motor behavior.

Overview of Theoretical Concepts

Best for Explaining Tasks With Slow Movement Times	*Best for Explaining Tasks With Fast Movement Times*
➤ Cognitive psychology	➤ Cognitive and ecological psychology
➤ Neuroscience	➤ Dynamic systems
➤ Constraints-led perspective	➤ Constraints-led perspective
➤ Memory	➤ Sensation and perception
➤ Problem solving	➤ Optic flow
➤ Decision making	➤ Invariances
➤ Motor learning and performance	➤ Motor learning and performance
➤ Consciousness	➤ Subconsciousness
➤ Anticipation and attention	➤ Direct perception
➤ Pattern recognition	➤ Affordances
➤ Skill development	➤ Self-organization
➤ Degrees of freedom	➤ Degrees of freedom
➤ Quiet eye	➤ Quiet eye
➤ Focal vision	➤ Focal and ambient vision
➤ Ventral system	➤ Dorsal system
➤ Closed-loop control	➤ Open-loop control
➤ Top-down processing	➤ Bottom-up processing

Gaze Control in Action

Go to www.kin.ucalgary.ca/nml/ and check out these Web sites for information on how the gaze is recorded and examples of how the quiet eye is used in a variety of sports.

➤ Visit www.pbs.org/saf/1206 to see a *Scientific American Frontiers* television show titled "On the Ball" with Alan Alda. This show illustrates how gaze data are recorded in a number of sports. It also features interviews with elite athletes who have used the quiet eye successfully in competition.

➤ Go to the *Golf Digest* Web site at http://golfdigest.com/search/index.ssf?/instruction/gd200401quieteye.html to find out how the quiet eye is used in putting.

Visual Perception, Cognition, and Action

In part I the theoretical foundations of the book are presented using selected concepts from cognitive psychology, ecological psychology, dynamic systems, and the constraints-led perspective. Each of these theories provides valuable insights into how athletes use vision to control their movements, although no theory alone is adequate to explain the control of both fast and slow movements. In many respects, it is the capacity of one theory or another to explain both slow and fast movements that separates the various theories. Current research shows that slow movements are controlled or influenced more by a combination of focal vision, top-down processing, ventral stream, and closed-loop control, while fast movements are informed best by ambient vision, bottom-up processing, dorsal stream, and open-loop control.

In the Introduction, the constraints-led perspective as proposed by Newell (1986) and Newell & McDonald (1994) was used as a springboard for taking into account the many factors that influence visuomotor behavior, including those that come from the environment, the organism, and the task. These are developed in chapter 1, which concentrates on the visual system and motor control within an ever changing brain. Since this is a book centered primarily on vision, chapter 2 covers the two methods used to record and analyze the gaze of athletes: the visual search and vision-in-action methods. Of the two approaches, the vision-in-action method (which is also called perception–action coupling studies) is emphasized more because this method always requires the participants to perform physically as the gaze is recorded, thus enabling a description of the gaze, attention, and other factors during sport success and failure.

Chapter 3 concentrates on the relationship of gaze control to attention. Prior to recent research, it was difficult to make a direct link between shifts of gaze and attention, but new evidence shows that under certain conditions explained in this chapter, a shift in gaze is invariably linked to a shift in attention.

At the conclusion of the introduction and part I, students should be able to do the following:

- ➤ Name and describe four main theories of visuomotor coordination, including being able to list their main strengths and weaknesses.

- ➤ Define the quiet eye, including its four major characteristics as they apply to the location, onset, offset, and duration of critical fixation or pursuit tracking gaze.

- ➤ Describe the main parts of the visual system and brain, including being able to diagram the general flow of visual information from the retina to the brain to the motor system.

- ➤ Describe how the brain changes with exercise and important factors that influence this process.

- ➤ Describe two methods for recording and analyzing the gaze of athletes and their respective contributions to defining skill and performance differences in sport.

- ➤ Define what visual attention is and the relationship of shifts of gaze to attention.

- ➤ Be able to explain the relationship between reaction time, movement time, and open- and closed-loop motor control.

- ➤ Be able to define the major terms as shown in bold and in the glossary.

CHAPTER 1

Visual System, Motor Control, and the Changing Brain

CHAPTER OUTLINE

◄◄ *Where Have We Been?*

In the introduction, the theoretical basis of the book was presented. The focus of the book is on the visual system and how the gaze of sport performers allows new insight into psychological factors critical to success in sport. Previously, the visual world of the performing athlete was hidden, but with the advent of mobile eye trackers it is now possible to scientifically study how control of the gaze underlies sport success and failure. Selected findings from four dominant theories (i.e., cognitive, ecological, dynamics systems, and constraints-led theories) were collected into an adaptation of the constraints-led model, featuring gaze control and quiet-eye findings in three major categories of sport tasks where research has shown the perceptual-motor cycles differ in distinctive ways.

➤➤ *Where Are We Going?*

The focus of chapter 1 includes the visual system, the brain and **motor control**, and brain **plasticity**. The path of visual information is followed from initial input at the retinal level through the eyes to the neural areas used to plan, organize, and control motor actions. The chapter begins with the basic anatomy of the eyes and brain, and then moves on to functional issues related to types of eye movements, the focal and ambient visual systems, and binocular vision. The visual centers of the brain are described along with the critical roles played by the occipital cortex, ventral (slower) and dorsal (faster) systems, mirror neurons, as well as motor control. The chapter concludes with a description of brain plasticity, which shows that the brain changes over a lifetime. Evidence is also presented showing that participation in enriched physical activities where decision making is encouraged is beneficial to optimal neural development and processing.

Visual System

Figure 1.1 presents a cross section of the human eye and shows that light enters the eye through the pupil, an opening in the iris. The **pupil** adjusts with the amount of available light and becomes smaller in bright light and larger in low light. The lens is adjusted by the ciliary muscles, but the **cornea**, which is the transparent surface of the eye, is not adjustable. When light enters the eye, it is bent first by the curvature of the cornea and then by the lens.

Bending the light in this way positions objects or locations of interest on the **fovea,** an area at the back of the eye in the **retina** that is responsible for visual acuity, or the ability to resolve small details and thus see objects or locations clearly. The retina converts light into energy that results in neural activation. The retina is lined with two types of visual receptors, called *rods* and *cones.* Cones are located within the fovea and are responsible for the detection of color and light and for resolving detail. The proportion of rods increases in the periphery of the retina, which is specialized for detecting low light and motion. The line of sight must be aligned with the fovea in order for an object or other location in space to be viewed with acuity.

Due to the small area of the fovea, the area over which we are able to see clearly is actually very small, about 2° to 3° of **visual angle.** One way to estimate the size of this area is to hold your thumb out in front of you at arm's length. The width of your thumb is about 2° of visual angle projected into space. Most athletes are surprised that they are only able to see clearly over such a small area. They must move their gaze purposely in order to see the different aspects of a scene with full acuity.

Notice in figure 1.1 that the image of the key is inverted on the fovea of the retina. Any image projected on the retina is upside down and backward. It is important to know that the retina does not see a picture of a key, because "the retina alone cannot perceive anything" (Goldstein, 2007, p. 46). The retina transforms light energy from the "key" into signals that are then processed by the brain. It is also important to stress that researchers do not know completely how this electrical energy is transformed into our subjective experience of seeing a key or other visual images. There is also a blind spot within each eye where the optic nerve and blood vessels enter and exit the eye. Most of us are unaware that we even have a blind spot since the location is slightly different in each eye and thus is rarely a factor in vision.

Visual Field and Line of Gaze

The total amount of light that stimulates your eyes at any moment in time is called the **visual field** (Coren, Ward, & Enns, 2004). Figure 1.2 shows the left and right visual fields. A **line of**

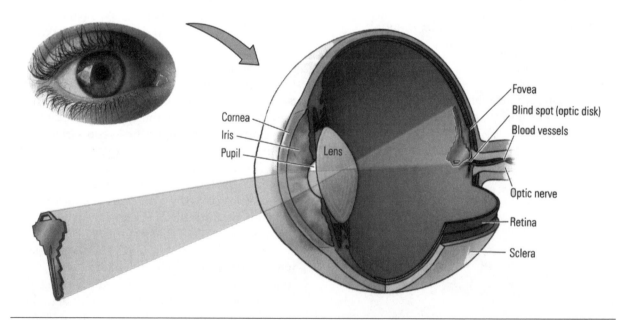

► **Figure 1.1**   Cross section of the eye showing the cornea, iris, pupil, fovea, sclera, retina, and blind spot.

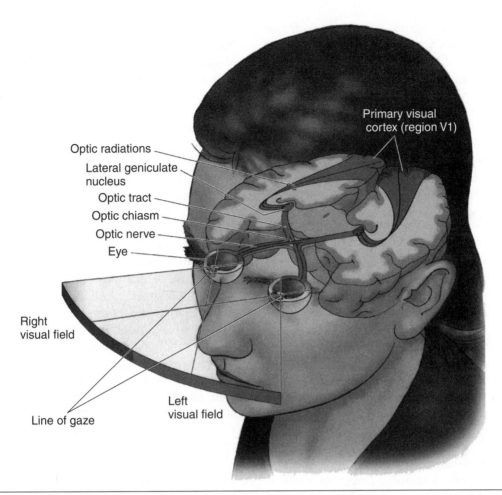

Primary visual
cortex (region V1)

Optic radiations

Lateral geniculate
nucleus

Optic tract

Optic chiasm

Optic nerve

Eye

Right
visual field

Line of gaze

Left
visual field

➤ **Figure 1.2**   The visual system, showing the visual fields of each eye, the line of gaze from the right eye and left eye, and the optic system, including radiations from each eye to the primary visual regions at the back of the brain.

gaze originates from each eye, passes through the appropriate field, and intersects in front. The line of gaze is defined as "the absolute position of the eyes in space and depends on both eye position in orbit and head position in space" (Schmid & Zambarbieri, 1991, p. 229). **Gaze control** is defined as the process of directing the gaze to objects or events within a scene in real time and in the service of the ongoing perceptual, cognitive, and behavioral activity (Henderson, 2003).

Figure 1.2 shows that information detected by the two visual fields (left and right) crosses over as it passes along the optic tract. Visual information flows along the **optic tract** through the lateral geniculate nucleus to the primary visual regions or occipital cortex, which are located at the back of the head. The passage of visual information along this route is continuous, and constant processing occurs within many parts of the brain.

Types of Eye Movements and Gaze Control

As one looks about a scene, the gaze alternates between periods of stability and periods when the gaze moves rapidly between objects and locations. Two types of gaze control are found: those that are maintained on objects or locations for a period of time sufficient for information to be processed by the brain, and those that move so rapidly that information cannot be processed in a conscious way.

Gaze That Permits Information Processing

A **fixation** occurs when the gaze is held on an object or location within 3° of visual angle for 100 ms or longer (Carl & Gellman, 1987; Carpenter, 1988; Fischer, 1987; Optican, 1985). The 100 ms threshold is the minimum amount of time needed to recognize or become aware of stimuli. Additional time is required to make a movement, with about 180 ms needed to actually see an object and initiate a simple movement, such as pressing a key. **Pursuit tracking** occurs when the gaze follows a moving object, such as a ball or a person. The 100 ms threshold is used for pursuit tracking for the same reason it is used for fixations; it is only when the gaze is stabilized on the moving object or person that the individual is able to process the information provided by that object or person.

Gaze That Does Not Permit Conscious Information Processing

Saccades occur when the eyes move quickly from one fixated or tracked location to another. For example, in golfing, saccades occur when the golfer looks from the hole to the ball and back during putting; in a team sport, they occur from one opponent to another. Saccades are rapid eye movements that bring the point of maximal visual acuity onto the fovea so that it can be seen with clarity. We average about 3 saccades each second when viewing a normal scene, and these range in duration from 60 to 100 ms. To see and comprehend a scene, we must move our eyes rapidly from one fixated location or object to another using saccades. During saccades, information is suppressed (Bridgeman, Hendry, & Start, 1975). Information gained during fixation or tracking is maintained across saccades so that a stable, coherent scene is viewed (Irwin, 1996; Irwin & Brockmole, 2004). We do not perceive the blur as our eyes move, nor are we able to see a new object that appears during a saccade. But we do possess an object-file transsaccadic memory (Irwin, 1996; Irwin & Brockmole, 2004) that allows us to perceive scenes that are cohesive and meaningful.

Blinks occur when the eyelid covers the eye. Blinking is essential for refreshing the cornea and lens and for maintaining vision. During blinks, information is also suppressed (Volkmann, Riggs, & Moore, 1981).

Focal and Ambient Systems

Performance in sport is affected by both the focal and ambient systems. In order for information to be processed by the focal system it must be detected by the fovea, a small area located at the back of the eye in the retina (see figure 1.1).

The focal system is used when fixated or tracked information falls on the fovea and aspects of an object or location are viewed with full acuity or detail. The **ambient system** includes the areas on the retina that are not within the fovea. The ambient system is specialized for motion, the rapid detection of information, and for perception during low light conditions. It has important properties that affect motor control. To illustrate how vital this system is, imagine you are an ice hockey goaltender. You are set to make a stop with your glove hand when suddenly the puck is redirected so fast that you simply cannot get your eyes on it. Miraculously, your glove hand adjusts just enough to make the stop. Were you just lucky, or is there evidence showing that humans possess a rapid perceptual system that works in well-practiced situations like this?

Critical to understanding how the ambient system functions in motor skills is the research of Pelisson, Prablanc, Goodale, and Jeannerod (1986). Participants wore an eye tracker and were required to point to a target that appeared on a computer screen within reach of their hand. They were unaware that the eye tracker was programmed to move the target to a second location when they made a saccade to see the target when it first appeared. Recall that information is suppressed during saccades; therefore they could not see the target move to the second location. Yet, their hand adjusted and moved accurately to the new target location! Although their focal system could not see the new target in its new location, the ambient system possessed properties that allowed the movement correction to be made. Therefore, it may be that an elite ice hockey goaltender, for example, can use information perceived in a fraction of a second by the ambient system.

The ambient system, however, has many limitations. The ambient system appears to be effective in contributing to accurate limb movements of very short durations (100 to 150 ms) (Bridgeman, Kirch, & Sperling, 1981; Pelisson et al., 1986; Rossetti, 1998), but when movements are longer or are novel, the ambient system is unable to process the information. Instead the focal system takes over and exerts cognitive control over the situation. The ambient system is therefore able to register the flow of information that contributes to rapid motor control in well-learned skills, but both the ambient and focal systems are needed when tasks are new or complex.

Properties of the Gaze in Space

We turn now to questions of the regulation of the eyes and head when an athlete orients the gaze to an object or location in space. A sequence of events occurs in which the eyes move before the head does (Guitton & Volle, 1987; Helsen, Starkes, & Beukers, 1997; Schmid & Zambarbieri, 1991; Zangemeister & Stark, 1982). The eyes localize the target first, followed by the head because of its greater size and inertia (Helsen, Elliott, Starkes, & Ricker, 1998; Helsen, Starkes, & Buekers, 1997). When athletes orient their gaze to a target requiring a large gaze displacement, there is a saccade to about 40° horizontal, which is the neural limitation for saccades from the central fixed position (Gauthier, Semmlow, Vercher, Pedrono, & Obrecht, 1991; Guitton & Volle, 1987; Helsen et al., 1997; Schmid & Zambarbieri, 1991). The movement of the eyes and head to the target is normally smooth, with the processing of information occurring within 100 ms of the eyes stabilizing on the new location.

Visual discrimination begins immediately and is maintained steadily on the target or other locations even though the head is moving. This is achieved through the vestibular ocular reflex (VOR), which induces a movement of the eyes in the opposite direction of head movement. It is easy to experience this reflex yourself by performing the following exercise. Look directly in front of you and fixate on a single location. Then move your head slowly from side to side while maintaining your gaze on the location. As your head moves in one direction, the VOR automatically compensates by producing a movement of the eyes in the opposite direction so that you can see a stable image.

Visual angle indicates the size of an image on the retina, and it is determined by extending lines from the edges of the object as viewed in space through the lens to the retina, as shown in figure 1.3. Here we see a soccer ball approaching from two distances, one near and the other farther away. The size of the object and its distance affect the visual angle, so a ball seen at a distance will subtend a smaller visual angle on the retina than one viewed from a shorter distance. Note also the second set of dotted lines, which show the part of the visual angle that is centered on the fovea. In the top picture where the ball is close, only a small part of the ball is located on the fovea, while in the picture at the bottom almost the entire ball is centered on the fovea. Does this mean that the edges of the ball will be seen as blurred in the top image but not blurred in the bottom? Although the edges of the ball in the top image are indeed blurred (as they are perceived by the ambient or peripheral system), players report that they see the ball clearly. This is because they use their memory system to build up the total image even though some aspects are not seen with full acuity.

Neural Centers of the Brain

This far, the anatomy of the eye has been presented along with a description of how spatial information is acquired using different types of eye movements. In this section, the parts of the brain used in visual processing are presented

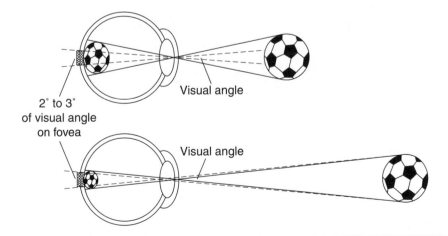

➤ **Figure 1.3**   Visual angle of a soccer ball as viewed at near (above) and far distances (below). Also shown is the portion of the visual angle located on the fovea.

and their role in **attention** and motor control explained. Figure 1.4 shows a view of the left posterior brain and the neural centers responsible for processing visual information. They include the optic nerve, the lateral geniculate nucleus, the optic radiations, which radiate back to the occipital lobe at the back of the head, the parietal lobe, the temporal lobe and inferotemporal cortex, and the frontal lobe. All of these areas are involved in processing the visual information needed to perform goal-directed actions.

Processing Visual Information in the Occipital, Parietal, and Temporal Lobes

In this section we look primarily at the processing of visual information in the visual cortex **(occipital lobe),** the **parietal lobe,** and the temporal lobe (see figure 1.4). Figure 1.4 shows that the occipital lobe is comprised of areas V1 to V5. Each of these areas is specialized for processing different visual inputs. Tong (2003, p. 219-220) states that V1 is "uniquely positioned as the primary distributor of almost all visual information that reaches other cortical areas. About

90% of projections from the eye are channeled through lateral geniculate nucleus (LGN) to V1." From V1, information is disseminated to various extrastriate visual areas for further analysis, including V2, V3/VP, V3A, V4, MT/V5, as well as most higher areas of the brain. V1 neurons are sensitive to orientation, motion direction, color, contrast, form, and ocular dominance (Kolb & Whishaw, 2001; Tong, 2003; Wong-Riley, Hevner, Cutlan, Earnest, Egan, Frost, & Nyugen, 1993). V2, V3, V4 and V5 receive inputs from V1 and V2 and are responsible for detecting form and motion. Outputs from V3A and V5 go to the dorsal stream and parietal lobe, while outputs from V3 and V4 go to the temporal lobe.

Binocular Vision and the Perception of Depth

Viewing an object with one eye is called **monocular vision,** and viewing it with two eyes is called **binocular vision.** We normally perceive the world using inputs from both eyes, but the brain creates one cohesive image. Let's imagine a ball approaching as in table tennis. We know that pursuit tracking occurs during the early part of

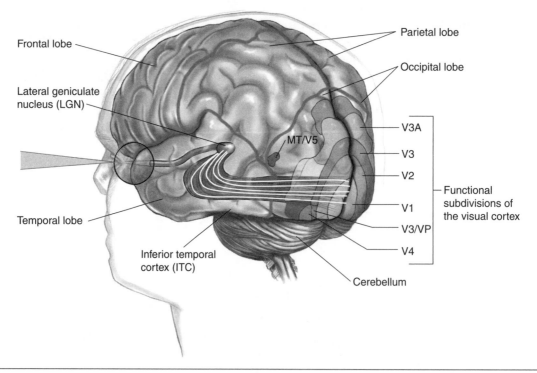

➤ **Figure 1.4**   The brain, including the subdivisions of the visual cortex of the occipital lobe, the parietal lobe, the frontal lobe, the inferotemporal cortex, and the temporal lobe.

ball flight (Ripoll & Fleurance, 1988; Rodrigues, Vickers, & Williams, 2002). At near distances, we also know that each eye has a slightly different visual field due to the spacing of the eyes in the head and direction of flight of the ball. As the ball is tracked, **binocular fusion** occurs, which is the merging of slightly different images from the two eyes into a single **stereoscopic perception,** simply called *fusion* or *binocular interaction.* The slight difference in the images, which arises from binocular disparity, is important because it provides the cue we use for depth, yet we still see a single, stable image. Gregory (1997, p. 60) states, "A remarkable thing about the visual system is its ability to combine the two somewhat different images into a single perception of solid objects lying in three-dimensional space (stereoscopic perception)."

Binocular disparity is the slight discrepancy between the two retinal images of a three-dimensional object or scene caused by binocular parallax. The basis for stereopsis or depth occurs in areas V1, V2, and V5 (MT) of the occipital cortex. Certain disparity selective cells are attuned to stimuli at specific distances. When too much disparity occurs, then double vision, or diplopia, occurs. Binocular disparity is usually expressed in terms of the difference in the visual angle subtended by points on the object or surface being viewed. The visual system is capable of responding with sensations of depth to disparities as small as 1/1,800 of 1° of visual angle, and near the fovea the maximum binocular disparity resulting in fusion corresponds to 1/6 of 1°. Gregory (1997) also states that stereo vision only functions for quite near objects, as differences between the images of each eye become too small to detect differences.

In addition to binocular cues for depth, there are many monocular cues, including interposition or occlusion, where one object is seen to be closer than another and therefore blocks the locations behind it. Shading and shadows also provide clues to depth, as do the size of an image on the retina and linear perspective. When objects are far away, they are smaller on the fovea. Linear perspective is evident when the lines on a tennis or volleyball court, for example, seem to converge as you look across the net, or when a vanishing point seems to exist in the distance as occurs when cycling along a long straight road.

Ventral and Dorsal Processing

Two forms of visual processing have been identified, dorsal and ventral (Milner & Goodale, 1995), that are specific to the separate regions of the brain shown in figure 1.5. The dorsal stream projects from the occipital lobe at the back of the head to the top of the posterior parietal lobe, while the ventral system projects forward along the sides of the head through the temporal lobes to the frontal areas.

The **dorsal stream** is the pathway that conducts signals from the occipital cortex to the parietal lobe and is responsible for orienting the gaze and sustaining attention at one location (Posner & Raichle, 1994). It is also responsible for the rapid processing and updating of information that is important for orientation in space and movement. The dorsal stream is also known as the *where pathway* because it directs attention to locations in space. Patients who suffer bilateral lesions of the parietal lobes (or Balint's syndrome) have problems processing information that defines the location of objects. The parietal lobes appear to contain the master map of locations that we use for navigating and for controlling our orientation in space (Treisman, 1999). The **ventral stream** is the pathway that conducts signals from the occipital cortex to the temporal lobe. It is also known as the *what stream* and is associated with the cognitive processing of information and higher executive processes. The ventral stream is responsible for assigning meaning to objects and events, and it

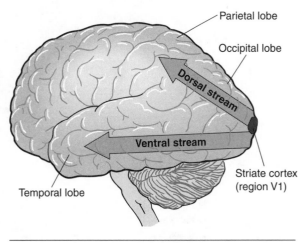

► **Figure 1.5**   The ventral and dorsal processing streams.

From An Introduction to Brain and Behavior by Bryan Kolb and Ian Q. Whishaw. © 2001 Worth Publishers. Used with permission.

guides the **anticipation** and planning of actions. The dorsal stream is adept at processing information of short duration, but the ventral system requires time to carry out its role.

Both the dorsal and ventral streams send information to the frontal lobes, where the billions of features are bound together into what the performer is perceiving and thinking. The **frontal cortex** is known as the executive of the brain and coordinates advanced thinking, planning, and **language**. The ventral and dorsal streams are closely associated with the somatosensory cortex, which is located at the top of the head between the parietal and motor cortices. The **somatosensory cortex** is responsible for the sense of touch, pressure, and feeling—capacities that are extremely important in all forms of movement.

Figure 1.6 shows the frontal, premotor, and motor areas of the brain in more detail. It is here where the brain accesses memories of performing a similar act in the past and where the commands to act are organized. The commands to move are then sent to the motor regions of the brain (the premotor and motor cortex), where specific movements are organized and executed.

Mirror Neurons

Central to the acquisition of motor skills is the ability to watch the performance of others and mimic the actions being observed. Humans are able to mimic the actions of others from the time they are born. This process occurs in a part of the brain called **mirror neurons.** Thus far, mirror neurons have been found in the frontal cortex and the parietal cortex as shown in figure 1.6. Mirror neurons were first discovered by Rizzolatti et al. (1996) through an accidental event in their lab. They were running experiments where a monkey was required to perform a grasping action with its hand. Recordings were made from different neurons that fired in response to whether the monkey picked up the object or performed another action. However, Rizollati et

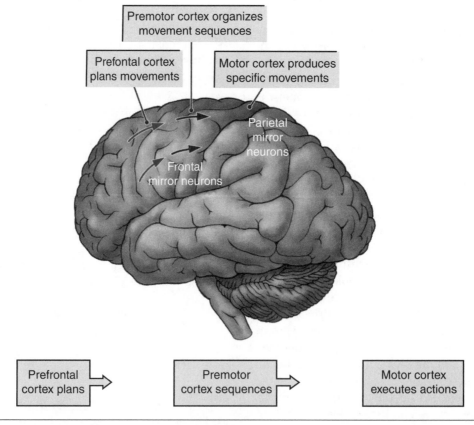

➤ Figure 1.6   The frontal areas of the brain, the premotor and motor cortex, and mirror neuron system, which is located in both the frontal and parietal lobes.

al. noticed that when they picked up the object while the monkey simply watched, the same neurons fired even though the monkey had made no movements. Ramachandran (2000) explained that "one might be tempted to think that these are motor 'command' neurons, making muscles do certain things; however, the astonishing truth is that any given mirror neuron will also fire when the monkey in question observes another monkey (or even the experimenter) performing the same action" (p. 6). Perhaps more interesting, if the experimenter used pliers to pick up the object, the monkey's neurons did not fire, which meant that the monkey did not know what pliers were or that they were used to grasp objects. The motor neuron system has since been shown to be highly integrated with the sensorimotor and motor cortices and is central to the preparation and production of head-orienting movements, as well as reaching, grasping, and the production of most object-oriented behaviors.

One of the first studies to identify mirror neurons in humans was by Ramachandran (2000), who studied patients with a rare disorder called **anosognosia,** where a stroke in the right hemisphere leads to a complete paralysis of the left side of the body. About 5% of the patients denied their paralysis even though mentally they were normal. In addition, they denied the paralysis of other patients whose inability to move was visible to them and to others. Ramachandran explained that "denying one's own paralysis is odd enough but why would a patient deny another patient's paralysis? We suggest that this bizarre observation is best understood in terms of damage to Rizzolatti's mirror neurons. It's as if anytime you want to make a judgment about someone else's movements you have to run a VR (virtual reality) simulation of the corresponding movements in your own brain and without mirror neurons you cannot do this" (p. 7).

Two types of motor neurons have since been identified (Iacoboni & Dapretto, 2006; Rizzolatti & Craighero, 2004). Strictly congruent motor neurons fire for observed and executed actions that are identical, while broadly congruent motor neurons fire when the observed action differs from an executed action that achieves the same goal. Both of these classes of motor neurons also fire in anticipation of an action being performed. Young children mimic the goals of an observed action and only later are concerned with developing specific actions; overall, they tend to simply copy the actions of adults in a mirror-like fashion. During this mirroring process, the mirror neurons in the frontal cortex are more active. The motor aspects of the observed actions are developed later, and there is more activation of the mirror neurons in the parietal cortex. Mirror neurons not only code the actions of others, but mirror neurons also are sensitive to the goals the person is trying to achieve, their intentions, and their emotional state. Damage of the mirror neuron system has been found to be one of the causes of autism (Dapretto, Davies, Pfeifer et al., 2006). Autistic children withdraw from the world and are unable to interact in normal contexts. **Autism** is a cognitive disorder characterized by greatly impaired social interaction; a narrow range of interests; deficits in language and communication; and fixed, repetitive movements.

Visuomotor Control

Visuomotor control is the process whereby visual (gaze) information is used to direct and control movements. The major steps in visuomotor control are summarized in figure 1.7, where we see a person acquiring the visual information needed to pick up a coffee cup. Eight steps are shown, beginning with the person (1) looking in order to locate the cup with the eyes and fixating it to register its shape, size, distance, and perhaps how full it is or if it is too hot to grab. This visual information is then (2) passed from the retina to the occipital lobes, and then through the parietal and ventral areas to the frontal lobe, where the reach and grasp commands are formulated. (3) Next, these commands go to the major **motor control neural areas** located at the top of the head (the primary motor cortex, the supplementary motor area, and the premotor area) and are responsible for the control of movements. Motor commands leave the motor areas and (4) go down the spinal column to the hands and arms, which carry out the action. Perhaps the person wants to grasp only the handle, wrap the hand completely around the cup, or move tentatively because the cup may be too hot to lift. (5) Receptors in the hand and fingers pick up sensory information such as heat, weight, and pressure, which are **feedback** signals that (6) race back up the arm and spinal cord to the motor cortex and frontal lobe, where it is confirmed that the cup is now grasped. Other brain regions such as the (7) **basal ganglia** and **cerebellum** modulate

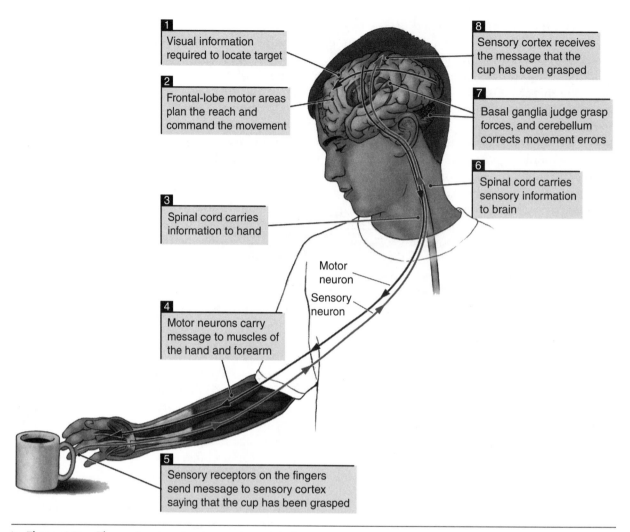

1 Visual information required to locate target

2 Frontal-lobe motor areas plan the reach and command the movement

3 Spinal cord carries information to hand

4 Motor neurons carry message to muscles of the hand and forearm

5 Sensory receptors on the fingers send message to sensory cortex saying that the cup has been grasped

8 Sensory cortex receives the message that the cup has been grasped

7 Basal ganglia judge grasp forces, and cerebellum corrects movement errors

6 Spinal cord carries sensory information to brain

Motor neuron

Sensory neuron

➤ **Figure 1.7**   The major steps in visuomotor control.

From An Introduction to Brain and Behavior by Bryan Kolb and Ian Q. Whishaw. © 2001 Worth Publishers. Used with permission.

the control of movement and make the necessary adjustments as the cup is raised to the lips or set down in a new location. The basal ganglia are a group of nuclei located deep in the forebrain that coordinate voluntary movement of the limbs and body. The cerebellum, also known as the hindbrain, is located at the back of the head and is involved in motor coordination and the timing of movement. In the final step, (8) the person prepares for the next movement by determining if the action was carried out in an adequate way.

Time Course of Visuomotor Processing

One of the remarkable things about the visual system is the extensive pathway along which information must pass. Figure 1.8 shows that

the visual pathway (1) begins when information is registered on the eye's retina by the focal and ambient systems, then (2) travels to the back of the head along the optic nerve and radiations to the (3) occipital cortex, where visual information is registered as billions of features. (4) These then race in parallel fashion both to the top of the head to the parietal cortex (dorsal) and along the sides of the head to the temporal (ventral) areas. There is an integration of information in the somatosensory cortex as (5) the information goes to the frontal cortex, where the goals and intentions reside and plans are formulated for the specific event that is occurring. (6) The flow of information then goes to the premotor and motor cortex at the top of the head before (7) going down the spinal cord to the effectors. Perhaps this is one of the reasons why vision is

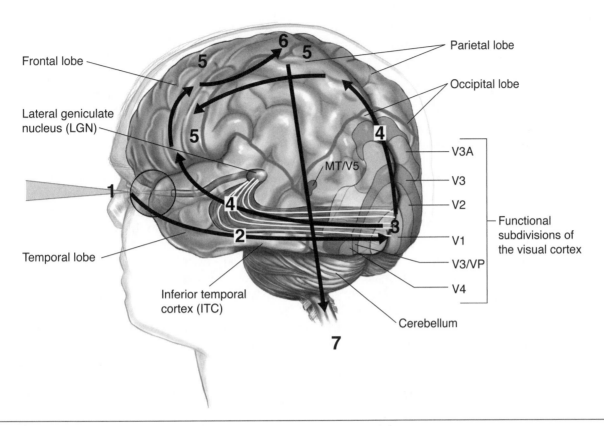

> **Figure 1.8**   An overview of the visual pathways used in motor control.
© 1999 Terese Winslow.

so dominant—its journey through the brain is so extensive that it reaches virtually all parts of the brain, and these parts all contribute to **motor control** in some way.

Although the main visual pathways are as shown in figure 1.8, a critical question is when visual awareness or **consciousness** occurs. When a person is visually aware they are conscious of what is being viewed; for example, they know an apple is red and not green, that a dog is black and not grey, or that a person is walking slowly rather than quickly. Does visual awareness begin immediately when information arrives at the retina, or does it occur first in the occipital area, or in the dorsal or ventral pathways, or later in the frontal cortex? Three models of visual awareness have been proposed based on animal lesion studies where sections of the brain have been surgically removed, as well as from studies of brain injury in humans (Tong, 2003). **Hierarchical models of visual awareness** propose that visual awareness occurs only when visual information reaches the higher cortical level areas (Crick & Koch, 1995). **Interactive models of visual awareness** propose that visual

awareness occurs in V1, that is, very early in the visual pathway (Buller, 2001; Pollen, 1999). **Alternative models** propose that visual awareness may be flexible and situation-dependent rather than hard-wired (Tononi & Edelman, 1998). Lesion studies of V1, as well as the parietal area, show that damage to the parietal or temporal regions greatly impairs visual awareness. The evidence also shows that V1 on its own is not sufficient for visual awareness. However, visual awareness can occur at V1 if inputs are received from the higher centers (Engel & Singer, 2001; Tong, 2003).

Overall, studies show that for a simple visual stimulus (for example, seeing a red dot on a computer monitor), it takes about 30 to 50 ms for the features of the stimulus to be registered in the occipital region, and it takes about 70 to 100 ms for them to reach the parietal, temporal, somatosensory, and frontal areas of the brain and for simple motor commands to be initiated. It then takes an additional 70 to 80 ms for the commands to travel from the motor centers to the muscles before the first observable movement, or a minimum of 180 to 190 ms in total. Although visual awareness may occur very early in the visual pathway, it takes at least this amount of time to see a visual stimulus and make a simple movement.

Changes in the Brain

The human brain is composed of two types of cells, called **neurons** and **glia,** which are shown in figure 1.9. When we are born, we have more neurons than at any other time in our lifetime, with estimates somewhere in the billions (Kolb & Whishaw, 2004). Neurons have a cell body, dendrites, a main axon covered with a myelin sheath, and terminal buttons that connect with other neurons. Neurons are responsible for carrying nerve impulses throughout the nervous system and for communicating with other neurons through synaptic junctions. Neurons acquire information from the sensory receptors (sight, hearing, touch, smell, taste) and pass this information to other neurons that send the information to the muscles to produce movements. Neurons communicate with one another through neurotransmitters and the transmission of electrical signals or action potentials. It is astounding how many inputs one neuron can receive, with estimates in the range of 1,000 or more converging inputs. These in turn diverge and affect other neurons; therefore, the synaptic influence can extend in some cases to millions of neurons (Fields & Stevens-Graham, 2002; Kalat, 2004; Kandel, Schwartz, & Jessell, 2000). There are many types of neurons, and each is specialized to optimize information transmission. The adult brain is capable of carrying messages in an infinite number of ways. Indeed, it is estimated that there are more than 1 trillion nerve cells in the brain, and each can make up to 10,000 connections.

The brain has nine times more glial cells than neurons (Fields & Stevens-Graham, 2002; Krebs, Huttman, & Steinhauser, 2005). Previously it was thought that their main purpose was to serve as a primary source of nutrients and sustenance for neurons, but new evidence shows they also are messengers, albeit in a different way than neurons. Glial cells lack the membrane properties required to fire action potentials, but they communicate with one another and with neurons chemically rather than through electrical signals. Glial cells play a major role in **information processing** in the nervous system, and they may one day provide a greater understanding of how information

is processed. During development "glia have a powerful role in setting up the basic scaffolding of the brain" (Fields & Stevens-Graham, 2002, p. 561) in that they extend the influence of **axons** and **dendrites** in forming synaptic connections. Axons are the parts of a neuron that conduct nerve impulses or messages over distances between neurons. Dendrites are branches of a neuron that greatly increase its area.

As with neurons, there are many different types of glial cells. Most numerous are astrocytes, which are shown in figure 1.9. Astrocytes not only supply neurons with nutrients, but they also absorb neurotransmitters and ensure that neurons are maintained in a balanced environment. In addition, astrocytes and other glia also communicate with one another and with neurons using the same neurotransmitters that neurons use. Neurons and glia differ in how they transmit information. Neurons use electrical signals while glia use chemical messages, which researchers have found are key in coordinating the activity of nerve cells in different parts of the brain at the same time.

This newly understood capacity, if upheld through research, offers hope to people suffering from disorders such as Parkinson's, Huntington's, and Alzheimer's. It is also important for those who participate in sport because it means that training leads to increased capacities in both

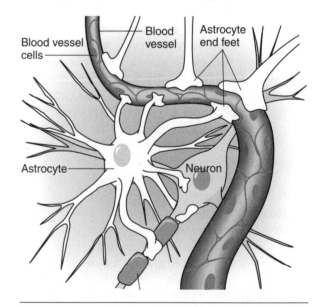

► **Figure 1.9**   Neurons and astrocyte, which is a type of glial cell.

From An Introduction to Brain and Behavior by Bryan Kolb and Ian Q. Whishaw. © 2001 Worth Publishers. Used with permission.

the body and the brain, with more permanent changes occurring in the brain when certain conditions prevail. Research shows that two processes called **synaptogenesis** and **neurogenesis** are facilitated in enriched environments that provide physical activity and decision-making opportunities.

Neurons undergo continual change as a result of maturation and experience. If the context of development is normal, then more and more neural connections are established while others die off as a result of disuse or understimulation. This process is called **neural plasticity** and is the capacity for neurons to change in response to experience and other influences. Neurophysical and neurochemical changes enhance the ability of the brain to compensate and adapt to environmental change and injury. In the next section, the processes involved in this process, synaptogenesis and neurogenesis, are explained.

Synaptogenesis

The human brain undergoes change continually from birth through a process called synaptogenesis. Our understanding of synaptogenesis goes back to Hebb (1949), who found that when one cell excites another repeatedly, a change takes place in one or both cells characterized by the growth of more dendrites, more synaptic connections, and a condition called arborization. A neuron that has been stimulated many times results in more synaptic connections or arborization, a longer axon, and more synaptic buds, while neurons that do not experience the same degree of stimulation are smaller and without the longer axon and dendrites. Continued stimulation between neurons causes the neurotransmitters to become more efficient. The structural properties of synapses show that they first undergo rapid change and then become stable during adulthood.

Neurogenesis

Not only is the brain capable of changing through synaptogenesis, but recent evidence indicates it also may be able to give birth to new neurons throughout life. It was generally believed that the human brain had no ability to repair itself by making new neurons and that the critical stem cells that underlie this process did not reside in the brain as they did in the muscles, skin, or

blood. If you cut yourself or break a bone, your body has an amazing ability to repair itself, but it was thought that this ability did not exist in the brain. The dogma of neuron death, also known as programmed cell death or cell fate, prevailed (Kandel et al., 2000, p. 1041).

Neurogenesis, or the birth of new neurons, was shown first in rats (Altman & Das, 1965), followed by songbirds (Nottebohm, 1985) and monkey primates (Gould, McEwan, Tanaput, Galea, & Fuchs, 1997). But no one believed that humans had the capacity to make new neurons until a 1998 study by Ericsson and colleagues. The evidence came from cancer patients, who, through the process of their diagnosis, had been given a marker called *bromodeoxyuridine (BrdU)* that had previously been used to detect the birth of new neurons in animals. BrdU becomes integrated into the DNA of dividing cells but is not retained by already established cells. Upon the death of the cancer patients and analysis of their brain tissue, it was found that they had produced new neurons after BrdU had been given, thus providing the first evidence that the human brain has the capacity for renewal over a lifetime. It is important to note that there is still considerable controversy surrounding whether neurogenesis occurs in humans, although it is widely accepted in animals and birds (Kalat, 2004).

Following Ericsson et al.'s findings, researchers set out to answer a number of new and exciting questions, which we will explore in the next section. For example, where in the brain are new neurons made? Are new neurons functional—that is, do they carry out the work they should? Are there specific conditions that foster the birth of new, functional neurons? What conditions increase the production of new neurons? And does the production of new neurons lead to improvements in motor behavior?

Where in the Human Brain Are Neurons Born?

The most active region in the brain for cell genesis is the **hippocampus** (see figure 1.10), which is highly responsive to enriched environments (Cao et al., 2004). The hippocampus is a large forebrain structure that is responsible for cell genesis, learning, and **memory** formation. New, undifferentiated neurons are born primarily in the hippocampus and then migrate to other areas

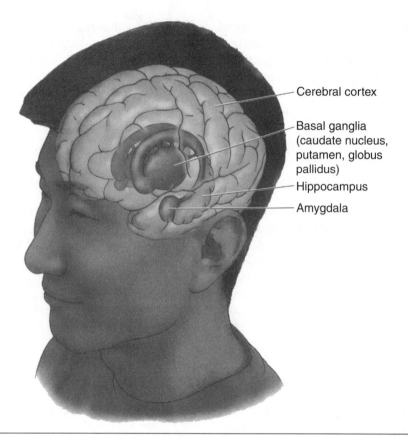

Cerebral cortex

Basal ganglia
(caudate nucleus,
putamen, globus
pallidus)

Hippocampus

Amygdala

➤ **Figure 1.10**   The cerebral cortex, basal ganglia, hippocampus, and amygdala of the human brain.

From An Introduction to Brain and Behavior by Bryan Kolb and Ian Q. Whishaw. © 2001 Worth Publishers. Used with permission.

of the brain that carry out specific functions. In mice and rats, it is estimated that 1,000 to 3,000 new cells are born each day. Mice and rats have 1 to 2 million neurons in total, so this means that 10% to 20% of rodent neurons are born through neurogenesis. It is not known what the comparable figures are for humans, but estimates runs to billions in early adulthood.

The hippocampus is located deep in the brain and looks a bit like the horns of a mountain sheep. The hippocampus is involved in learning and memory formation. Damage to the hippocampus prevents the retention and transfer of short-term memories to long-term memory centers that are located throughout the brain. An example of what life would be like with this condition is captured in a movie called *50 First Dates* (2004). Two people fall in love, but one of them has experienced hippocampal damage that prevents her from remembering that they had met. Her boyfriend conjures up ways to meet her every day, and they fall in love over and over again.

At the tip of the hippocampus is the **amygdala**, which plays a major role in emotional control and memory formation. The closeness of the amygdala to the center of memory formation partly explains why even one devastating experience seems to stay with us forever. Painful memories are laid down along with their emotional consequences. For instance, many people remember exactly where they were and what they were doing the day of the September 11, 2001 terrorist attacks. They remember their reaction to the events of that horrific day and the emotions it engendered within them. Similarly, when an athlete has a devastating experience, the emotions associated with the event are laid down in the hippocampus. The nature of these memories differs from person to person for reasons that are not understood. For example, one athlete can miss the winning free throw in the championship basketball game and have it affect his life forever, while another will carry no emotional scars at all. It is too soon to say if the strength of memories of such emotional events occurs because of the birth of new neurons or because of changes in existing neurons, but evidence presented in the next section suggests that the former may be the greater contributor.

Factors Affecting Neurogenesis and Synaptogenesis

A brain is functional only if it can learn new things and lay down memories that facilitate specific behaviors both in the present and future. Studies have shown that new neurons are indeed functional (Carlen et al., 2002; van Praag et al., 2002), but the degree of functionality depends on many factors. On the long list of possible influences are hormones, neurotransmitters, growth factors, transcription factors, aging, nutrition, physical exercise, environmental enrichment, stress, choice, and motivation (Brown et al., 2003; Kemperman, 2002).

Intriguing new evidence shows that physical activity is one of the main ways the brain improves, and the effect of physical activity on both neurogenesis and synaptogenesis is much greater than was previously thought (Draganski et al., 2004; Fabel et al., 2003; Gould, Beylin, Tanapat, Reeves, & Shors, 1999; Gould & Gross, 2002; Gross, 2000; Mirescu, Peters, & Gould, 2004; Sanes & Donahue, 2000; van Praag, Kemperman, & Gage, 1999, 2000). When physical activity occurs within an enriched environment involving extensive physical activity and decision training, the gains are even greater.

Because it is essential that changes in new neurons be measured from birth to adulthood, animals with short life spans, such as mice and rats, are used to research the influence of various factors on neurogenesis. Van Praag et al. (1999) attempted to separate the effects of (a) an enriched learning environment where toys were used to make the cages mentally challenging, (b) an enriched social environment where interaction was possible with other mice, and (c) an enriched physical activity environment where a running wheel permitted extensive exercise. They found that in the short term, the mice that ran daily on a running wheel had significantly more new neurons compared with the other groups, but these numbers declined once the running wheel was removed. Although running stimulated the production of new neurons, the maintenance of these neurons was no greater over the long term than that found in the other environments. A follow-up study by Brown et al. (2003) using the same living conditions found that voluntary exercise in which decision making was promoted in combination with an enriched environment produced the greatest permanent gains in both synaptogenesis and neurogenesis. Although these studies were not conducted on humans, there is emerging evidence that physical activity within cognitively stimulating environments enhances brain function by improving memory and reasoning skills.

Studies are also beginning to emerge that show neural changes as a result of **motor learning.** Draganski et al. (2004) used fMRI to determine if changes occurred in the brains of humans learning to juggle over a span of 3 mo. They were divided into two groups (jugglers and nonjugglers) and had their brains scanned three times: before learning to juggle, when they were able to juggle for 60 s, and after 3 mo of no juggling. High-resolution magnetic resonance scans were taken at the three intervals and the percent change in gray matter determined. No significant differences were found between the jugglers and nonjugglers at the beginning of the study, but during the second scan, which was taken at the end of 3 mo, a significant increase in gray matter was detected in the occipital cortex and visual areas of the jugglers. In addition, these changes in gray matter persisted for those who learned to juggle for an extended amount of time, while the nonjugglers showed no changes in gray matter over the duration of the study.

Gaze Control in Action

Coaches of sport have always known that the training they provide changes the bodies of their athletes—muscles become stronger, a greater amount of oxygen is taken up by the blood, there is more energy available, technical skills become more efficient, and more can be done with less effort. These physiological and biomechanical changes are well known, but less well known is the fact that physical training also leads to positive changes in the brain. Cao et al. (2004) state that just as "intensive muscular activity drives myogenesis and improves muscular size and strength; similarly robust hippocampal activity may drive neurogenesis and increase hippocampal size and cognitive strength." New insights into the nature of the brain and especially synaptogenesis and neurogenesis reveal four things that are important for teachers and coaches of sport:

➤ Training environments that are physically and mentally enriched stimulate the development of the brain in positive and productive ways.

➤ Athletes of all ages need to be physically engaged in exercise that is psychologically stimulating.

➤ Exercises should have meaning and be performed in environments where high levels of cognitive effort and decision making are required.

➤ Voluntary exercise where decision making is promoted produces greater long-term gains in learning than does enforced exercise.

Measuring What Athletes See

◄◄ *Where Have We Been?*

The previous chapter presented the visual and neural systems, with a focus on the anatomy of the visual system, types of gaze, properties of the focal and ambient systems, and ventral and dorsal processing. We also saw that the brain continually changes through two processes, synaptogenesis and neurogenesis, both of which are enhanced through physical exercise and training in cognitively enriched environments.

➤➤ *Where Are We Going?*

In this chapter, two methods of researching the role of vision and attention in sport are presented: the visual-search and vision-in-action paradigms. When the visual-search method is used, the eye movements of athletes are recorded as they view videotapes, photographs, computer simulations, or other simulated content from their sport. When the vision-in-action method is used, the gaze of the participant is recorded while they perform in real-world sport settings. The visual-search method is only briefly reviewed here because it has been presented extensively elsewhere (see Ripoll, 1991; Smeeton, Ward, & Williams, 2004; Williams, Davids, & Williams, 1999; Williams & Grant, 1999; Williams & Ward, 2003; Williams, Ward, Knowles, & Smeeton, 2002). The majority of this chapter is devoted to describing the vision-in-action method.

What Do Athletes See?

Have you ever wondered what you look at when you perform a skill, when putting in golf, for example, or when shooting a basketball, or when trying to get open on the soccer field? Have you also wondered if your teammates or competitors see a different world than you? Maybe they see the critical cues sooner, or for longer periods of time, or at just the right moment. As mentioned, this chapter describes the two main methods for recording the eye movements or gaze of athletes. These methods allow us to answer many of the questions that have intrigued researchers for decades. Do elite performers see the same **locations** and **objects** as nonelite performers? Does control of the gaze affect how well an athlete performs a sport task? If gaze control is important in sport performance, and if we understand how elite performers control their gaze, can we train those with lower skill levels to control their gaze in a similar way? And will this control help them achieve higher levels of success? In order to answer these questions, we first need to look at the technology used to record the gaze of athletes.

Eye-Tracking Technology Today

Most modern eye trackers are corneal-reflection systems that record the participant's eye movements on video using a camera mounted on a headband or glasses, as shown in figure 2.1. The figure shows a light eye tracker upon which are mounted two video cameras and electronics that permit the measurement of the eyes as they move. Corneal-reflection eye trackers direct a small, bright spot on the cornea of the eye while at the same time the optics of the system determine the center of the pupil. Since the position of the corneal reflection remains constant relative to the headband but the center of the pupil moves whenever the eye moves, the system is able to measure the difference between the center of the pupil and corneal reflection, and from this it determines the point of regard. The scene camera, also mounted on the headband or glasses, provides a video of what the athlete is looking at. An example of this type of gaze data is presented later in this chapter in figure 2.9, which shows the gaze of a basketball player taking a free throw.

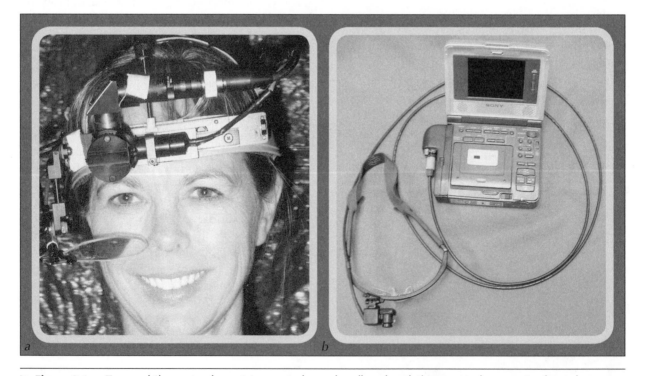

➤ **Figure 2.1**   Two mobile eye trackers: *(a)* mounted on a headband and *(b)* mounted on a pair of goggles.

Photo *b* with permission of Applied Sciences Laboratories, Bedford, MA.

Visual-Search Paradigm

The **visual-search paradigm** is the older of the two paradigms and dates back to the beginning of psychology (James, 1890/1981). The term **visual search** is defined as "the process by which one locates a target in a cluttered scene" (Zelinsky, Rao, Hayhoe, & Ballard, 1997, p. 448). It has also been described as "the scan of an environment for particular features—actively looking for something when you are not sure where it will appear" (Sternberg, 2003, p. 83). The visual-search paradigm has a long history of use in reading, art, mathematics, and chess, and for the past 20 y it has also been used extensively in sport.

Figure 2.2 shows an early visual-search setup used in a study designed to determine whether athletes with different skill levels attended to the same technical elements in lower skill levels of gymnastics (Vickers, 1988). Two groups of gymnasts (high and low skilled) had their eye movements recorded while observing a series of slides taken from a videotape of compulsory balance beam moves. The figure shows a participant with her head resting in a chin rest (to ensure accuracy) while her eye movements are recorded by the two cameras located on the floor. Her gaze is indicated by the x–y coordinate on the VCR videotape. The results showed that the highly skilled gymnasts used fewer fixations of longer duration than those with lower skill levels. They also directed their gaze to the torso region of the athletes being observed, whereas the lower-skilled gymnasts viewed the athletes' head, feet, and hands. The elite gymnasts seemed to be more aware of the role that the center of gravity (or the torso region) plays in performing the complex movements.

Figure 2.3 shows how visual-search studies are carried out today (Williams, Davids, Burwitz, & Williams, 1994; Williams et al., 1999). In the figure, a soccer player is standing on pressure-sensitive pads while viewing videotapes of tactical plays presented on a life-size screen. This setup has been used extensively in many sport activities where the goal is to identify differences in eye movements,

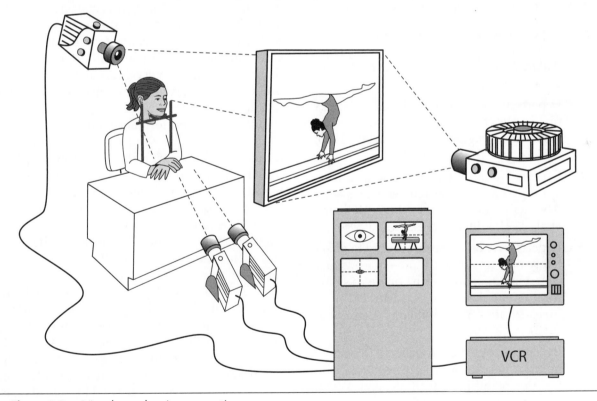

➤ **Figure 2.2**   Visual searches in gymnastics.

Reprinted from Human Movement Science, Vol. 7, J. Vickers, "Knowledge structures of elite-novice gymnasts," pp. 47-72, Copyright 1988, with permission from Elsevier.

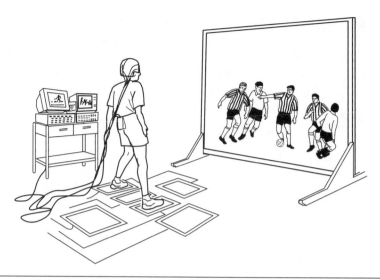

➤ **Figure 2.3**   The visual-search paradigm as used in soccer.

Reprinted, by permission, from A.M. Williams, K. Davids and J.G. Williams, 1999, *Visual perception and action in sports* (London: E & FN Spon), 149.

attention, and decision making between nonelite and elite performers. Considerable progress has been made in defining how novices and experts differ. Williams and Ward (2003, p. 221-222) summarize some of the major findings as follows:

➤ Experts have superior recall and recognition of sport-specific patterns of play (e.g., Allard & Starkes, 1980; Starkes & Deakin, 1984; Williams & Davids, 1995).

➤ Experts are faster in detecting and recognizing objects, such as a ball within the visual field (e.g., Allard & Starkes, 1980; Millslagle, 1988; Starkes, 1987).

➤ Experts are more efficient and use more appropriate visual-search behaviors (e.g., Abernethy, 1991; Vickers, 1992; Williams et al., 1994; Williams & Davids, 1998).

➤ Experts have an enhanced ability to effectively pick up advance (pre-event) visual cues, particularly from an opponent's postural orientation (Allard & Starkes, 1991; Jones & Miles, 1978; Williams & Burwitz, 1993).

➤ Experts have greater attunement to relative motion information when presented in the form of point-light displays (e.g., Ward, Williams, & Bennett, 2002).

➤ Experts have more accurate expectations of likely events based on the refined use of situational probabilities (Williams & Ward, 2003).

The visual search paradigm has provided valuable insights into how novice and expert athletes differ, but it has two main limitations. Because the physical skills in a sport are rarely, if ever, performed during a visual search study, no insight is gained into the gaze, attention, and decision-making characteristics of athletes when they succeed and fail. Although the visual search paradigm is very good at detecting skill differences (expert versus novice), it is not able to determine how differences in gaze control and cognition affect performance outcomes.

In visual search studies, participants are required to look straight ahead at displays presented directly in front of them. In the real world of sports performance, athletes carry their head and gaze in ways dictated by the inherent constraints of the task. For example, when golfers perform a putt, they look down at the green and their head swivels from the ball to the hole (or other areas of the green) and back. At least two visuomotor workspaces are used, one in the vicinity of the ball and the club and the other in the vicinity of the hole. In soccer, ice hockey, basketball, and other team sports, players not only look straight ahead, they also look left, right, up, down, and all around. In all forms of goaltending, the gaze is oriented upward and located at a distance on the object being shot, kicked, or thrown; and then as the object approaches the gaze moves downward as the object is stopped, caught, hit, or otherwise controlled. In some sports, such as basketball shooting and dart throwing, the athlete's limbs actually occlude the visuomotor workspace as the skill is performed (see chapter 5). The visual-search paradigm, by design, often negates or ignores the task and **organismic constraints** inherent in sport tasks. So, although the visual-search paradigm tells us much about sport expertise and provides intriguing insight into the perceptual and cognitive characteristics of elite performers compared with novices, it does not identify the specific characteristics of gaze control under all **task constraints**, nor does it identify the gaze and attentional characteristics that are found when an athlete is successful or fails.

Vision-in-Action Paradigm

The **vision-in-action paradigm** (Vickers, 1996a) differs from the visual-search paradigm in several ways. First, an athlete's gaze is recorded as he or she physically performs in a manner that is very similar to that found in the sport; therefore, there is always a coupling of perception and action. Second, the athlete performs a well-known sport task that, whenever possible, has published international standards of achievement (e.g., race times, shots made, goals saved). In this way athletes can be grouped into skill categories based on objective standards of achievement. Third, the athlete performs the task until an equal number of successful and unsuccessful trials are accomplished.

The vision-in-action paradigm therefore recognizes many of the factors found in the constraints-led model: the task, the environment, the organism, and perception–action coupling within sport perceptual-motor workspaces. In vision-in-action studies, the nature of the task and the athlete determine the field of view as the task is performed. The orientation of the head and gaze therefore exists as a function of both the task and the skill level of the athlete. The gaze is recorded in three-dimensional space; therefore the participant's gaze behaviors are studied over the full length, breadth, and depth of the visuomotor workspace. Since the ability to handle depth is important in all sports, the vision-in-action approach reveals how the athlete acquires information in all three dimensions. In the section below the evolution of eye tracking research in sport is presented. The early studies often did not possess all the characteristics listed above due primarily to limitations in technology.

Early Eye-Tracking Studies in Sport

It was not until the 1980s that researchers were able to record the eye movements of athletes in the live sport setting. Beginning in the early 1980s, a flurry of eye-tracking studies emerged in roughly the following order:

➤ Ice hockey goaltending (Bard & Fleury, 1981)

➤ Basketball shooting (Ripoll, Bard, Pailliard, & Grosgeorge, 1982; Ripoll, Bard, & Pailliard, 1986)

➤ Baseball hitting (Bahill & LaRitz, 1984)

➤ Pistol shooting (Ripoll, Papin, Guezennec, Verdy, & Philip, 1985)

➤ Badminton (Ripoll & Fleurance, 1988)

➤ Golf putting (Vickers, 1992)

These early studies provided a first glimpse of the eye movements of athletes as they performed well-known tasks from their sport.

Bard and Fleury (1981) recorded the eye movements of elite and novice ice hockey goaltenders on ice using an eye tracker that did not permit any movement of the head. A Plexiglas shield was placed in front of the goaltender for safety, and fixations were determined relative to the shooter's body, stick, or puck. A trial ended when the goaltender made a movement with the glove hand or stick, signifying when a stopping action might occur in a game. The results showed that although both experts and novices focused the majority of their fixations on the puck and stick, the gaze of the expert goaltenders was more consistent than the gaze of the novice goaltenders across both the slap and wrist shot. The expert goaltenders were also faster in initiating a response than the novices. Because the eye tracker limited the movements of the goaltenders, it was not possible to determine their gaze during saves and goals. Recent research in ice hockey goaltending is presented in chapter 7.

Ripoll et al. (1982) and Ripoll et al. (1986) carried out two studies in basketball shooting. Their focus was to not only determine expertise differences, but also gaze differences during hits and misses. They found that expert shooters oriented their head toward the basket sooner and maintained their gaze in the region of the hoop longer than did nonexpert players. One of the main characteristics related to both expertise and accuracy was the rapidity with which the visual acquisition of the target was achieved. The elite shooters looked to the target sooner and then took more time to anchor the head in terms of eye–head stabilization before shooting. No significant differences were found in the duration of eye movement. Since these two studies, a number of others have been completed in basketball, and these are presented in chapter 5.

Bahill and LaRitz (1984) recorded the gaze of baseball players as they tracked a ball that was pulled toward them using the pulley device, shown in figure 2.4, at speeds up to 90 mph (145 kph). A camera was placed above the head that recorded the hitter's head movements, and an integrated electrooculography system recorded the movements of the eyes. The results showed that the players tracked the ball using

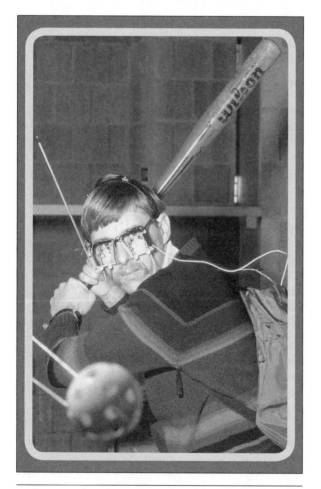

► **Figure 2.4**   The eye-tracking system used by Bahill and LaRitz (1984) to determine the tracking ability of baseball players.

Reprinted, by permission, from A.T. Bahill and T. LaRitz, 1984, "Why can't batters keep their eyes on the ball?," *American Scientist* 72: 249-253.

a combination of head and eye movements as the ball approached. Both the college players and a professional player began tracking the ball immediately and continued to track it to a point 2.6 m from the plate, at which point their gaze fell behind the ball. The professional player tracked the ball longer than the others, within 1.5 m of the plate. Pursuit tracking of the college players comprised 50°/s for the eyes and 20°/s for the head, resulting in a combined gaze velocity of 70°/s, while the professional player tracked the ball with the eyes at 120°/s and 30°/s for the head, resulting in a combined peak gaze velocity of 150°/s. Because the ball passed the players at a speed that exceeded 1,000°/s, continuously tracking the ball to the plate was not possible.

Bahill and LaRitz also found that the professional player used an anticipatory saccade on some trials, where his gaze raced ahead of the ball to the point of ball–bat contact. Since no hitting movements were allowed due to technical limitations, it was not possible to determine if the reported gaze control characteristics occurred on hits, misses, or both. It was also not possible to determine if a similar type of gaze control occurred when a player brought the full force of a baseball swing to bear. It would not be until a cricket study by Land and McLeod (2000) that additional insight would be gained into the gaze control of higher- and lower-skilled batsmen. This study is presented in chapter 7.

Ripoll et al. (1985) recorded the gaze of five international elite pistol shooters who hit a perfect 200 out of 200 targets in a recent competition and then compared their gazes with five national-level near-elite shooters who hit 193 out of 200 targets in the same competition. The shooters performed pistol shots to a stationary target as shown in figure 2.5, which shows the gaze control of the near-elite shooters on the left and the elites on the right. The near-elite shooters shifted their gaze, arm, and weapon as a unit to the target, while the elite shooters first fixated the target and then brought the pistol into line with the gaze before aiming and pulling the trigger. The national-level shooters were slower aligning the arm and gun, but they took less time fixating the target once in position. The elite shooters used the opposite strategy; they brought the weapon quickly to the target and then took more time to aim and complete the shot.

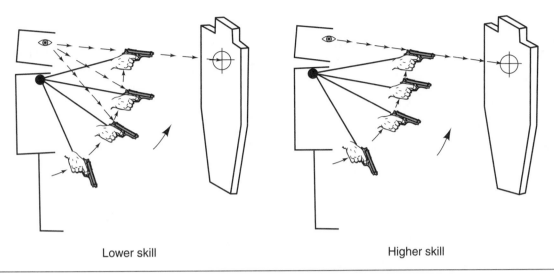

Lower skill   Higher skill

➤ **Figure 2.5** Gaze control of national-level near-elite shooters (left) and international elite shooters (right).

Reprinted from H. Ripoll et al., 1985, "Analysis of scanning patterns of pistol shooters," *Journal of Sport Sciences* 3(2): 93-101, by permission of Taylor & Francis, Ltd.
http://www.tandf.co.uk/journals

Vickers (1992) recorded the gaze of high-skilled golfers (mean handicap 6.2) and low-skilled golfers (mean handicap 14.1) as they performed 10 ft (3 m) putts on a flat surface (Vickers, 1991a, 1991b, 1992). Figure 2.6 shows a frame of data that is similar to that recorded in the study.

Figure 2.7 shows the mean duration of fixations during the preparation, during the backswing and foreswing (stroke), and after contact. The high-skilled golfers fixated the hole longer (~ 2 s) and used slow saccades of about 500 ms between the hole and ball. They did not spot-sight along the green (that is, direct their gaze to an imaginary line or spot on the green to and from the hole); instead they directed two to three fixations to the hole and then to the ball or club, with saccades linking the fixations. During the stroke, they maintained a steady fixation on the top or back of the ball. This final fixation occurred in 93% of all putts. For elite golfers, there were no fixations on the club-head as it moved through the backswing into the foreswing. At contact, the quiet eye remained on the putting surface for upward of 250 ms.

In contrast, the low-skilled golfers had a higher frequency of gaze, shorter fixations on the hole, and faster saccades between the hole and ball, and they often used spot-sighting, fixating on the green along an imaginary line between the ball and hole. Their final fixation was significantly shorter, and they often tracked the club on the backswing, resulting in the gaze being off the ball at contact in 31% of trials. Irrespective of skill level or accuracy,

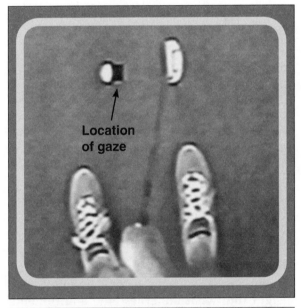

➤ **Figure 2.6** A frame of gaze data similar to that recorded in Vickers (1992) that shows the golfer's gaze as indicated by the square black cursor shown located on the back of the ball. Also visible are the putter, the golfer's hands, and the golfer's stance.

the final fixation, which consequently is called the **quiet eye** (see chapter 6), was a significant determiner of both accuracy and skill and had a duration that began before the backswing and was maintained at this location until after ball contact.

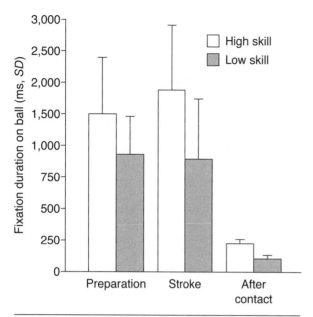

> **Figure 2.7**   Mean fixation duration of high- and lower-skilled putters during the preparation, during the backswing and foreswing (stroke), and after ball contact.

Mean values derived from Table 2 of Vickers, 1992.

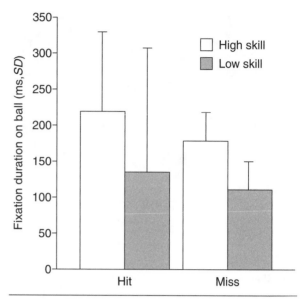

> **Figure 2.8**   Mean duration of fixation of high- and lower-skilled golfers on hits and misses during the contact phase of the putt.

Derived from Figure 6 of Vickers, 1992.

Figure 2.8 shows the duration of the golfers' fixations on hits and misses. Regardless of skill level, accuracy was significantly better when the final fixation extended beyond contact for more than 200 ms. (This final fixation has subsequently been called the quiet-eye dwell time.) A number of more recent studies on golf are presented in chapter 6.

Recent Vision-in-Action Studies

These initial attempts to record the gaze of performers in the live sport setting provided new insight into what underlies elite and nonelite performance, but by the mid-1990s several problems still stood in the way of efficiently and accurately determining the gaze of the performing athlete. Researchers needed a more efficient way to couple the gaze and motor behaviors so that both were synchronized in space and time. The importance of coupling the gaze with the motor behavior can be illustrated through figure 2.6. Although this frame of data provides very accurate data about where the gaze is located in the visuomotor workspace, it does not provide an indication of the golfer's movements at the same time. In golf you can get some idea of the stroke from the movement of the club as seen

from the golfer's perspective, but this is not a reliable source of stroke data, as golfers often look toward the hole at the moment of contact and so this critical moment is often missed. In addition to coupling the athlete's movements with his or her gaze, it was also necessary to find a way to code and analyze the coupled gaze and motor data so that meaningful findings could be derived for use by practitioners in the field.

A study on basketball shooting by Vickers (1996a) provided a solution to many of these problems. It coupled the athletes' gaze with their ocular and motor behaviors, as illustrated in figure 2.9. The figure shows a frame of vision-in-action data as recorded in the basketball free throw. Each frame of vision-in-action data is comprised of four parts: an eye image (A), a gaze image (B), a motor image (C), and a time code (D) that records time synchronized in all three images.

Image A in figure 2.9 shows the shooter's eye as detected by a miniature camera on the eye tracker. It is from the surface of the eye that corneal-reflection data originate. Two sets of crosshairs are superimposed on the eye. One records the center of the pupil and the second records the corneal reflection, which originates from a low-light source on the headband. By measuring the differences between the two crosshairs,

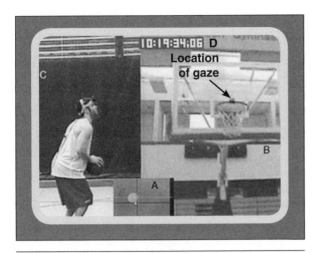

> **Figure 2.9**   A frame of data in vision-in-action data in basketball shooting, showing the eye image (A), gaze image (B), motor image (C), and time code (D).

the system is able to determine where the gaze is located in space. Image B in figure 2.9 is the image produced by the miniature scene camera, also on the headband, and it shows the scene in front of the athlete and where the athlete looks. The location of the gaze is indicated by the black cursor, which is located on the front of the hoop. The accuracy of this cursor is 1° of visual angle, which is approximately the size of the cursor as shown. Recall that the limit of foveal vision is 3° of visual angle; therefore the location of the cursor tells you what the athlete is looking at with the focal system anywhere in the scene. From this, it is also possible to infer what might be perceived in the periphery by the ambient system.

Image C in figure 2.9 was recorded by an external camera that recorded the shooting movements as the shots were taken. The perspective shown in the figure is in the sagittal plane. From this view the duration of the motor phases of the shooting action can be determined. Image D in figure 2.9 shows the time-code generator that records time in all three images synchronized at a rate of 30 frames each second (33.33 ms each frame), or at the rate of 60 fields each second (16.67 ms each field). The time-code generator shown here records time at the rate of 30 frames each second, but time-code generators may display time in milliseconds, frames, or fields of video data. Each frame of vision-in-action data therefore shows where the athlete's gaze is located in the scene being viewed and when this occurs relative to the different phases of the shooting action.

Interpreting Vision-in-Action Data

Vision-in-action data provide a rich source of coupled gaze and motor data that is analyzed in a series of steps. First, it is important to determine when the trial begins and ends. Second, the different motor phases are defined and their temporal durations recorded. Third, the gaze is coded in terms of the type of gaze used (fixations, pursuit tracking, saccades, blinks, and other). Fourth, the locations and objects of interest to the athlete are coded as found in the visuomotor workspace. Fifth, statistical analyses are carried out on the coded data and skill, and performance differences are determined for trial duration, motor phase duration, and percent of gaze to specific locations or objects; and for frequency of gaze, duration of gaze, quiet-eye duration, and other variables of interest. Because the motor and gaze data were synchronized when collected (as shown in figure 2.9), it is possible to determine the significant perceptual-motor characteristics underlying sport expertise and performance.

Defining Trial Onset and Offset

It is first necessary to identify the onset (beginning) and offset (end) of each trial. A consistent method must be found so that the onset and offset are the same on every trial. One method that has proven to be effective is to set a constant period of time prior to the onset of a critical movement in each trial. For example, if the task is the basketball free throw then the onset of the trial could begin 5 s before the release of the ball from the shooter's hand (Vickers, 1996a). A similar example in ice hockey goaltending would have the onset of the trial be 1 s before the puck leaves the shooter's stick (Panchuk & Vickers, 2006). The offset of the trial also should be a constant that occurs in each trial. In the free throw, the offset of the trial may occur when the ball hits the rim of the hoop (Vickers, 1996a) or when it is released from the fingertips (Oudejans, van de Langenberg, & Hutter, 2002). The offset of the trial in ice hockey goaltending was when the puck passed the plane of the net (Panchuk & Vickers, 2006). When setting both the onset and offset, it is very important that a total duration be selected that includes all the critical gaze and motor information required.

Defining the Motor Phases

Next it is important to define the **motor phases** or movement kinematics that make up each trial. **Movement kinematics,** "as applied to movement behavior, describes the movement of the limb, the entire body, or both. The locations of the various parts of the body during movement, the angles of the various joints, and the time relations between the movement of one joint and the movement in another are examples of the many ways movement kinematics that can be recorded" (Schmidt & Lee, 2005, p. 36). In the vision-in-action method, it is important to define the motor phases found in each task investigated. The motor phases of a task are derived from biomechanical sources, motor control sources, and the technical literature in each sport. These motor phases "describe the temporal structure of a sequence" of movements (Schmidt & Lee, 2005, p. 466). Table 2.1 presents the motor phases as identified in a number of studies. The first phase is a **preparation phase,** which is common to all the studies listed. It is during this time that the movement is organized; therefore it is akin to the reaction-time phase, which will be described in chapter 3. The second phase has many names, including the **impulse phase** (Abrams, Meyer, & Kornblum, 1989), the initiation phase (Helsen, Starkes, & Beukers, 1997), and the first observable movement (Schmidt & Lee, 2005; Schmidt & Wrisberg, 2004). The **error correction phase** is a period of time when feedback may affect movement (Abrams, Meyer, & Kornblum, 1990). This final phase also has different labels, such as *execution, contact,* and *follow-through,* that are more task specific. Note that a number of studies listed in table 2.1 have adopted the technical language widely used in the sport, for example, backswing and foreswing in golf and flexion and extension in table tennis (Bootsma & van Wieringen, 1990; Ripoll & Fleurance, 1988; Rodrigues, Vickers, & Williams, 2002; Vickers, 1992, 1996a; Vickers, Rodrigues, & Edworthy, 2000).

Temporal data in the vision-in-action paradigm, as in the visual-search paradigm, is expressed in both absolute (ms, s) and relative (%) time. Schmidt and Lee (2005) point out that even though we are able to change many aspects of a movement, such as overall movement time or amplitude, movements have invariant qualities that remain the same across selected conditions. One motor invariant is **relative time,** which is

Table 2.1   Phases of Motor Tasks as Identified in Various Studies

Study	Type of skill	Phases of targeting skills		
Abrams et al. (1990)	Fitt's aiming	Preparation	Impulse	Final correction
Helsen et al. (1997)	Fitt's aiming	Preparation	Initiation	Movement time
Bootsma (1991)	Table tennis	Preparation	Backswing	Foreswing/contact
Rodrigues et al. (2002)	Table tennis	Preparation	Backswing	Foreswing/contact
Janelle et al. (2000)	Rifle shooting	Preparation	Trigger pull	
Vickers et al. (1999)	Rifle	Preparation	Trigger pull	
Vickers (1992)	Golf	Preparation	Backswing	Foreswing/contact
Vickers (1996a)	Basketball	Preparation	Preshot	Shot
Vickers et al. (2000)	Darts	Preparation	Flexion	Extension
Vickers et al. (1997)	Volleyball	Preparation	Flexion	Extension
Williams, Singer et al. (2002)	Billiards	Preparation	Flexion	Extension
Martell et al. (2004)	Ice hockey	Pattern recognition	Situation assessment	Execution

defined as the "fundamental temporal structure, organization, or rhythm of a movement . . . this structure remains the same even when people decide to make changes in the flexible features of the pattern (Schmidt & Wrisberg, 2004, p. 157). Schmidt and Wrisberg (2004) further explain that a more precise way to look at relative time is as a set of ratios or percentages that defines the durations of several phases of the movement, or time intervals. In the vision-in-action method, the relative time of each motor phase is determined by dividing the duration of the phase by the total trial time, thus expressing each component as a percentage or ratio of the whole. Similarly, the relative time of the gaze is determined. Since the gaze and motor behavior are coupled and synchronized perfectly in time, the coordination of the gaze and motor behavior is determined in normalized units.

Once the onset and offset of the trial and motor phases have been identified, the next step is to identify each gaze used within and across these phases. Four gaze behaviors (fixations, pursuit tracking, saccades, and blinks) were defined in chapter 1. These definitions are used to code the type of gaze data as shown in figure 2.9. Here we see that the athlete's gaze is located on the front of the hoop. If he maintains his gaze at that location within 1° of visual angle (the width and depth of the cursor) for a minimum of three frames of gaze data (or 99.99 ms), then this gaze would be coded as a fixation. If his gaze moves from one location to another in a minimum of two frames (or 66.66 ms), then this would be coded as saccade. If after the ball was released from his fingertips, he tracked the ball within 1° of visual angle for a minimum of three frames of data (or 99.99 ms), then this would be coded as pursuit tracking. If the athlete should shut his eyes so that the gaze cursor disappeared for at least three frames of data (or 99.99 ms) and the eye image showed that his eyes were closed, then this would be coded as a blink. Finally, if the gaze data is blurred due to rapid head movements, or the athlete's gaze moves completely out of the visuomotor workspace so it cannot be coded, then the gaze would be coded as "other," meaning it was not possible to code it using one of the pre-established coding rules as indicated above. Normally, each gaze in a trial is coded so that a full understanding of how the gaze is controlled can be obtained.

Defining What Athletes Look At

After the onset and offset of the trial are determined, as well as the onset and offset of each motor phase, the next step is to code what the athlete is looking at. Athletes look at both objects and locations within the **visuomotor workspace**. Objects differ from locations and are defined from a psychological perspective using the definitions provided by Treisman (1986a, p. 1):

An object in the real world is a physical entity that has, at any given time, a defined location, mass, volume, shape, and other physical properties. It may reflect or generate light, sound waves, or chemical stimuli; it may move or be moved, it has some degree of temporal continuity. A perceptual object is a psychological representative of a physical object that is currently affecting the sensory receptors of the perceiving organism. This psychological representative may vary in the specificity of the information that it carries. At one extreme only the existence of the object may be registered, so that the representation functions as an individuated and countable placeholder. At the other extreme, the object may be identified and may generate predictions and causal inferences about its past and future behavior. Perhaps the only prerequisite for perceiving an object is some minimal temporal or spatial continuity of the stimulus. It must maintain its integrity over movement or other transformations.

Using this definition, objects within the performance environment include balls, pucks, shuttles (or similar), rackets, and all other equipment, as well as opponents, teammates, officials, coaches, judges, spectators, and all other persons. Objects may also have subcomponents, such as a player's head, torso, or feet, or a specific part of a piece of equipment (e.g., stick handle, stick blade).

Locations are distinct from objects in that they are topographically defined and therefore rarely move, but they are similar to objects in that they are psychological representatives affecting the sensory receptors of the performing player. The perception of locations allows the performer to determine the relative position of the body and other objects in space. The spaces within which locations occur can span 360° around the performer and are three-dimensional in nature, possessing height, width, and depth.

Spatial locations in sport therefore include all the surfaces that athletes perform on, whether horizontal, vertical, or possessing depth (e.g., ice, snow, grass, greens, floors, walls). Locations also include lines or other marks on playing surfaces, goals, hoops, nets, and similar equipment. Locations define the spatial and environmental constraints within which the performer competes, and in sport these are usually clearly defined by the rules of the game. Objects possess temporal information that dictates how spatial locations are used. For example, a tennis serve that is delivered at a slow speed allows an easier perception of the lines on the court, whereas a serve delivered at a fast speed pressures the gaze system and makes it more difficult to discern the relationship between the object and the location of lines on the court. Each object and location provides unique information important to understanding how the visual system contributes to motor learning and control.

Defining Dependent and Independent Variables

The dependent variables of a vision-in-action study include trial onset, offset, and duration as well as motor phase onset, offset, and duration. In terms of the gaze, the dependent variables include the location, frequency, onset, offset, and duration of the different types of gazes. Normally fixation and pursuit tracking of objects and locations are of primary interest, as little difference has been found in saccadic times across participants, tasks, and conditions. The primary independent variable in the visual-search paradigm is expertise (novices versus experts), whereas the vision-in-action paradigm always determines both expertise and performance differences. Vision-in-action studies also always include trials as an independent variable, therefore determining if learning or practice effects are present. Trial effects are also used to determine the consistency and stability of the gaze and attention over time.

Vision-in-action research also tries to specify the skill level of participants using external sources. One of the conveniences of sport is that independent statistics are kept on many aspects of most sports and it is easy to obtain this information from official sport Web sites. Whenever possible, the level of expertise is determined using data acquired independently during competitions, as well as in the experimental setting. As briefly covered in the introduction, two skill levels are used whenever possible in vision-in-action studies: elite or expert, and near-elite or near expert. An elite or expert performer is one who has attained the highest statistics in competition in the sport task being investigated. These individuals should also show that they can perform at a similarly high level during the experiment. A **near-elite** or near-expert performer has significantly lower statistics in the sport task being investigated and also performs at a lower level during the experiment.

One of the goals in selecting athletes using the elite–near-elite comparison is to hold constant as many of the physical attributes and training conditions as possible. The ideal participants are elite and near-elite athletes who play on the same team and therefore compete in the same league, have the same coaches, take part in the same practices, play the same positions, and are close in age. They do not significantly differ on any of the main physiological measures used to define physical prowess in the sport, but they differ significantly in terms of accuracy or another objective performance indicator in the task being investigated. The overall goal in the elite–near-elite comparison is to determine the extent that the athletes' gaze and attention contribute to performance, all other aspects held relatively constant. This strategy recognizes that physiological and biomechanical measures often do not predict who will be best in a contest. A long history of research in exercise physiology has shown that there is no guarantee that the athlete who has the best physiological measures (e.g., aerobic or anaerobic capacity, lactic tolerance, strength, flexibility) will be the athlete who excels in the end (McArdle, Katch, & Katch, 2001). The search for what underlies elite performance in sport is therefore an elusive one and still one of the most fascinating problems in science.

Gaze Control in Action

Check out the article "Spark: 'Quiet Eye' Helps Elite Athletes" at http://edition.cnn.com/2005/ TECH/03/21/spark.quiet.eye/index.html for information on how the gazes of athletes are recorded. The article shows how eye-tracking technology has evolved to provide new insights in sport.

CHAPTER 3

Visual Attention and Gaze Control

◄◄ *Where Have We Been?*

In the last chapter, the visual-search and vision-in-action methods were presented as two ways to determine how the gaze is controlled in sport. Both methods have contributed to our knowledge about expertise in sport, but only the vision-in-action method provides insight into how the gaze is controlled during sport success and failure.

►► *Where Are We Going?*

In this chapter, visual attention and its relation to control of the gaze are described. The fractionated reaction-time paradigm is presented, along with the thresholds for visual, auditory, and kinesthetic reaction time. Open- and closed-loop motor control are described, as well as the relationships of these two systems to the processing of feedback and the effect these have on motor behavior. Attention is defined, as are bottom-up and top-down processing. The relationship between shifts of gaze and attention is then explored. It will be shown that under certain conditions, a shift of gaze is always accompanied by a shift in attention to the object or location being viewed. These concepts provide important insight into how sport performers temporally organize and control their movements.

Information-Processing Time

One of the oldest areas of research in psychology is the study of information-processing time. The sensory systems of vision, audition, and touch have been studied extensively since the 19th century in terms of the average amount of time it takes to perceive a stimulus and make a simple movement. Table 3.1 shows the average reaction times for visual, auditory, and touch stimuli as reported by Ladd and Woodworth (1911). It shows the results obtained by eight different researchers, with the means for visual, auditory, and touch stimuli at the bottom. The mean reaction time is 189.5 ms for a visual stimulus, 146 ms for an auditory stimulus, and 150 ms for touch stimulus. Since these results were published, countless studies have been carried out confirming that vision is the slowest of the sensory systems, with an average reaction time between 180 and 200 ms (depending on the task conditions). **Auditory reaction time** is next, with mean values between 140 and 160 ms, and **kinesthetic reaction time** is the fastest, averaging between 120 and 140 ms, or slightly faster than the average of 150 ms shown in table 3.1 (the difference being due to improved sensing technology since the research presented in the table was carried out).

Fractionated Reaction-Time Paradigm

Historically, the amount of time it takes to prepare a movement is called **reaction time,** and the amount of time it takes to actually produce the movement is called **movement time.** But how much of the reaction times reported in table 3.1 were expended during the movement phase—that is, how long did it take to press a key, push a handle, or perform some other behavior as opposed to cognitively preparing the movement? Most psychological accounts of reaction time combine the reaction time and movement time within the reaction-time phase, because the tasks performed are usually simple ones where the movement time is both minimal and constant across participants. However, when real-world motor skills are studied, the movements are often more complex, have distinct phases, and have longer movement times; therefore, it is important to understand in these situations how reaction time and movement time are defined in order to produce a total response time.

Both reaction time and movement time are explained through the **fractionated reaction-time paradigm** (Ladd & Woodworth, 1911; Magill, 2004; Posner, 1980; Schmidt & Lee, 2005), which is diagrammed in figure 3.1. Four temporal components are shown: (1) a warning signal to get ready; (2) a signal to start the movement, or "go" signal; (3) the first moment of observable movement; and (4) the time when the movement ends. Once the warning is given, the reaction-time period follows. This period consists of two components, called **premotor time** and **motor time.** Figure 3.1 shows that these two periods are defined by the amount of electrical activity being generated by the muscles using **electromy-**

Table 3.1   Time Relations of Mental Phenomena

Researcher	Visual stimulus (ms)	Auditory stimulus (ms)	Touch stimulus (ms)
Hirsch	200	149	182
Hankel	225	151	155
Donders	188	180	154
Van Wittich	194	182	130
Wundt	175	128	188
Exner	150	136	128
Auerbach	191	122	146
Von Kreis	193	120	117
Mean reaction time	189.5	146	150

From G.T. Ladd and R.S. Woodworth, 1911, *Elements of Physiological Psychology* (New York, NY: Charles Scribner's Sons), 470-499.

ography (EMG). During the premotor time, no movement of the muscles can be detected, but during the motor time, the muscles have begun to contract. Since it is often impossible to secure EMG recordings due to the complexity of these measures, the movement-time period usually begins with the first observable movement that can be detected. The combination of reaction time and movement equals the **total response time**.

In order to better understand how reaction time and movement time function in a sport skill, let's follow what happened to the sprinter Linford Christie in the final of the 100 m race at the 1996 Olympics. Christie was the favorite to win the race, but he had two false starts, which led to his disqualification. His faults can be explained using the fractionated reaction-time paradigm and the well-known limits of auditory reaction time, as presented in table 3.1. The rules of sprinting in 1996 stated that the racers must not take their foot off the back block for at least 100 ms after the gun sounded. If a racer's foot left the back block sooner than 100 ms, it meant that the racer had started before the gun, according to the well-known

threshold for auditory reaction time, which dates back more than 100 y (as shown in table 3.1). Although the average threshold for auditory reaction time is between 140 and 160 ms, the 100 ms standard was adopted by the international track community because reaction time can be decreased with training (Carlton, 1981a, 1981b).

Once the racers were situated in the blocks, a warning or "ready" signal was provided by the starter in the form of a verbal direction. On this command, the sprinters rose into position and waited for the gun or "go" signal. It was during this reaction-time period that Christie made an error and left the blocks too soon. A sensor in the back block under Christie's foot was activated between 80 and 90 ms after the sound of the gun, and so the race was stopped. Each start block was also fitted with a speaker so that the racers could clearly hear the starter's commands and the sound of the gun. Christie twice made the decision to go too soon and was disqualified from the biggest race of his career.

Christie and many other elite track athletes have since argued that they can respond legally to

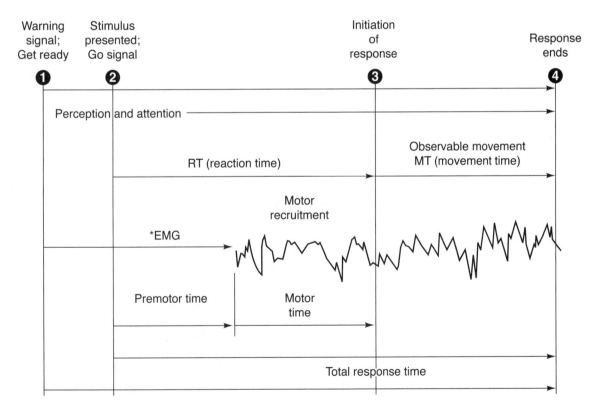

➤ **Figure 3.1**   The fractionated reaction-time paradigm shows the time course of information flow before and during a movement.

an auditory signal in times faster than the 100 ms allowed by the rules. But is it really possible for a superbly trained sprinter to move the entire body in response to an auditory signal in less time than 100 ms? It's highly unlikely, and this is reflected in the recent ruling by the international track community that actually increased the amount of time the athletes must delay their exit from the blocks, from 100 to 120 ms. The 120 ms threshold now means that sprinters have to wait even longer before leaving the blocks.

Hick's Law

Reaction time varies according to many factors, and the law that explains how these factors affect information-processing time is **Hick's law** (Hick, 1952). Hick's law states that the amount of time it takes to prepare a response is dependent upon the number of stimulus–response (SR) alternatives that are present. "Choice reaction time is linearly related to the Log_2 of the number of stimulus-response alternatives, or the amount of information that must be processed in order to choose a response" (Schmidt & Lee, 2005, p. 464). In order to understand how Hick's law functions in the real world, let's again consider a sprinter in the blocks for the 100 m race. Several stimuli are present, including the sound of the starter's voice, the sound of the gun, the sound of the racers on each side, the crowd, the beating of the racer's heart, the feel of the surface under the feet, the temperature, and the presence of the racers on each side, to name but a few. The motor responses that could be paired with one or more of these stimuli include getting into position, getting set, the pressure on the hands, the motion over the arms, the push from the front foot, the push from the back foot, the angle of the head, and so on. Hypothetically, each of these movements could be paired with each stimulus. It is easy to see how a racer's head could be filled with a great deal of information that might interfere with the start. In general, reaction time increases when more muscle units must be prepared; when movements are more complex, are of longer duration, or involve more limbs; or when the person is a novice.

The effect of so many SR alternatives on **visual reaction time** is shown in figure 3.2. Hick's law states that reaction time increases in a linear way when the number of stimuli and response pairs increase. When a person is in a complex setting,

such as an airplane cockpit, where there are numerous dials and digital readouts and where both the hands and feet perform specific actions, reaction time can approach much higher values, with the upper limit being around 700 ms. It is also important to emphasize that with practice, the number of SR alternatives decreases and there is a corresponding decrease in reaction time.

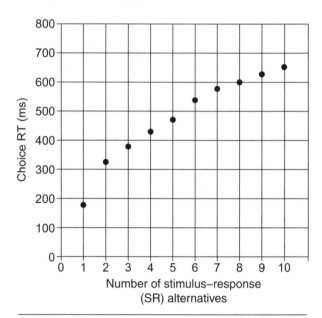

> **Figure 3.2**   Hick's law, showing the relationship between the number of SR alternatives and visual reaction time (ms).

Is the Reaction-Time Period Always Brief?

The discussion thus far has focused on defining the average thresholds for reaction time. Traditionally, the term *reaction time* has been applied to skills that are performed very quickly. For example, Schmidt and Lee (2005) define it as "the interval between the presentation of an unexpected stimulus and the initiation of the response" (p. 466). The unanticipated designation is critical when performing laboratory experiments and also when performing many real-world skills (e.g., sprinting) in order to prevent guessing. But the idea that the reaction time is always brief is incorrect. We saw in the previous section that Hick's law allows for reaction times that can be very long. Some sport skills also have long reaction times; for example, the preparation phase of the golf putt averages about 10 s for most golfers. Reaction times in this book will therefore vary by task, and in some cases they will be brief and in others they will be longer.

Interpreting the Reaction-Time Period

The preparatory or reaction-time phase of a movement is interpreted differently by cognitive, ecological, and **dynamic systems** theories. If one is a cognitive scientist, then the reaction-time period describes the time when the brain organizes the neural networks that plan and control the movement. During this phase, cues are perceived and attended to, a plan of action is developed, and the decision to act in a certain way is made. If one comes from the ecological or dynamic systems perspective, then the equivalent interval of time is not defined in terms of the internal flow of information through the brain and other cognitive structures, but as time when information may be picked up by the moving system.

One act of information pickup reported extensively in the literature and presented in the introduction to this text is **optic flow** (Gibson, 1979). An important example of optic flow is called time-to-contact, or tau, (Lee, 1980; Lee, Young, Reddish, Lough, & Clayton, 1983) and occurs when a ball or other object is thrown or hit toward a person at high speed. Not only does the individual have to anticipate the speed of the object as it approaches, but he or she also has to determine the most optimal moment to make contact. When the object is far away, the size of the object on the retina is small, but as it approaches it becomes larger (see figure 1.3). Lee (1980) found that the changes in the size of the object on the retina appeared to trigger the required action without the internal processing described by cognitive scientists.

Gibson and Pick (2001, p. 150-151) also state that when a skill is learned, specific visual attractors are defined through a "process of education of attention," a process in which there is a "narrowing down from a vast manifold of information to the minimal, optimal information that specifies the **affordances** of an event, object or layout." Once the visual attractors are learned, the system is able to function automatically without any need for conscious processing.

As is evident, there are a number of theoretical ways to interpret the reaction-time phase. In the next section, the Schmidt model of motor learning and control is presented (Schmidt, 1991; Schmidt & Wrisberg, 2004) as a useful framework that incorporates many of the information-processing and motor control stages emphasized in this book.

Schmidt Model of Motor Learning and Control

One of the most comprehensive models from a cognitive-behavioral perspective is the Schmidt model (Schmidt, 1991; Schmidt & Lee, 2005). Figure 3.3 shows that the Schmidt model is made up of 14 information-processing events. The amount of time it takes for events 1 through 7 to occur is the reaction-time period, which can vary greatly depending on the task, the conditions present, and the skill level of the person. These seven events describe how we (1) identify information about the stimulus, (2) select the program needed to perform an action, and (3) program that action. These three steps are influenced by the information we already have stored in (4) memory and in the (5) motor programs we have developed. A **motor program** is "an abstract representation," that when initiated, results in the production of a coordinated movement (Schmidt & Lee, 2005, p. 466). Less variable than these events (in healthy individuals) is the amount of time it takes for movement commands to race down the spinal cord to the muscles (6-7).

Events 8 through 12 then describe how four feedback loops (M1, M2, TR, and M3) influence the movement once it has begun. Each of these loops is defined by time intervals that enable the use of feedback arising from the movement to help maintain the action or modify it as necessary. The **M1 (monosynaptic) loops** are brief (30-50 ms) and relay sensory information from the muscles to the spinal cord. They automatically maintain balance and stability without conscious awareness. The **M2 loop** is longer (50-80 ms) and goes from the muscles up the spinal cord to the brain to stored plans and programs for the actions we are performing. We are also not aware of this feedback; the time period is too fast to permit conscious awareness.

The third loop, or **triggered reaction** (TR), has a latency of 80-120 ms and takes into account feedback that is received when we act against an object or location in the environment. Imagine trying to hit a baseball and having your foot slip, or skiing down a slope and hitting a patch of ice. When this occurs, feedback from your foot races

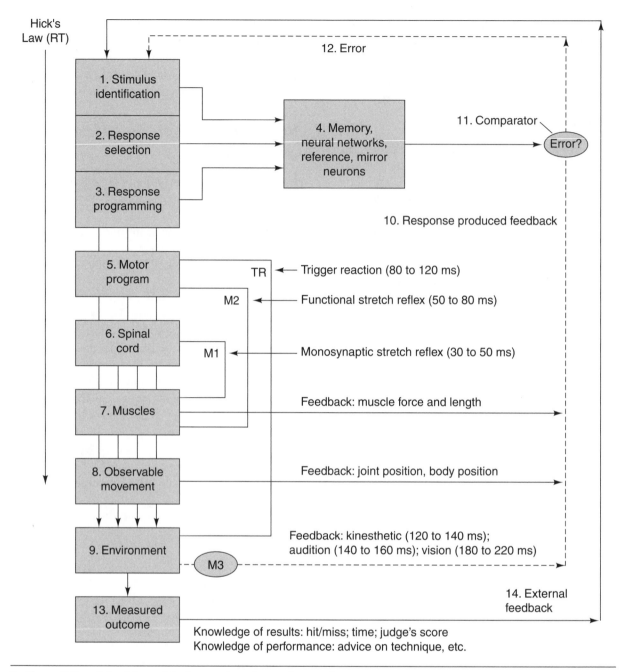

Hick's Law (RT)

12. Error

1. Stimulus identification

2. Response selection

3. Response programming

4. Memory, neural networks, reference, mirror neurons

11. Comparator

Error?

10. Response produced feedback

5. Motor program

TR ← Trigger reaction (80 to 120 ms)

M2 ← Functional stretch reflex (50 to 80 ms)

6. Spinal cord

M1 ← Monosynaptic stretch reflex (30 to 50 ms)

7. Muscles

Feedback: muscle force and length

8. Observable movement

Feedback: joint position, body position

9. Environment

Feedback: kinesthetic (120 to 140 ms); audition (140 to 160 ms); vision (180 to 220 ms)

M3

14. External feedback

13. Measured outcome

Knowledge of results: hit/miss; time; judge's score
Knowledge of performance: advice on technique, etc.

➤ **Figure 3.3**   Schmidt model of motor learning and control.

Adapted, by permission, from R.A. Schmidt and C.A. Wrisberg, 2004, *Motor learning and performance*, 3rd ed. (Champaign, IL: Human Kinetics), 315.

up to the brain and, depending on your skill level, you may be able to correct the movement automatically. The TR loop is modified by the skill level and experience of the person. The last loop, called the **M3 loop,** is the longest loop. It requires conscious perception and attention to what we feel, see, hear, or otherwise sense. The latency of the M3 loop varies by the sensory system being used. The fastest is that of kinesthetic reaction time, which, as we saw in table 3.1, has a latency

of about 120 ms; next is the auditory reaction time, which requires 140 to 160 ms; and the slowest of all the reaction times is vision, which requires 180 to 220 ms to see a stimulus and produce an action.

Notice that the M1, M2, TR, and M3 loops represent a feedback system, where one loop is nested within another and all are able to integrate their information and send a common message back to the brain. These loops encompass events 7 though 12 and comprise the final common pathway of signals that emerges at a reference of correction (event 11) stored in memory, where the feedback is assessed relative to past and present experiences. The movement is corrected if an error has been perceived; otherwise it is maintained without correction.

Finally, events 13 and 14 deal with how external forms of feedback affect our movements. Two basic forms of external information are shown, called **knowledge of results** and **knowledge of performance**. Knowledge of results arises from the outcome of the movement (hit or miss, a fast time or a slow one, a good judges' score), while knowledge of performance is usually concerned with technique and form. Knowledge of results is often self-evident, while knowledge of performance usually comes from a coach or teammate who provides guidance about the quality of the movement. These final two sources of feedback have a great effect on how well humans learn and perform motor skills, a topic that will be dealt with in detail in chapters 9 through 12, when the decision-training model is presented.

Open- and Closed-Loop Control

In all actions it is important to know how the reaction time interacts with and influences movement time. The concepts of open- and closed-loop motor control provide a time-based system for understanding the interaction of these two events (James, 1890/1981; Posner, 1980; Schmidt, 1991; Schmidt & Lee, 2005; Ladd and Woodworth, 1911). Whether a movement is under **open-** or **closed-loop control** is usually defined by the extent to which it can be organized in advance and carried out prior to the feedback from the muscles influencing the movement. If the movement time is very short, then the system is considered to be under open-loop control; there is simply not enough time during movement time for feedback arising from the M1, M2, and TR loops to affect the movement. Examples of skills organized in advance and performed in times shorter than 200 ms are the forward swing in baseball, the forward stroke in tennis, the forward stroke in billiards, the pulling of the trigger on a rifle or pistol, the forward slap shot in ice hockey, the final extension of the hand in the dart throw, and the boxing punch. These movements are organized in advance at the higher levels and run off so quickly that there is normally not enough time for feedback to change how the action is performed.

When the duration of a movement exceeds about 200 ms, the movement is considered to be under closed-loop control. There is time for the feedback arising from the muscles, the joints, and the visual and other sensory systems to affect the movement as it occurs. Feedback flows to the brain and is assessed by the higher centers in terms of what needs to be maintained as planned or changed. If a change is made, then essentially a second reaction-time phase is enacted and the movement reorganized and corrections made in light of the new information. For example, the movement time of a golf drive is between 900 and 1,400 ms, so a golfer theoretically has enough time to make three or four changes to the swing in this period of time. Perhaps the new information comes from the hand slipping on the club, or from an inner voice that says "Keep the elbow in, shift the weight, keep the eye on the ball," and so on. The closed-loop system is susceptible to the intrusion of our thoughts, or any other feedback that may arise. When golfers state that they prefer to swing without thinking, they are essentially attempting to control a motor skill that is inherently under closed-loop control in an open-loop manner—they do not want their thoughts to affect their swing once it is initiated. Instead, they have decided to organize the movement in its entirety during the reaction-time phase (events 1-7) before the swing begins and perform it without any feedback. In order to do this, they have to have a singular focus that prevents any intrusion of unwanted information. Finally, athletes can control the same skill using open-loop control, closed-loop control, or a combination of both systems. Having a good working understanding of the concepts of reaction time and movement time and of open- and closed-loop control provides insight into how performers use time to organize and control their movements.

What Is Visual Attention?

Thus far we have seen that it takes time to attend to information in the environment. More time is needed when that information is complex, when we are in a new situation, or when we have not yet learned to attend to what is most important in the environment. In this section we now look at the relationship between control of the gaze and visual attention. When we perform a motor task, the vast amount of information normally available in the environment is ignored in favor of specific information that is processed to the exclusion of all else. The process whereby this occurs is called attention. We possess a limited attentional capacity, meaning we can only concentrate or focus on relatively small amounts of information at any one time. We use selective attention to orient our mental energies to what is most important while ignoring or blocking out all else (Driver, 2001; Neisser, 1979, 1983).

All athletes face vast arrays of visual information in diverse perceptual workspaces. The spaces over which attention must be oriented and controlled in sport are extensive and include a rich assortment of stimuli, all of which can command both the gaze and the attention of the performer. Skilled performers have learned to control their gaze so that the optimal information is perceived or attended to at the right time. William James (1890/1981, p. 381-382) provided the most enduring and vivid description of this process:

> Everyone knows what attention is. It is the taking possession by the mind, in a clear and vivid form, of one out of what seem several simultaneously possible objects or trains of thought. Focalization, concentration of consciousness are of its essence. It applies withdrawal from some things in order to deal effectively with others, and is a condition which has a real opposite in the confused, dazed, scatter brained state which in French is called *distraction*, and *Zerstreutheit* in German.

Feature Integration Theory and the Spotlight of Attention

In chapter 1 it was shown that the brain does not process whole pictures; instead, billions of features are registered by the visual system and processed by specialized centers in the occipital lobe and higher brain areas. These features specify the color, shapes, edges, motion, and other properties of the objects and locations being viewed. Specific features are then bound together in the higher centers located in the parietal, temporal, somatosensory, and frontal cortices to create our perception of the world, and this occurs during the process of attention.

A comprehensive theory that explains how the billions of features are registered and then bound together into objects and locations is **feature integration theory,** as proposed by Treisman and Gelade (1980) and Treisman (1999). When an object is fixated, the stimulus properties are encoded into separate neural pathways, each of which generates a feature map for color, orientation, size, distance and stereo distance, and other factors, as shown in figure 3.4. Selected features from these maps are then integrated into a master map where one object or location among many becomes the **spotlight for the attention** and pops out more than anything else. Attention at that location permits the identification of the object integrated with memory processes. The notion of a spotlight of attention has a long history (Cave & Bichot, 1999; Hernandez-Peon, 1964; Posner, 1980; Treisman, 1999; Treisman & Gelade, 1980; Treisman, Cavanagh, Fischer, Ramachandran, & von der Heydt, 1990) and is one of the dominant theories of visual attention today.

Bottom-Up and Top-Down Processing

How an object or location is processed by the visual system depends on whether bottom-up or top-down processing is used. **Bottom-up processing** proceeds in a "single direction from sensory input, through perceptual analysis, towards motor output, without involving feedback information flowing backwards from 'higher' centers to 'lower' centers" (Corbetta & Shulman, 2002, p. 201). During bottom-up processing, the features and details present in an object or location are perceived, most often subconsciously, and then used to direct motor behavior. The extent to which one or both of these properties occurs governs athletes' control over their gaze and visual attention.

The bottom-up aspects of an object or location are the features that pop out without any need for conscious processing and include the color, textures, motion, edges, and other properties inherent in the image. An important aspect of bottom-up processing is saliency. **Salient features** are those that are intrinsically conspicuous (Itti & Koch, 1999) in a given context and that preattentively affect the orientation of attention. A salient feature also tends to be "independent of the nature of a particular task, operates very rapidly, and is driven in a bottom-up manner, although it can be influenced by contextual,

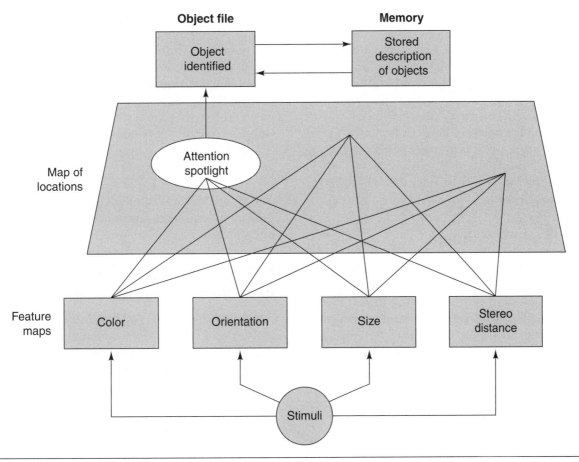

➤ **Figure 3.4** Feature integration theories and the spotlight of attention.

Illustrations from pages 101 and 127 from IMAGES OF MIND by Michael I. Posner and Marcus E. Raichle. © 1994 by Scientific American Library. Reprinted by permission of Henry Holt and Company, LLC.

figure-ground effects. If a stimulus is sufficiently salient it will pop out of a visual scene. This suggests that saliency is computed in a pre-attentive manner across the entire visual field . . . the speed of this saliency is on the order of 25-50 ms per item" (Itti & Koch, 2001, p. 194). When salient features are novel or occur in events that are unusual, they command immediate attention. Examples of salient features in various sports are the spin of a ball, the change in size as a ball approaches, the orientation of a racket, the directional properties of a defensive player, the shadows found on a golf green, the icy luminance of a ski course, or the swirl of an eddy in kayaking. These types of bottom-up features pop out of the visuomotor workspace and will be used effectively depending on whether the athlete is also able to use top-down processing.

During **top-down processing,** "the flow of information is from the 'higher' to 'lower' centers, conveying knowledge derived from previ-

ous experience rather than sensory stimulation" (Corbetta & Shulman, 2002, p. 201). Top-down processing is affected by our memories, our goals and expectations, and the amount of knowledge and experience we have in a given situation. Top-down processing often occurs rapidly and has qualities linked to awareness, insight, and the degree of experience the person has in a sport. Top-down processes originate from the higher cortical areas and provide the deeper understandings that are required in all sport. We therefore see that **motor performance** is affected by both bottom-up factors, such as novelty and unexpectedness, and top-down factors, such as anticipations, expectancies, goals, and intentions. The extent to which bottom-up processing dominates over top-down processing or vice versa is a controversial question that is important to consider in sport.

Context plays a major role in top-down processing, and when viewed within Newell's (1986) and Newell and McDonald's (1994) constraints-led model, it includes organismic constraints such as mental set, goals, and expectations, as well as environmental and task constraints. In sport, the elite performer learns to ignore many bottom-up stimuli (such as the pushes of an opponent, inclement weather, crowds) and to maintain a top-down focus, while novices tend to see everything or nothing. They have not yet developed the ability to discriminate and assign meaning and higher-order rules that make actions easier to perform.

The Binding Problem

Treisman (1999, p. 105) explains that the **binding problem** "concerns our capacity to integrate information across time, space, attributes and ideas . . . . [it is] required when we select an action to perform in a particular context. We must, for example, reach in the right direction, lift the glass with the correct muscle tension, and drink the water it contains rather than eat or inhale it." In many respects the binding problem is similar to the notion of **chunking** as proposed by Miller (1956) and more recently by Wheeler and Treisman (2002). Through learning and experience, seemingly diverse pieces of information are grouped together into fewer but more meaningful ideas or concepts that enhance the control of action. For example, a figure skater who learns to perform up to 80 different moves in a program of 3 to 5 min does not try to remember 80 separate moves, but instead chunks or binds these together into a few sequences that are easier to remember and perform.

Hypothetical Sport Application of Feature Integration Theory

Figure 3.5 presents an adaptation of Treisman's feature integration theory as it might apply to the basketball free throw. At the bottom is the visual field of the athlete, which is oriented toward

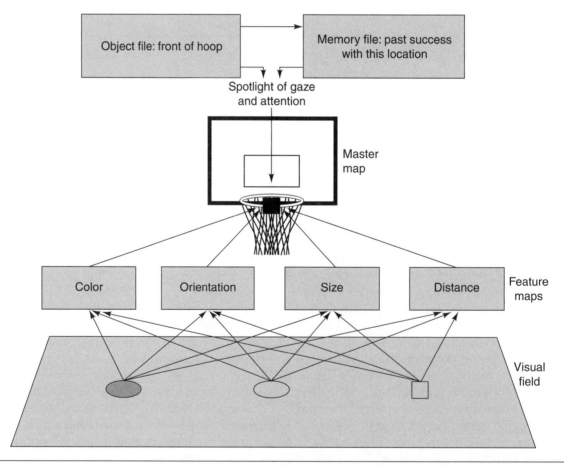

➤ **Figure 3.5**   Treisman's feature integration theory and the spotlight of attention adapted to the basketball free throw.

the basket. Specialized areas in the brain record the color, orientation, size, distance, and other features of the hoop and the backboard. Some of these features will pop out and become the spotlight for attention; for example, a shooter may select the shiny spot on the front of the hoop, or the middle back of the hoop, or even a location on the backboard. The spotlight is also affected by the existence of an object file for the hoop as stored in memory. The memory file also contains a record of past success with this location. Evidence that basketball athletes do indeed orient their gaze and attention to specific locations on the hoop that differ according to shooting success or failure will be presented in chapter 5.

Topographical Mapping

The process whereby certain spatial relations among locations are preserved in the brain is called **topographical mapping**. The relative distance between two locations is accurately preserved, while others undergo transformations that lose the absolute qualities that are present. The concept of topographical mapping means that absolute distances and directions are lost, while relative distances and directions are preserved. For example, the basketball hoop in figure 3.5 appears to be elliptical, but in absolute terms the hoop is a perfect circle. We can speculate that a skilled shooter ignores the elliptical appearance of the hoop and treats it as a large space that the ball can pass through with ease, while a novice may see the elliptical shape and imagine the ball passing through the space with greater difficulty.

A second example of topographical mapping is found in singles badminton and involves the athlete's perception of the back alley of the court during the serve. A perfect serve is one that drops vertically directly on the back line. The elite player knows that the shuttle has aerodynamic properties that cause it to stall and fall vertically if it is hit hard in an upward direction toward the back of the court. He or she therefore sees the back alley as an upward-rising column within which the stalled shuttle will invariably fall. All that is needed is to hit the shuttle hard in an upward direction and accuracy is virtually ensured. In contrast, the novice will try to control the speed, distance, and directional velocity of the shuttle, which is difficult to do consistently.

Control of the Gaze and Overt and Covert Attention

Thus far attention has been defined within the context of feature integration theory, bottom-up and top-down processing, the binding problem, and topographical mapping. We now consider the extent to which the focus of attention is defined by the locus of the gaze, or how we orient our gaze relative to the objects and locations in space. Two forms of attention are presented. During the **overt orienting of attention**, or overt attention, both the location of the gaze and the locus of attention are directed to the same location or object in space. For example, a basketball player using overt attention will look directly at the player and think about passing the ball to that player. In contrast, during the **covert orienting of attention**, or covert attention, the gaze is located on one object or location and the attention on another. Think of a basketball player looking in one direction as a pass is made in another. This is a case of covert attention—the gaze is in one direction and the focus of attention and resultant pass in another.

Relationship Between Shifts in Gaze and Locus of Attention

The extent to which a shift in the gaze indicates a shift in attention has gone through two major schools of thought. Until recently, it was thought that it is easy to separate, or dissociate, the locus of the gaze from the locus of attention, and therefore eye-movement data were not considered to be a strong indicator of the locus of attention. Lately, however, there has been a major shift in the literature. New evidence shows that, under certain conditions, a shift in the gaze is invariably preceded by a shift in attention (Corbetta, 1998; Deubel & Schneider, 1996; Henderson, 2003; Kowler, Anderson, Dosher, & Blaser, 1995; Kustov & Robinson, 1996; Shepherd, Findlay, & Hockey, 1986). These studies show that when participants shift their gaze to a specific part of the perceptual-motor workspace, a shift in attention also occurs under certain conditions. In the next section, we look at the evidence that favors a complete dissociation of the locus of gaze and attention and that which shows how shifts of gaze and attention are invariably linked.

Evidence of a Dissociation

It is easy to look at one location and attend to something else. For example, a football quarterback may be looking at one receiver but attending to another on a different part of the field. When this occurs, the locations of the gaze and of attention are dissociated or separate. Posner (1980) and Treisman and Gormican (1988) have all shown that the locus of the gaze can easily be dissociated from the locus of attention. Studies typically include conditions requiring both the overt and covert control of attention. During the covert-orienting trials, the participants were required to keep their gaze on a central fixation point and press a reaction-time key when they first perceived targets located in the periphery. In the overt condition, they were required to shift their gaze to the stimulus as soon as it appeared and press the key. On some trials an arrow would appear, accurately signaling where the target would appear, and on others it would not be present. On occasion the arrow would direct attention to the wrong location, thus giving an erroneous cue. In all cases, an eye tracker was used to ensure that fixation was initially maintained centrally, and to record the time course of saccades to the peripheral locations. The goal was to determine if differences in reaction time occurred as a result of the use of overt or covert attention. Reaction times during both overt conditions did not differ; attention could be shifted quickly with or without a shift in gaze. Indeed, attention could be shifted faster to the new locations than either the gaze or the motor response, the general temporal order being that the attention shifted first, the gaze moved second, and the motor response occurred last.

In addition, shifts of attention were facilitated by the presence of the arrow cue. When the location of the target was cued in advance, reaction times were faster than when they were not cued, highlighting the importance of planning and anticipation on both the shifting of attention and on making saccades to that location. Unexpected cues almost always attracted a rapid shift of gaze and attention. Finally, once attention had been directed to a new location, there was a reluctance to return to that location again. This phenomenon is called *inhibition of return* and will be discussed in greater detail later in the chapter. Based on these results, Posner (1980) and many others concluded that the neural systems that control attention and eye movement are separate. Since it was easy to move attention to other locations and objects while the gaze was directed to a different location, knowing where the gaze was in space contributed little to knowing where attention resided. Eye movements and gaze shifts per se were therefore given less weight since the internal processes of attention were thought to be most important.

Evidence Against a Dissociation

The view that the eye movements and attention can be easily dissociated has prevailed until recently and has dominated the literature in eye movements, cognition, and motor learning and control. But a number of studies provide new and convincing evidence from multiple sources (cognition, neuroscience, and motor behavior) that, under certain conditions, a shift of the gaze invariably predicts a shift in attention (Corbetta, 1998; Deubel & Schneider, 1996; Henderson, 2003; Kowler et al., 1995; Shepherd et al., 1986).

Shepard et al. (1986) used the same basic setup as that used by Posner and others, but they manipulated spatial attention by varying the probability (50/50, 80/20, and 20/80) that a peripheral stimulus would appear in a position that was the same as or opposite to the actual target location. The cue arrow served the purpose of generating expectancies of the target location. In the 50/50 condition, the cue provided no information about which side the cue would appear and had little effect on reaction times. In both the 80/20 and 20/80 conditions, the cue provided accurate spatial information and a clear advantage was found for the cued position. The longer the elapsed time between the onset of the cue and the onset of target, the faster was reaction time.

Reaction times were also similar during overt- and covert-orienting conditions, with one exception. When the participants were required to saccade in the direction of the cued arrow but still maintain their attention on the central fixation point, they could not do so. This result showed that when a saccade was made, there was a corresponding shift in attention in the direction of the saccade and a slowing of the resultant reaction time. Additional support comes from many studies (Deubel & Schneider, 1996; Henderson, 2003; Kowler et al., 1995), including studies on brain imaging that show that common neural structures are involved in moving the gaze and shifting visual attention in the parietal and frontal lobes (Corbetta, 1998).

Illustration of Overt and Covert Attention

This section presents an exercise that will aid understanding of covert and overt attention as they apply in a sport task. Figure 3.6 shows a frame of vision-in-action data taken of a golfer performing a putt. Image A shows the golfer's eye with x–y coordinates. Image B presents his visual field with the green, ball, putter, and stance visible. The location of his gaze is shown by the cursor, which is located on the back of the ball. Image C shows his putting stroke.

Now let's apply the concepts of overt and covert attention to this skill. Imagine you are the golfer in figure 3.6 and perform the following series of exercises. First, hold your gaze on the ball and then shift your attention to the hole. You will find this task easy—maintaining fixation on the ball as you think about the hole is an easy dissociation of the gaze from attention. You are using covert attention and there is a clear dissociation between where your gaze is fixated (ball) and where your thoughts have gone (hole). In the second exercise, maintain your gaze on the ball and also direct your attention there. You might be attending to the dimples on the ball, or

the trademark on the ball, or the orientation of the clubface. Again, this is easy to do. There is a complete association between the locus of your gaze and locus of overt attention. In the third critical exercise, try to fixate the ball and maintain your focus of attention on the ball 100% of the time as you shift your gaze to the hole. Do not shift your attention from the ball even as you shift your gaze to the hole. You will find that you cannot keep your attention on the ball; instead it will move to the hole when you shift your gaze (saccade) there. Your attention will be drawn to the hole even though you fully intended to keep it on the ball.

This exercise shows that there is a much greater degree of entrainment between shifts of gaze and shifts in attention than previously realized. When athletes shift their gaze to a new location, it means that they have also shifted their attention to that location. But it is important to stress that once the gaze and attention have arrived at the new location, the **duration of fixation** is not always an indicator of sustained attention. Athletes can covertly divert their attention elsewhere even as fixation remains on that location; that is, they can maintain their fixation on the hole and be thinking about something else.

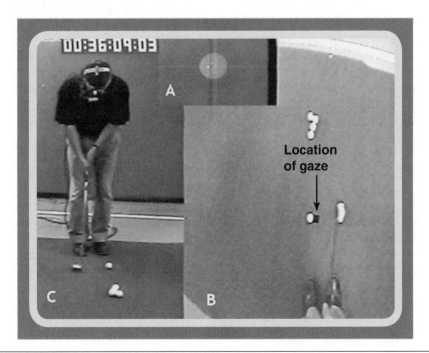

➤ **Figure 3.6**   A frame of vision-in-action data of a golfer as recorded during the putt. Image A shows the eye of the golfer; image B is of the visual field and black cursor, which shows the golfer's gaze on the back of the ball; and image C shows the movements of the golfer as he performs the putt. The time-code generator measured time in all three images at the rate of 30 frames/s (33.33 ms/frame).

Visual Attention and Representation of the World

Thus far the visual attention system has been presented as a reliable system that provides an accurate depiction of our world. The idea that we create a stable representation, or picture, of the world, has until recently been a major assumption of perception, cognition, and memory research and accords nicely with our subjective experience of the world. We feel strongly that we know what to expect in most situations, and we look for predictable qualities in well-known events. There is also a sense that this representation depends on the storage of images that are built up across shifts of the gaze, and that each fixation is responsible for updating or revising our representation in real space and time. But are we really able to store images that are true representations of our world? A growing number of studies show that our subjective experience of the world exerts such a powerful influence on us that there is much that we miss, even when it is right before our eyes.

Inattention and Change Blindness

Our perception of the world is often dominated by internal representations that may prevent us from attending to events that are fully present (Neisser, 1979, 1983; Rensink, 2002). **Inattention blindness** "denotes the failure to see highly visible objects we may be looking at when our attention is elsewhere" (Mack, 2003, p. 180). **Change blindness** is a phenomenon that often occurs when humans fail to notice critical changes in their environment. Change blindness is defined as "the failure of observers to detect large, sudden changes in a display. Although such changes are readily seen under normal conditions, change blindness is easily induced if the changes are made simultaneously with an eye movement, film cut, image flash, or other transient that masks the motion signals normally accompanying the change" (Rensink, 2002, p. 1469).

Research on change blindness has shown that we do not see changes in images and can be impervious to cues that are highly salient. Large changes in pictures of real-world scenes often go unnoticed for up to 50 s, even if the change is made repeatedly and even if the observer knows in advance that a change is to be made (Henderson & Hollingsworth, 2003).

Change blindness normally occurs when there is a complete change in the location, color, or other properties of an object or person. For example, Simons and Levin (1998) asked people on the street for directions. A few seconds after the conversation began, workers carrying a large board passed between the (unwitting) participant and the experimenter, permitting the experimenter to switch with another person. Observers often missed the fact that the person they were talking to had switched, but they were much more likely to notice the change when the experimenter was a member of their social class, indicating a high-level influence on the representations used during the interaction.

Werner and Theis (2002) determined whether observers of American football games noticed changes inserted in well-known scenes. They found that experts in the sport were quicker to spot changes, regardless of whether or not the changes affected the meaning of the scene. Rensink (2002) explained that this is consistent with the proposal that experts code the scene in a way that allows them to spot changes in meaning relatively quickly, and that their familiarity with the domain allows them to scan meaningful scenes more efficiently.

Certain qualities of the human visuomotor system appear to compensate for aspects of change blindness. Chapter 1 presented the special properties of the focal and ambient systems, as well as those of the ventral and dorsal systems. We saw that the dorsal system is the faster system and is specialized for the automatic control of action, while the ventral system is concerned with more time-demanding cognitive processes and slower conscious motor control. Bridgeman, Kirch, & Sperling (1981) and Pellison et al. (1986) showed that the special properties of the ambient or dorsal system might protect people from some aspects of change blindness that may occur in motor settings. The displacement of an object during a saccade was not consciously perceived, but a corrective saccade was still made to the new location. Pellisson et al. (1986) further showed that if a target is displaced during a saccade, not only is a corrective saccade made subconsciously, but participants also correct the trajectory of the hand so that it accurately points to the target even though they never consciously noticed its displacement.

These findings indicate that the visuomotor system is able to detect changes in the movement of objects, even though these may not be attended to or overtly seen or processed by the focal system. Change blindness may therefore not be as great a factor in motor skills as it is in purely cognitive tasks. The sport performer may be more impervious to aspects of change blindness and therefore better able to respond to what is occurring in real space and time.

Inhibition of Return

Inhibition of return is the process whereby a currently attended location is prevented from being attended to later on. If an object or location is viewed on one occasion, then there is a lower probability that an attempt will be made to fixate that location again. Itti & Koch (2001)

explain that inhibition of return has many uses. First, it allows a performer to "rapidly shift the attentional focus over different locations with decreasing saliency, rather than being bound to attend only to the location of maximum saliency at any time" (Itti & Koch, 2001, p. 200). Second, a performer who views a location one time is less likely to return to that location later, making the ability to correctly understand what is occurring the first time a critical one.

Inhibition of return is a crucial characteristic of human visual attention and may have ramifications for sport performance. For example, highly skilled athletes may not need to revisit an area once attended as often as those with lower skill levels. This is indeed what was found in a study of elite and near-elite ice hockey players (Martell & Vickers, 2004). The elite players had a greater capacity to quickly see what was important and didn't need to revisit that area again (see chapter 8 for more details).

Gaze Control in Action

For a number of years I had students in my class study Mark McGwire's final hits of the 1998 season. During the 1997-98 season, Mark McGwire hit 70 home runs, thus breaking Roger Maris' record of 61 that had stood for more than 30 y. As part of the laboratory exercise, students determined McGwire's reaction time, movement time, and total response time from video footage taken during his final hits, 32 to 70, of the 1998 season in an effort to understand how his reaction time or movement time may have contributed to his performance. After they studied the footage and compiled data, they were required to answer the following question: Was McGwire's performance due to his exceptional reaction time, his exceptional movement time, or some combination of both?

You can complete a similar laboratory exercise to determine how reaction time, movement time, or a combination of both affect performance in the baseball swing. To carry out this laboratory exercise, follow these steps:

1. Read the text below on conducting research as well as the data on Mark McGwire.

2. Find a video of a baseball player attempting to hit a ball on 10 or more pitches. You can use a video of yourself or of a famous player.

3. Play the video on your computer or on a DVD or VHS player in real time and then frame by frame. Be sure you use a video that has not been compressed. (In North America, 1 s of video usually comprises 30 frames. Each frame then consumes 1,000 ms / 30 frames, or 33.33 ms/frame.)

4. Use the definitions for reaction time, movement time, and total response time described in the text applied to baseball that follows. Count the number of frames of video that occurred during each period. For each swing, record the numbers of frames in the data recording sheet. You will need to determine the number of ms per frame for each swing (1 frame = 33.33 ms).

5. Determine the mean reaction time (ms), mean movement time (ms) and total response time (ms) in absolute and relative time (see chapter 2).

6. Discuss the following questions: Using your reaction time, movement time, and total response time means, did the player you analyzed have a mean reaction time, mean movement time, or mean total response time that was similar to or different from the elite players described below? (Consider how well the person you analyzed hit the ball in answering this question.) In your opinion, was the hitter's performance (% hits) due to the optimal or nonoptimal use of reaction time, movement time, or total response time? Finally, using your results, identify two ways you would coach this person to improve.

Data Recording Sheet

Swing number	Reaction time (RT): Frames from release of ball to initiation of swing	Movement time (MT): Frames from initiation of swing until ball hits bat	Total response time (TRT) = RT + MT	Relative time percent (%) of total time = TRT / RT (or MT)
Swing 1				
Swing 2				
Swing 3				
Swing 4				
Swing 5				
Swing 6				
Swing 7				
Swing 8				
Swing 9				
Swing 10				
Mean				

Whenever you do a research project, it is first necessary to look at the available literature and determine what has been done previously. A number of studies have broken this period of time into a reaction-time phase and movement-time phase using film and video analysis (Breen, 1967; Hay, 1985). It takes 460 ms for an 89 mph (143 kph) baseball pitch to travel from the pitcher's hand over the 60.5 ft (18.4 m) to the pitcher's mound (Schmidt & Wrisberg, 2004).

The reaction-time period is defined as the amount of time from when the ball leaves the pitcher's hand until the final forward movement of the bat to hit the ball, while the movement-time period is the final forward swing of the bat (also called *swing time*). The timing of each period can be easily calculated from a video of the swing. In North America, 1 s of video usually comprises 30 frames. Each frame then consumes 1,000 ms/30 frames, or 33.33 ms/frame. Table 3.2 shows the reaction times, movement times, and total response times reported by Breen (1967) of several baseball players. We see that across a number of great hitters, reaction times ranged from a high of 350 ms to a low of 310 ms, and movement times ranged from a high of

Table 3.2   Reaction Times, Movement Times, and Total Response Times
of Great Baseball Hitters

Athlete	Reaction time	Movement time	Total response time
Ted Williams	310	230	540
Mickey Mantle	330	210	540
Willie Mays	330	210	540
Hank Aaron	350	190	540
Ernie Banks	320	220	540
Other 300 hitters	317	223	540
Average	326	214	540
Mark McGwire	311	157	468
Mark McGwire (out of 540 ms)	362	178	540

230 ms to a low of 190 ms. Note that all of these times have been normalized to 540 ms. By normalizing reaction time and movement time to one value, in this case 540 ms, the hitters can be compared with one another.

Table 3.2 shows that McGwire's reaction time for his final 38 homeruns was 311 ms, his movement time was 157 ms, and his total response time was 468 ms. When these times were normalized to 540, his reaction time was 362 ms, and his movement time was 178 ms. During the reaction-time phase he therefore had more time to track the ball than any player in history, and he also swung the bat faster than any player in history. However, it is important to remember that although we can speculate that McGwire did track the ball longer, his gaze was not recorded; therefore we do not know if this was the case for him or any of the other hitters. A number of studies are presented in chapter 7 that describe the gaze control of elite athletes during interceptive timing tasks like baseball hitting. From this research we can surmise that McGwire probably tracked the ball longer than anyone, especially when the ball moved erratically. (A baseball gaze control study has yet to be done *in situ* to determine exactly what baseball players see as they hit or miss the ball.)

We also know that McGwire's performance was not due to his exceptional vision—he actually had poor acuity in one eye and had to wear contacts when he played. That he performed so well with relatively poor vision is not unusual in sport; there is little or no evidence to suggest that performance is due to any hard-wired aspect of our visual system (e.g., acuity, stereopsis, contrast sensitivity, dynamic acuity) (see Abernethy & Woods, 2000; Applegate & Applegate, 1992). Instead, the available evidence suggests that the ability to perform at the top of a sport requires the combination of a long reaction-time during which the gaze is controlled optimally on critical information, followed by a movement-time phase that is also optimal given the skill being performed.

PART II

Gaze Control and the Quiet Eye in Sport

Part II begins in chapter 4 with the presentation of a unique gaze control framework that has been derived from the available gaze research in sport and other motor skills. The framework shows that humans control their gaze in a distinct way within three major categories of tasks: targeting tasks, interceptive timing tasks, and tactical tasks. Each of these is defined, along with their subcategories and research exemplars. Gaze control within each category is affected by four factors: the number of perceptual-motor workspaces that define the task, the locations and objects in each workspace, the spotlight of attention, and gaze-in-action coupling.

Chapter 5 provides specific information about the control of the gaze and quiet eye in tasks where the targets for the gaze are fixed in space (e.g., basketball free throw and jump shot, rifle shooting), while chapter 6 explains how the gaze and quiet eye are controlled in tasks where the focus of the gaze is more complex, as is found in abstract- and moving-target tasks (e.g., pass to a moving receiver). Chapter 7 concentrates on interceptive timing tasks (e.g., baseball batting, table tennis, volleyball serve reception, goaltending), and explains how the gaze and quiet eye are used to anticipate the flight of objects with both predictable and unpredictable flight paths. In chapters 5, 6, and 7, quiet-eye training studies

are also presented in selected sports. Chapter 8 then concentrates on tactical tasks and how control of the gaze and decision making occur in these types of tasks. Exemplars include walking through a cluttered environment, speed skating, soccer and ice hockey tactics, and ice hockey and soccer goaltending.

At the conclusion of part II, students should be able to do the following:

➤ Diagram the gaze control framework, including its three major categories of tasks, the subcategories of each, and the four gaze control factors that define each.

➤ Define the quiet eye in at least one targeting task, one interceptive timing task, and one tactical task.

➤ Describe how quiet-eye testing and training are done.

➤ Carry out at least one quiet-eye training exercise, as described at the end of each chapter.

➤ Describe the Setchenov phenomenon and a potential link between an external quiet-eye focus and the ability to do more physical work.

➤ Define the major terms as shown in bold and in the glossary.

Gaze Control Framework

◄◄ *Where Have We Been?*

In the last chapter, attention was defined and feature integration theory presented. We looked at the relationship between shifts of gaze and shifts of attention and saw that when the gaze shifts to a new object or location in space, a shift in attention precedes the saccade. The chapter concluded with a description of change blindness and inhibition of return.

►► *Where Are We Going?*

In this chapter, a gaze control framework is presented that has been derived from the current gaze research in sport. Rather than each sport having unique gaze and attention characteristics, current research shows that the gaze and attention are controlled in distinct ways within three main categories of tasks: targeting tasks, interceptive timing tasks, and tactical tasks. Within each of these categories, the gaze is affected by the number of perceptual-motor workspaces over which the gaze is controlled; the number and type of locations and objects that exist within each visuomotor workspace; the spotlight of attention within each visuomotor workspace that contributes to higher levels of performance; and gaze-in-action coupling, or how the gaze and spotlight of attention are optimally timed to permit a high level of motor performance. This framework provides a much simpler way of understanding how the gaze and attention function in sport compared with treating each task separately in terms of the gaze and attentional requirements needed to perform at the highest level.

Three Categories of Gaze Control

When we first learn to play a sport, we not only learn the movements in the sport, but also how to orient and control our gaze and attention as we perform. Current gaze research in sport shows that when a high level of skill is attained, not only is the gaze directed to the most important locations and objects in the performance space, it is also timed so that the critical cues underlying optimal performance are perceived and attended to at the right time.

Figure 4.1 presents the **gaze control framework** that describes the control of the gaze in three major categories of motor tasks (i.e., targeting, interceptive timing, tactical). These were first described in the introduction within the constraints-led model of motor coordination as proposed by Newell (1986); Newell and McDonald (1994); and Williams, Janelle, & Davids (2004). In figure 4.1, the three categories are displayed as three overlapping circles. This arrangement shows that all three types of gaze control are often found within a single sport, although this is not always the case. Also shown are the primary purpose of the gaze in each of the three categories, the subcategories found within each category, the number of visuomotor workspaces, the spotlights for the attention that are normally found, as well as a number of exemplars that will be presented in the following chapters. Whenever possible, research exemplars are presented for each subcategory. For some of the listed studies, the quiet eye has already been confirmed in the literature, while in others this has not yet occurred. Also note that in a few cases a research study has not yet been published and only pilot data have been collected. As the number of gaze studies in each subcategory increases, there will most likely be changes in the gaze control framework. In the next section, each category and subcategory of gaze control is explained in detail in terms of the role the gaze plays in the task, the number of visuomotor workspaces used, the spotlight of attention, and perception–action cycle. Whenever possible the information presented has been gained from the study of elite performers.

Gaze Control in Targeting Tasks

In **targeting tasks,** the function of the gaze and attention system is to locate a target in space and control the aiming of an object to the target area. Within targeting tasks, there are three subcategories of tasks: gaze control to **fixed targets,** to abstract targets, and to **moving targets.** In these tasks an object is usually propelled with the hands or feet away from the body in an aiming movement toward a target. Accuracy and consistency in performance are the ultimate goals. Exemplars are shooting a basketball, performing a golf putt, throwing a dart, shooting a rifle, and throwing to a receiver. Although the motor behaviors differ markedly in each case, the problem for the gaze and attention system is the same: to focus on the most critical part of the target and time the acquisition of information so that there is an optimal coupling between the gaze and aiming movements, thus leading to successful completion of the task.

➤ *Gaze control to fixed targets.* The target for the gaze and aiming is fixed in space, and its location is stable and predictable in nature (e.g., basketball hoop, rifle target). Accuracy depends on fixating a specific location on the target before the aiming action is carried out. A high level of focus is required to perform well. Studies underlying this subcategory are presented in chapter 5.

➤ *Gaze control to abstract targets.* The targets for the gaze and aiming are fixed in space, but they are often multiple and abstract in nature (e.g., golf putting on a sloped green, billiards). In order to perform accurately, the visual workspace has to be interpreted, complex patterns determined, and an optimal sequence of gaze made to critical locations and objects before aiming occurs. Studies underlying this subcategory are presented in chapter 6.

➤ *Gaze control to a target in motion.* The target for the gaze and aiming is in motion and a ball or other object is thrown toward it, where it is caught or otherwise controlled by a receiver or other player (e.g., throw in football, pass in soccer). Anticipation of the target motion is critical, along with focus. To date, a gaze control study has not been completed in this category, although pilot studies have been done.

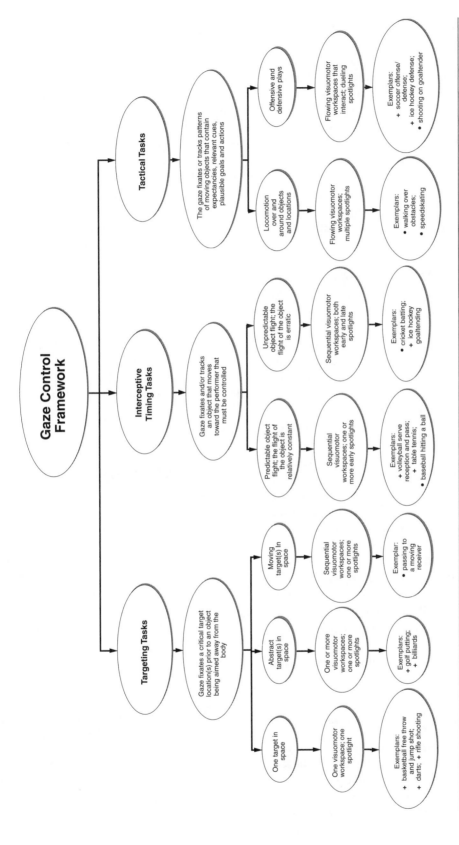

▲ **Figure 4.1**   Gaze control framework for targeting, interceptive timing, and tactical tasks. + = Quiet eye has been identified; • = Quiet eye yet to be identified.

Gaze Control in Interceptive Timing Tasks

In **interceptive timing tasks,** an object travels toward the performer and the gaze and attention systems are used to read the object as it is delivered, track it as it approaches, and then control it as it is received.

Interceptive timing tasks have three sequential phases in common: object recognition, object tracking, and object control. During the object-recognition phase, fixations and pursuit tracking are used to study the movements of the object and the individual propelling the object as it is pitched, bowled, kicked, shot, or otherwise propelled toward the receiver. During the object-tracking phase, smooth pursuit-tracking gazes are used to maintain the image of the object on the fovea in order to detect if it spins; accelerates or decreases in speed; changes direction; or is affected by wind, sun, or a host of other factors that can occur. During the object-control phase, the object is caught with the hand, kicked to a teammate, hit as in baseball or cricket, passed to a teammate as in volleyball, and so on. Many interceptive timing tasks in sport require the object to be directed to a secondary target at contact. There are two subcategories of gaze control in interceptive tasks, and these depend on whether the flight of the object is predictable or unpredictable. Gaze control during **predictable object motion** occurs when the flight of the object is relatively constant. Gaze control during **unpredictable object motion** is used when the flight of the object spins, slides, curves, or moves erratically. When object flight is predictable, early tracking of the object is usually sufficient to ensure accuracy. However, when it is unpredictable, early tracking, plus saccadic movements and late tracking of the object, are also critical. Representative studies are presented in chapter 7.

Gaze Control in Tactical Tasks

Tactical tasks often subsume the gaze behaviors found in targeting and interceptive timing tasks, and they also include a third category of gaze control—reading complex patterns of moving objects (e.g., players, balls, pucks). Think of reading the offense or defense in a team sport such as basketball or baseball, or trying to discern the open part of a net where you want to make a shot in field hockey, or reading a race course

as in skiing, kayaking, or mountain climbing. In each of these cases the motor behaviors differ greatly, but the problem for the gaze is always the same—to detect the most important cues present in an environment full of moving objects and make the best decision, often under severe time constraints. The performer has to understand the meaningful relationships between locations and objects that contain expectancies, relevant cues, plausible goals, and actions (Klein, 1999). Again, the physical movements of tactical tasks differ greatly, but the problem for the gaze is similar in and across a number of tactical contexts. **Pattern recognition** and tactical awareness are not only important in sports like basketball, volleyball, ice hockey, and football, they are also critical in speed skating, ski racing, and similar activities.

Two subcategories are presented: gaze control during locomotion and gaze control during offensive and defensive plays in sport. Currently there are fewer gaze studies in the tactical tasks category than any other. With more research, this is the category that will probably change the most. Representative studies are presented in chapter 8.

Four Factors That Affect Gaze Control

Within each of the categories shown in figure 4.1, four major factors affect the control of the gaze: the number of visuomotor workspaces over which the gaze is controlled; the number and type of locations and objects that exist in the perceptual-motor workspace; the location of critical cues and spotlight of attention; and gaze–action coupling, or optimally timing the gaze, spotlight of attention, and specific phases of the motor behavior.

Number of Visuomotor Workspaces Over Which the Gaze Is Controlled

The first factor that affects gaze control is the number of visuomotor workspaces over which the gaze and attention must be controlled. The visuomotor workspace is the spatial environment within which objects and locations exist that command the performer's gaze and attention and upon which specific motor behaviors are enacted. When the gaze of sport performers are recorded in real-world settings, it is soon apparent that performers do not always look straight ahead and direct their gaze to one visuomotor workspace only, as is often the perspective found in visual-search studies; instead, they direct their gaze to multiple visual fields that can exist all about them depending on the task. Generally, the number of visuomotor workspaces increases from targeting tasks to interceptive tasks to tactical tasks. During targeting tasks with one fixed location (e.g., dart throwing or basketball), there is one visuomotor workspace (the board or basket). In golf or billiards there are often two or more visuomotor workspaces, and in interceptive timing tasks the number of visuomotor workspaces is sequential and dictated by the speed of the object, the size of the area over which the object travels, and the relative position of the athlete. Tactical tasks have the greatest number of visuomotor workspaces, and the gaze is controlled over both large and small spaces. For example, in ice hockey the athlete has to detect the movement of a puck that may be high or low, to the left or right, or in front of or behind the athlete, as well as moving quickly, slowly, or erratically (Martell & Vickers, 2004). As the number of visuomotor workspaces increases, decisions have to be made about how to control the gaze and attention given the overall goal. A decision has to be made about which visuomotor workspace fields are most important and in which order information should be acquired prior to performing.

Number of Objects and Locations Within Visuomotor Workspaces

The second factor that affects gaze control is the number of locations and objects viewed when a task is performed. Recall from chapter 3 that objects are distinct from locations (Treisman, 1986a) in that they are normally in motion, while locations are spatial and topographical in nature and do not have the capacity to move. Objects in sport include balls, pucks, shuttles, people (opponents, teammates, officials, coaches, judges, spectators, and all other persons), rackets, and mobile equipment. Locations range in complexity from a single target in space that is relatively easy for the gaze and attention system to locate and perceive (e.g., a fixed basketball hoop), to multiple target locations that provide more challenge for the gaze, attention, and motor systems

(e.g., abstract targets), to whole fields of play, as found in tactical tasks.

Controlling the gaze relative to objects and locations in the performance space is important in the gaze control framework. But, is there evidence that athletes fixate or track specific objects and locations when they perform? Perhaps they center the gaze and look into empty spaces where the movement of players can be more globally perceived, as has been suggested by Tenenbaum (2003) and Williams, Davids, and Williams (1999). These authors have suggested that athletes use a central fixation point or a visual pivot to keep track of events using the ambient system rather than the focal system.

The number of fixations or pursuit-tracking gazes were determined in selected targeting tasks, interceptive timing tasks, and tactical tasks. Table 4.1 shows the percent of fixations or tracking gazes to objects, locations, or open spaces as found in studies on the basketball free throw (Vickers, 1996a), the golf putt (Vickers, 1992), the volleyball serve pass and reception (Vickers & Adolphe, 1997), and ice hockey tactics (Martell & Vickers, 2004).

Objects included balls, the puck, the golf club, and offensive and defensive players, and locations included the hoop, backboard, floor, green, hole, and setter area. Spaces were classified as negative or positive and were adapted from definitions used by Bard et al. (1980) and Williams et al. (1999). A positive space was one where information relevant to the task was acquired, while a negative space was outside the field of play and irrelevant to the task goals.

Table 4.1 shows the following:

➤ Objects and locations were fixated or tracked more often than spaces.

➤ High- and low-skilled performers differed in the percentage of gaze devoted to objects, locations, and spaces, but these differences often were not significant.

➤ Percentage of gaze was influenced most by the category of the task performed. In targeting tasks such as the basketball free throw, more fixations were directed to a fixed location (the hoop, backboard), and fewer were directed to objects (ball) or open spaces. In the golf putt, more fixations were directed to objects (ball, club), followed by fixed locations (hole, breakpoint on the green); they were directed

Table 4.1 Percent of Fixations and Pursuit Tracking to Locations, Objects, and Spaces in Targeting, Interceptive Timing, and Tactical Tasks

Category	ELITE ATHLETES			NEAR-ELITE ATHLETES		
	% objects	Locations	Spaces	% objects	Locations	Spaces
Targeting task						
Free throw	11	89	0	11	89	0
Golf putting	71	29	0	61	39	0
Interceptive timing task						
Volleyball serve	87	0	13	85	0	15
Tactical task						
Ice hockey defense	69	0	31	67	0	33

Studies were Vickers (1996a); Vickers (1992); Vickers & Adolphe (1997); Martell & Vickers (2004).

least to open spaces. In the interceptive timing task of volleyball, more fixations or pursuit tracking were allocated to the moving object (ball) and fewer to open spaces, while in the tactical sport of ice hockey, about two-thirds of fixation and tracking were directed to objects (puck, offensive players) and one-third to open spaces located between opposing players (positive space) or downward on the ice during fast skating (negative space).

Table 4.2 shows the percent of fixations, pursuit trackings, and saccades found in each of the studies shown in table 4.1. Recall that information can be processed during fixations and pursuit tracking, but during saccades information is suppressed as the gaze moves rapidly from one location or object or space to another.

➤ In the target task of basketball, fixations were used more and were directed to the hoop and backboard.

➤ In golf putting, the percent of fixations and saccades was more evenly distributed.

➤ In the interceptive timing task of volleyball, fixations were directed to the server and ball, followed by pursuit tracking on the ball. Saccades were used to regain tracking.

➤ In tactical tasks, fixation and tracking gaze were most prevalent, followed by saccades and fixations to positive and negative spaces.

In terms of the relative percent of fixations, saccades, and pursuit tracking, the nature of the task appeared to play the largest role in determining the use of the different types of gaze. These results therefore provide support for the constraints-led model, as well as the three categories of gaze control presented in figure 4.1.

Spotlights of Attention Within Visuomotor Workspaces

The third factor that affects gaze control is the spotlight of attention. Within each visual field, one or more spotlights of attention are found. Optimal sport performance is defined not only by an ability to temporally control the gaze across visual fields, but also by an ability to define what is most important within and across each visuomotor workspace. Both bottom-up and top-down processes define the spotlight for the attention. During bottom-up processing, salient aspects of an object or location pop out and command the performer's gaze and attention. In top-down processing, the athlete brings previous expectancies and plans that dictate how the environment is perceived. Elite performers function with both capacities, while novices may be controlled more by bottom-up or top-down processes (Treisman, 1986a; Williams et al., 1999; Starkes & Ericsson, 2003). The quiet eye is an example of the spotlight of attention in a number of tasks.

Table 4.2 Percent of Fixations, Pursuit Tracking, and Saccades Found in Targeting, Interceptive Timing, and Tactical Tasks

Category	ELITE ATHLETES			NEAR-ELITE ATHLETES		
	Fixations	Tracking	Saccades	Fixations	Tracking	Saccades
Targeting skill						
Free throw	89	1	11	85	1	14
Golf putting	47	7	46	45	8	4
Interceptive timing						
Volleyball serve	30	46	24	29	45	26
Table tennis	30	46	24	29	45	26
Tactical task						
Ice hockey defense	57	43		57	43	

Gaze–Action Coupling

The fourth factor that defines how the gaze is controlled is the timing of critical gaze with the phases of the movement. The quiet eye is one example of the spotlight of attention. In each category of tasks, research shows that some gaze locations (spotlights, quiet eye) are more important than others and that the ability to focus on the right object or location at the right time is a factor in both sport expertise and performance.

Evidence that the gaze must be optimally timed with motor behavior is provided by a study in darts (Vickers, Rodrigues, & Edworthy, 2000). Skilled players took shots to the bull's-eye of a regulation dartboard until they made five hits and five misses. The goal was to determine the characteristics of the gaze, and in particular the quiet eye, during hits and misses. Imaging software (NIH Image) was used to determine the location and timing of the gaze relative to the bull's-eye during three phases of the throwing action: alignment, arm flexion, and extension.

During the alignment phase, the players aimed the dart at the bull's-eye using their preferred technique, during the flexion phase the arm flexed toward the body in preparation for the throw, and during the extension phase the hand propelled the dart forward to the board. Analysis showed that the final fixation, or quiet eye, was the most important gaze, and that the onset of this fixation occurred well before

extension of the forearm. The results are shown in figure 4.2 across the final 90 fields, or final 1,500 ms of the hits and misses (1 field = 16.67 ms). The durations of the flexion and extension phases were similar on hits and misses, so these were collapsed, as shown by the vertical dotted lines. The location of the gaze relative to the target center is shown in radial error units. A radial error (RE) of zero indicated that the center of the gaze cursor was located on the center of the bull's-eye, while an RE of 13.5 (the horizontal line) indicated that the gaze had moved off the target.

Three results, shown in figure 4.2, are important. First, the gaze was fixated on the center of the bull's-eye during the preparation of the throw and then moved progressively off the target during the flexion and extension phases of both hits and misses. Second, during the extension phase, there were no fixations on the target, so the critical quiet-eye fixation occurred earlier, during the alignment and flexion phases. Third, during misses, the final fixation (or quiet eye) occurred early and was of a shorter duration than during hits. These results show that although it is necessary to know where to look and for how long, it is just as important to know when to look at a target. Target information gained too soon or too late does not lead to the same levels of accuracy as information that is obtained optimally, which in the dart throw was just before extension of the forearm in the aiming action.

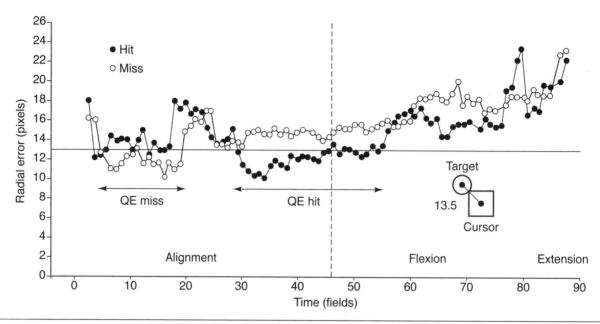

➤ Figure 4.2   Displacement of the gaze (in RE pixel units) from the bull's-eye during hits and misses. The inset target and gaze cursor show that the distance from the center of the bull's-eye to the center of the gaze cursor was 13.5 pixels. If the gaze had remained on the bull's-eye, the radial error would have been zero.

From J.N. Vickers, S.T. Rodrigues and G. Edworthy, 2000, "Quiet eye and accuracy in the dart throw," *International Journal of Sports Vision* 6: 30-36.

Gaze Control in Action

Given the gaze control characteristics of targeting tasks, interceptive timing tasks, and tactical tasks presented in this chapter, classify the following five sport tasks as either a targeting task (fixed, abstract, or moving), an interceptive timing task (predictable or unpredictable), or a tactical task (locomotion, offensive play, or defensive play).

Task	Category of gaze control
➤ Rugby field goal kick	➤ _____
➤ Short track speed skating (pass inside)	➤ _____
➤ Fast break in basketball (3 vs 1 defender)	➤ _____
➤ Pistol shooting (one target)	➤ _____
➤ Pass in football	➤ _____

CHAPTER 5 ▸▸

Gaze Control to a Single Fixed Target

◂◂ *Where Have We Been?*

In the last chapter, three major categories of gaze control were presented as found in targeting, interceptive timing, and tactical tasks. Four gaze control characteristics were presented that affect how the gaze is controlled within and across each of these categories: the number and type of locations and objects that need to be fixated, the number of visuomotor workspaces over which the gaze must be controlled, the spotlight of attention, and optimal gaze–action coupling.

▸▸ *Where Are We Going?*

In this chapter, research on gaze control when aiming at a single fixed target is presented. Representative tasks are basketball shooting (free throw and jump shot) and rifle shooting (standing shots and biathlon). Although the motor behaviors required in each of these tasks differ, the demands placed upon the gaze control and attention systems are similar. The quiet eye is introduced as a gaze that underlies higher levels of expertise and performance accuracy in these tasks. Two training studies (Harle & Vickers, 2001; Oudejans, Koedijker, Bleijendaal, & Bakker, 2005) are presented. These studies show that training a quiet eye leads to unusually large increases in performance, which is also accompanied by **self-organization** of the skill. The final part of the chapter shows how the quiet eye may insulate athletes from choking under pressure.

Has Targeting Contributed to a Bigger Brain?

The ability to locate a target with the gaze and perform an aiming movement that places an object consistently on or near that target may be uniquely human. This is the thesis of William Calvin (1983), who states that humans throughout time have exhibited a fascination with targeting that is not found to the same degree in primates. Although primates may display some rudimentary targeting abilities—for example, they use rocks to open nuts or other sources of food—they never spend countless hours throwing at a far target just for the fun of it. Aiming at targets is a pursuit of many humans around the world, young and old, male and female, high and low skilled. Children will throw rocks at targets for hours, and adults continue to engage in targeting activities throughout their lifetime. Indeed, many adults make this their profession, as is the case with professional athletes in basketball, golf, ice hockey, and soccer, to name but a few sports where hitting targets with a high degree of accuracy is important.

Calvin states that aiming to hit targets led to the development of the bigger human brain. He explains that our ancestors first discovered how to hit food targets with rocks and passed this knowledge down from generation to generation. A hunter throwing at a distance is a lot safer than one close in, so special targeting implements were developed. Targeting implements evolved from those held in the hand (stones, knives), to those thrown (spears), to those propelled over great distances using bows and arrows, to rifles and missiles. A small human can fell a very large animal if the right target is hit (the heart or another vital organ) with the right implement.

As advances in targeting occurred, Calvin states that the temporal and frontal lobes developed to levels not seen in primates or other species. Of course, modern humans do not have to hunt for food, so targeting in this sense is no longer required. Instead, we have developed complex sport and computer games that stimulate and challenge the human mind to be accurate and consistent.

Humans have evolved all manner of targeting pursuits that require the placing of objects in or on specific locations, most often under difficult conditions. As mentioned, sport is one of the main arenas where this occurs. Think of the targets in golf, basketball, darts, bowling, sky diving, ski racing, kayaking through gates, hitting a receiver, playing the piano, and video games. These activities all contain targets of some kind. It often takes many years of practice to be good at a targeting activity. Furthermore, in order for a targeting skill to find a place in a sport, it has to be challenging for most humans to perform. The best field shooters in basketball hit only 50% of their field shots (or chance), the best shooters in ice hockey or soccer rarely score more than once each game, and the best golfers still take 1.8 putts each hole.

Gaze Control in the Basketball Free Throw

The free throw is taken with a clear line of sight to the hoop without opposition. The player stands behind the free-throw line, which is located 15 ft (4.57 m) from the basket, and shoots at a hoop located directly in front at a height of 10 ft (3.04 m). Accuracy in this skill averages 76% for the best men and women players in the world (www.nba. com). Free-throw shooting percentages below 65% are considered low, and top performers shoot above 90% in competition. From a motor control perspective, the free throw is classified as a closed or self-paced skill because opponents do not interfere with the shooter during performance. Oudejans, Koedijker, Bleijendaal, and Bakker (2005) state that although there is a good deal of literature on the kinematics, biomechanics, and physics of basketball shooting (e.g., Brancazio, 1981; Elliott, 1992; Elliott & White, 1989; Hay, 1993; Hudson, 1985; Kirby & Roberts, 1985; Knudson, 1993; Knudson & Morrison, 1997; Miller & Bartlett, 1996; Penrose & Blanksby, 1976), no study has isolated a single quality that improves shooting performance. Techniques differ from player to player, with many biomechanical styles being equally effective (Knudson, 1993; Wissel, 1994; Wooden, 1988).

Location and Frequency of Fixations

During the preparation of an accurate shot, the gaze is directed to a single location on the hoop and fixation is maintained on that location for an optimal duration (Harle & Vickers, 2001; Vickers,

1996a, 1996b, 1996c). Most shooters select the front of the hoop, although other locations are equally effective, such as the back center of the hoop, middle of the hoop, or backboard center (Vickers, 1996c). It does not matter which location is fixated as long as only one target location is the focus of the gaze and attention.

Elite shooters have a lower **frequency of fixations** during each shot than do novices or near-elite athletes, and the number of fixations is lower on accurate shots than on inaccurate shots. The area over which the gaze is controlled on the target is also smaller, in agreement with Treisman's notion of a smaller spotlight for attention (Treisman, Cavanagh, Fischer, Ramachandran, & von der Heydt, 1990; Treisman, 1993; Treisman, 1998). The elite shooter directs the gaze to a narrower location on the hoop, while the near-elite player lets the gaze wander to more locations. This is illustrated in figure 5.1, which shows the fixation locations of two players during five free throws. Both athletes played on the same elite team, but player A's accuracy was 82% during the previous season of competition, while player B's percentage was 65%. Shooter A focused on only one location during each free throw, which was the front of the hoop, while player B directed his gaze to three locations during the shot: the front rim, the back rim, and the backboard, for a mean frequency of 2.3 fixations each shot. Recall that a shift of gaze is preceded by a shift in attention (Corbetta, 1998; Deubel & Schneider,

1996; Kowler, Anderson, Dosher, & Blaser, 1995; Shepherd et al., 1986); therefore it seems that player A not only controlled his gaze with more precision, but also focused his attention on only one location during each shot, while player B did not exhibit the same level of control over his gaze and attention.

Quiet Eye in the Free Throw

In addition to having a lower frequency of fixation on the hoop, elite shooters fixate the hoop at the optimal time during the preparation and execution of the shot. This ability to maintain focus and concentration on one location as the shot is prepared and executed is called the quiet eye (Vickers, 1996a). The quiet-eye period of elite basketball players has four spatial–temporal qualities that together contribute to the players' higher levels of accuracy. First, the quiet eye is a fixation directed to a single location on the hoop. In order to be coded as a fixation, the gaze must be held on one location within 3° of visual angle or less for a minimum of 100 ms. Second, the quiet-eye period has an onset that occurs before the final movement of the skill. Third, the quiet eye has an offset that occurs when the fixation deviates from the location by more than 3° of visual angle for longer than 100 ms; therefore the quiet-eye period can carry through and beyond the final movement. Finally, a longer quiet-eye period is a characteristic of higher levels of both skill and

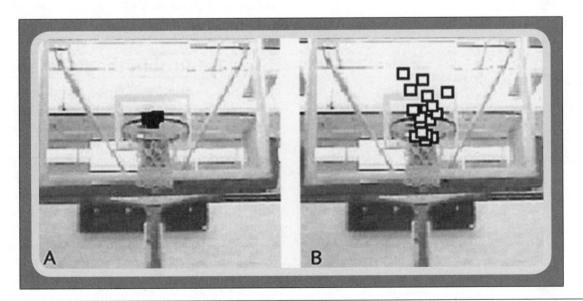

➤ **Figure 5.1** Fixation locations of an elite free-throw shooter (left) and a near-elite shooter (right) during five consecutive free throws.

accuracy. Figure 5.2 shows the quiet-eye period from Vickers (1996a). On hits, the elite shooters had a quiet-eye duration that averaged almost 1 s on hits and 800 ms on misses, while the near-elite shooters had a quiet duration that was shorter than 350 ms on both hits and misses.

Vickers (1996a) also suggested that optimal gaze control in the free throw is explained through a hypothesis of location suppression. During the location phase, the athlete focuses on the most critical location on the target for about 1 s before the shot is initiated. Fixation is held at that location until the ball enters the athlete's visuomotor workspace, during which time the close proximity of the ball and hands is suppressed in order for the shot to be performed accurately. Vickers also found that it is rare for a new fixation on the hoop to be initiated after the ball enters the visuomotor workspace; the optimal fixation onset occurs before the shot is taken. The final shooting action should be performed quickly under open-loop control. Recall from chapter 3 that open-loop control is used when movements are so fast that there is no time for feedback to affect the shooting action.

The longer quiet-eye period has been described as "a critical period of cognitive processing during which the parameters of the movement such as force, direction, and velocity are fine-tuned and programmed" (Williams, Singer, & Frehlich, 2002, p. 205). This explanation suggests that all the planning and organization of the shooting action is done in the higher neural networks before the shot is executed. Alternatively, researchers from the ecological perspective (Oudejans et al., 2002; Oudejans et al., 2005) have proposed that the long-duration quiet eye allows the system to receive critical visual information that is vital to controlling the skill until the moment of release of the ball. In other words, these authors propose that visual feedback is critical up to the moment the ball is released from the fingertips.

These two opposing views have major ramifications not only in terms of theories of motor control, but also in terms of how athletes are trained. If a cognitive perspective is followed, then the optimal form of training is one where the athlete is taught to fixate the hoop early and organize the action before the final shooting action. Athletes would also be taught to perform the shot without initiating a new fixation on the hoop as the shot is taken. In the second perspective, athletes would be trained to continually acquire information about the hoop until the ball leaves the fingertips since this information is critical to success. In the following section we explore these two views in the case of the basketball jump shot.

Gaze Control in the Jump Shot

The jump shot differs from the free throw in that it is a dynamic shot taken from any part of the floor, most often under pressure from one or more defenders. The jump shot is therefore classified as an open skill because external factors such as defenders and distance from the basket often affect performance. The shooting percentage of top players is around 45%, with some higher than 50% (www.nba.com). Oudejans et al. (2002) determined the effects of viewing time on the jump-shot accuracy of 10 highly skilled basketball players using the experimental setup shown in figure 5.3. The figure shows an athlete wearing a pair of PLATO liquid-crystal goggles. These goggles were opened or closed in less than

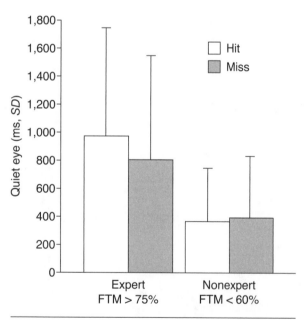

▶ **Figure 5.2**   The quiet-eye duration of elite and near-elite basketball players on hits and misses.

From J.N. Vickers, 1996, "Visual control when aiming at a far target," *Journal of Experimental Psychology: Human Perception and Performance* 22(2): 342-354. Reprinted by kind permission of the Experimental Psychology Society.

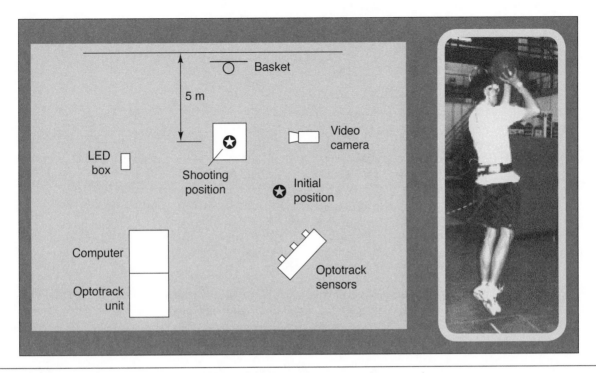

> **Figure 5.3** Experimental setup used by Oudejans et al. (2002) in the jump shot.

Reprinted from Human Movement Science, Vol. 21, R.R.D. Oudejans, R.W. van de Langenberg and R.I. Hutter, Aiming at a far target under different viewing conditions: visual control in basketball jump shooting, pp. 457-480, Copyright 2002 with permission from Elsevier.

5 ms by the movement of the shooting hand as it passed the level of the eye.

Four viewing conditions were used. In the early vision condition, the athletes could see the hoop early in the shot, but they could not see it during the final 350 ms due to the goggles shutting as their shooting hand activated sensors located above their eye (see *m*1 and *m*2 in figure 5.4). In the late-vision condition, the players could see the hoop late during the final 350 ms, but not early. In the no-vision condition, the players had to shoot without being able to see the hoop at all, and in the full-vision condition, the jump shots were taken without any obstruction of vision. The players also performed the shots dynamically, taking a step and one dribble before shooting from the same location near the free-throw line.

Oudejans et al. (2002) found that two shooting styles were used, one high and one low. They defined the high style as one where during the final extension of the forearm and hands the participants could see the rim in the ready position, as shown in figure 5.4. Here the ball is located above the head before release. In the low style, players released the ball from in front of their foreheads before the ball reached the ready position. In the study, only two athletes used a low

style. These athletes had high levels of accuracy during the early-vision condition, but low accuracy when vision was occluded during the last 350 ms. The remainder of the high-style athletes performed best during the late-vision condition and poorer during the early-vision condition. It was clear that the type of shooting technique affected when the basket could be fixated, and this in turn affected accuracy.

For the high-style shooters, accuracy was highest in the full-vision condition (61.5%), followed by the late-vision condition (60.5%), and last by the early-vision (30%) and no-vision (17.5%) conditions. In addition, during the late-vision condition, when only 350 ms were available to see the hoop, the high-style shooters increased the period of time the goggles remained open before release of the ball by an average of 50 ms. These athletes therefore created a longer period of time during which they could see the hoop, which Oudejans et al. (2002) argued was a lengthening of the quiet-eye period. This study showed that in the jump shot, basketball players who used the high-style shooting (but not the low) defined a quiet-eye period that appeared to be much later and briefer than what Vickers (1996a) found in the free throw.

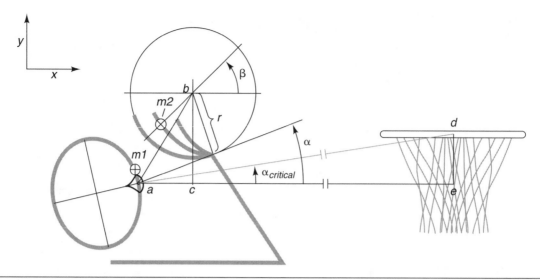

➤ **Figure 5.4**   Schematic display of positions in the ready position of the ball; the rim; and the shooter's hand, head, and eye. $m1$ = marker on goggles; $m2$ = marker on shooting hand.

Reprinted from Human Movement Science, Vol. 21, R.R.D. Oudejans, R.W. van de Langenberg and R.I. Hutter, Aiming at a far target under different viewing conditions: visual control in basketball jump shooting, pp. 457-480, Copyright 2002 with permission from Elsevier.

Quiet Eye in the Free Throw and Jump Shot

A limitation of the Oudejans et al. (2002) study was that the gaze of the athletes was not recorded as the jump shots were taken. Vickers et al. (in progress) therefore recorded the gaze of 11 elite male basketball players in both the free throw and the jump shot in an effort to determine which type of gaze control contributed to higher levels of accuracy. The players performed the jump shots from behind the free-throw line in the same location as used by Oudejans et al. (2002).

This study identified three shooting phases—preparation, ball-up, and extension. The preparation phase was a constant period of 1 s back in time from the onset of the ball-up phase. The ball-up phase began with the first observable upward movement of the ball, during which time the angle at the elbow of the shooting arm remained constant or decreased as the ball was brought to the ready position, as shown in figure 5.4. The extension phase occurred as the ball was propelled toward the basket and released; during this time the angle at the elbow increased.

Next, Vickers et al. identified the quiet-eye period. By definition, the quiet eye must begin

before the final movement or impulse phase. In order to compare their results to Oudejans et al. (2002), they selected the extension phase as the final movement. Note that Vicker's study (1996a, p. 345), used an earlier final movement, which was "the first upward motion of the ball until the ball left the fingertips of the player," which in the current study was the ball-up phase.

Table 5.1 presents the mean durations of the phases of the free throw and the jump shot. In the free throw, the ball-up phase averaged 677.24 ms (SD = 156.13 ms) on hits and 650.51 (SD = 148.87 ms) on misses, while in the jump shot, the ball-up phase averaged 471.84 ms (SD = 89.72 ms) on hits and 483.90 (SD = 89.29 ms) on misses. In the free throw, the mean duration of the extension phase was 139.39 ms (SD = 26.52 ms) on hits and 152.48 ms (SD = 61.28 ms) on misses, while in the jump shot, the mean was 108.77 ms (14.81 ms) on hits and 109.15 (SD = 17.74 ms) on misses. The study therefore confirmed, as expected, that the jump shot is a quicker shot than the free throw. Recall that the preparation phase was held constant at 1 s, so the average duration in each free throw was 1816.63 ms on hits and 1802.99 ms on misses, while the mean duration of the jump shot on hits was 1580.61 ms and 1593.05 ms on misses.

Table 5.1   Mean Durations of the Motor Phases of the Free Throw and Jump Shot

Phases	FREE THROW		JUMP SHOT	
	Hit	Miss	Hit	Miss
Preparation (ms)	1000	1000	1000	1000
Ball-up (ms)	677.24 ± 156.13	650.51 ± 148.87	471.84 ± 89.72	483.90 ± 89.29
Extension (ms)	139.39 26.52	152.48 ± 24.50	108.77 ± 14.81	109.15 17.74
Total (ms)	1816.63	1802.99	1580.61	1593.05

Accuracy was not affected by the duration of the trial or of the ball-up or extension phases in either shot.

Occlusion Period

In both the free throw and the jump shot, Vickers et al. (in progress) found that there was a period of time when the ball and hands entered the visuomotor workspace and occluded the basket. Figure 5.5 shows an elite shooter performing a jump shot. The top photo shows the final fixation or quiet eye on the basket before the player begins his jump with his gaze on the hoop front. The middle photo shows the **occlusion period**, where the gaze is located momentarily on the hand. The bottom photo shows the athlete in the ready position prior to the extension phase. At this time his gaze is not on the hoop. In the free throw, the mean occlusion period averaged 230.30 ms on hits (*SD* = 127.70 ms) and 239.72 (*SD* = 129.96 ms) on misses. In the jump shot, the mean occlusion period was 179.17 ms (*SD* = 104.56 ms) on hits and 190.85 ms (*SD* = 109.56 ms) on misses. The duration of the occlusion period was not a factor in accuracy in either shot. Also note that two athletes did not have an occlusion period because they moved the ball laterally to the side, thus allowing them to see the hoop during the complete shooting action. These players were among the most inaccurate of the group.

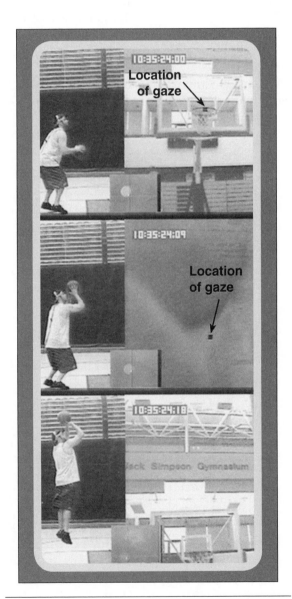

➤ **Figure 5.5**   Three frames of vision-in-action data in the basketball jump shot, showing the A) ball-up phase, B) the occlusion period, and C) the extension phase.

Quiet-Eye Duration in the Free Throw and Jump Shot

The mean quiet-eye duration in the free throw is shown in figure 5.6. It was significantly longer on hits than on misses, averaging 448.15 ms (SD = 281.03 ms) on hits and 304.26 ms (SD = 205.55 ms) on misses. Figure 5.7 then shows the quiet-eye duration for each player on hits and misses. The x-axis shows the percent accuracy during the experiment, as well as during the season. Missing percentages were for players who did not actively play that season. A longer quiet-eye period was a characteristic of hits for 8 of the 11 players, whether determined in absolute time (ms) as shown or in relative time (%).

It was also important to determine if any fixations were initiated after the extension phase began. In the free throw, this occurred in 15 shots out of 110 total shots. The mean duration of these late fixations averaged 116.67 ms on hits (SD = 25.20) and 128.57 ms (SD = 29.99 ms) on misses. The duration of these fixations was not a factor in accuracy.

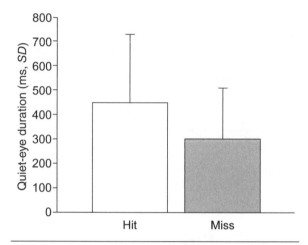

➤ **Figure 5.6**   Mean quiet-eye duration on hits and misses of 11 players in the free throw.

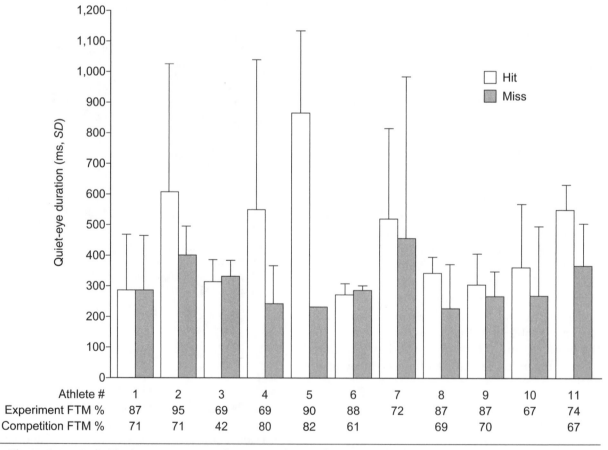

➤ **Figure 5.7**   Individual mean quiet-eye duration on hits and misses in the free throw. FTM = free throws made.

Figure 5.8 shows that the quiet-eye duration in the jump shot was significantly longer on hits (293.94 ms, SD = 176.4 ms) than on misses (238.56, SD = 122.09 ms). Figure 5.9 shows the mean quiet-eye duration for each of the 11 players, revealing that the duration was longer on hits for 8 of 11 players. Their accuracy in the experiment is shown on the x-axis and ranged from a low of 64% to a high of 96%, compared with a low of 35% and high of 57% in games. Fixations after the quiet-eye period were also determined. Very few were found (4 out of 110); therefore the jump shot is too quick and dynamic to permit the onset of a new fixation on the onset of the extension phase, or during the final 120 ms.

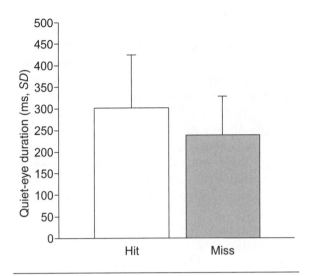

➤ **Figure 5.8**   Mean quiet-eye duration on hits and misses in the jump shot.

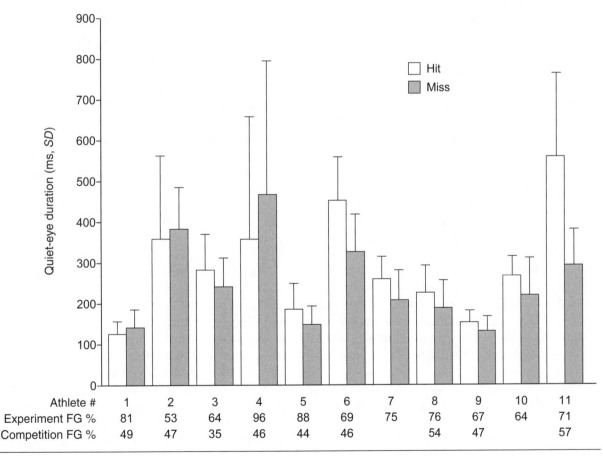

Athlete #	1	2	3	4	5	6	7	8	9	10	11
Experiment FG %	81	53	64	96	88	69	75	76	67	64	71
Competition FG %	49	47	35	46	44	46		54	47		57

➤ **Figure 5.9**   Quiet-eye duration in the jump shot on hits and misses. FG = field goal.

Effect of Shooting Style

Vickers et al. (in progress) determined the shooting style of the athletes by using the definitions of Oudejans et al. (2002). Recall the high style was one where the athletes could see the hoop during the final 350 to 400 ms of the shot, and the low style was one where fixation on the target occurred before the ball was released from in front of the forehead. The study found that participants used both the low and high styles as well as the lateral style where the ball was moved to the side, thus allowing the player to see the hoop continuously while taking the shot. The study also determined whether using one style or another was a factor in accuracy. Percent accuracy in the free throw and the jump shot did not differ for the low or high styles, but the lateral style was not as successful. It appears that bringing the ball up through the midline of the body is an important characteristic of elite shooters. During the preparation, they align the midline of their body to the hoop so that their gaze, the ball, and the front of the hoop are in a straight line.

Optimal Timing of the Quiet Eye

Thus far we have seen that both the free throw and the jump shot had significantly longer quiet-eye durations on hits than on misses, and that using a high or low style was preferable to using the lateral style. In this section, we now look at how the quiet eye was timed with the phases of the jump shot. Figure 5.10 shows the mean quiet-eye duration of each athlete in the jump shot relative to the mean onset of the extension phase (time 0 ms on the y-axis). The right axis shows, in descending order, the mean ball release time (bold line), the onset of the extension phase (time 0 ms), the final 350 ms as used in Oudejans et al. (2002), the mean occlusion period, and the mean onset of the ball-up phase. Quiet-eye onset, offset, and duration for each player is shown on hits and misses.

The following results are important. First, most of the players initiated the quiet-eye period during the ball-up phase, but there was tremendous variability in when this occurred. Second, most of the athletes maintained their gaze on the same location on the hoop from

the occlusion period to the ready phase, thus providing support for the suppression aspect of the **location–suppression hypothesis** of Vickers (1996a). Third, an earlier onset of quiet eye was a characteristic of hits. Finally, 6 of 11 athletes maintained fixation through to the extension phase and 2 athletes until release of the ball, thereby providing support for Oudejans et al. (2002, 2005) and the efficacy of a longer quiet-eye period.

Quiet-Eye Training in Basketball Shooting

In order for a psychological intervention to be successful in a motor task, four conditions must be met (Gopher, 1993; Williams and Grant, 1999). First, it must be shown that control over the allocation of attention in the task leads to higher levels of performance. Second, individuals must be identified who have difficulty controlling their attention. Third, there must be evidence that these individuals have the ability to improve their attention and performance with proper training. And fourth, it must be shown that the training of attention contributes to improvements not only in the experimental setting but also in the real world of competition.

Two of these conditions have been met in the studies in basketball presented thus far. First, it has been established that the ability to control the gaze and attention while preparing and executing the shot leads to higher levels of accuracy. Highly skilled players have a lower frequency of fixation on the hoop, and their final fixation or quiet eye is significantly longer on hits than on misses. Second, near-elite players have a higher frequency of gaze and a shorter duration of quiet eye in both the free throw and the jump shot. With these two conditions met, two training studies are now presented that show that training athletes' visual attention, specifically the quiet eye, leads to changes not only in their gaze control, but also to higher levels of performance in both the experimental and competitive settings. The first study is in the basketball free throw (Harle & Vickers, 2001) and the second in the jump shot (Oudejans et al., 2005).

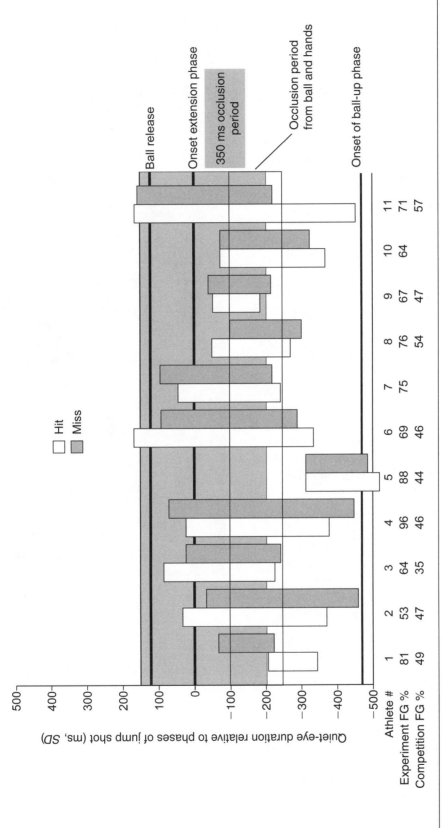

▶ **Figure 5.10** Quiet-eye duration in the jump shot on hits and misses. The left *y*-axis shows time (in ms) before and after the onset of the extension phase (time 0 ms). The right *y*-axis shows the mean release time of the ball, the onset of the extension phase, the occlusion period, and the 350 ms period as defined by Oudejans et al. (2002).

Quiet-Eye Decision Training in the Free Throw

Harle and Vickers (2001) trained the members of an elite university team over two seasons of league play and compared their shooting percentages post hoc with those of two control teams who competed at the top of the same league but did not receive similar training. A program of **quiet-eye training** was developed from the results shown thus far. Quiet-eye training involves using both video modeling and video feedback to help athletes develop the same quiet-eye focus and motor control found in elite performers. During the training sessions, the athletes were shown their gaze on video, which was compared with the gaze of an elite model similar to that shown in figure 5.11. In order to train a quiet eye in the basketball free throw, the following points were stressed:

➤ Take your stance at the line and orient your gaze to the hoop as soon as possible, as shown in the top photo of figure 5.11. Fixate the hoop even as you carry out your preshot routine.

➤ Hold the ball in front and fixate a single location on the hoop (front, back, or middle) for about 1 s. Stability of the quiet eye on one location is crucial. Visualize the ball going in the basket.

➤ When ready, perform the free throw so that the ball and your hands travel up through the midline of your body. The ball will briefly occlude the basket as it enters your visuomotor workspace. Learn to suppress seeing the movement of the ball and your hands at this time. Do not move the ball to the side.

➤ Shoot using a quick, fluid action.

In part III of this book, the decision-training model is presented as a new coaching method. **Decision training** is used in training the quiet eye as follows. In order for nonelite players to learn to use the type of attention employed by elite players, they must make a decision to change their focus of attention in a specific way. The first step is to show them the quiet-eye control of an elite player, such as in figure 5.11.

Using frame-by-frame control, each of the important cues is pointed out and explained

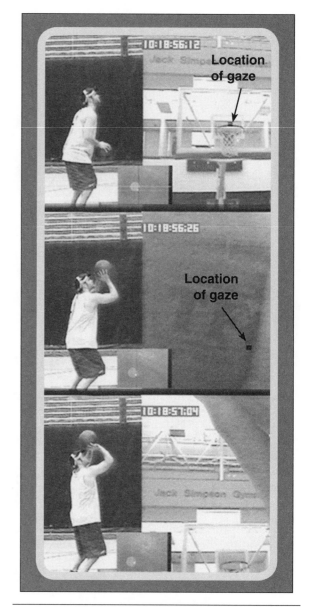

➤ **Figure 5.11**   Three vision-in-action frames showing the gaze of an elite player in the free throw during the preparation phase (top), during the occlusion period (middle), and just before the extension phase (bottom). Refer to figure 5.5 to compare this information with similar phases in the jump shot.

to the players. Next, players look at their own vision-in-action data and identify how their gaze control, quiet eye, and attention are the same or different from the elite player. During this process there should be no coaching of technique. The players should be encouraged to use the frame-by-frame controller in order to identify how their gaze and attention differ from that of the high-skilled shooter. Most athletes are adept at identifying the differences, and they are also surprised at how erratic their control of gaze and attention is compared with the elite player. The third step is to ask the athletes to decide which aspect of their gaze they will change in their next practices. Usually the first decision the athlete makes is to reduce the frequency of fixation to only one quiet-eye location on the hoop. In follow-up sessions, the next decision is usually to change the timing of the onset of the quiet eye so that it occurs earlier, before the occlusion phase.

The results showed that in a posttest after season 1 the quiet-eye trained team improved significantly in quiet-eye duration, from a mean of 300 ms to 900 ms. The team also changed in terms of the relative duration of the free throw, even though this was not overtly trained. After quiet-eye decision training, they took longer to prepare the shot (to allow for the longer quiet eye) and less time to perform the shooting action. Their accuracy also improved by 12% in the posttest, but there was no significant improvement in game accuracy, which still remained low (54.1%), as shown in figure 5.12. However, in the second season, the team improved their accuracy to 76.7% in games, an increase of 22.6%. This increase was significantly more than the increase seen for teams A (66.18%) and B (74.05%), who did not receive similar training but ranked 1st

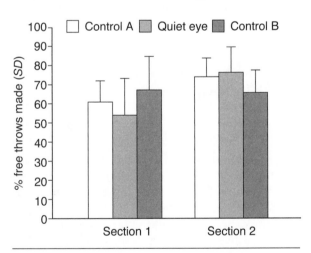

➤ **Figure 5.12** Percent improvements over two seasons of the quiet-eye trained group and two control teams (A and B).

Reprinted, by permission, from S.K. Harle and J.N. Vickers, 2001, "Training quiet eye improves accuracy in the basketball free throw," *The Sport Psychologist* 15(3): 289-305.

and 3rd nationally. The quiet-eye trained team also improved its ranking from 17th nationally to 2nd in season 2.

Goggle and Screen Training in the Jump Shot

Oudejans et al. (2005) investigated the effects of visual control training on the performance of basketball jump shooting by expert male players. Their participants were 10 elite male basketball players who played in one of the top leagues in the Netherlands. All played either at the guard or forward position and were the best shooters on their teams. Average free throw and 3-point shooting percentages during games prior to the study were 78% and 38%, respectively. The goal of the training was to improve the athletes' pickup of information during the final period just before ball release. Two methods were used over a training period of 8 wk. The players wore the liquid-crystal goggles, shown in figure 5.3, which occluded the hoop so that players were able to see the hoop only during the final 350 ms. These goggles forced the players to attend maximally to the hoop during the short amount of time it was visible. In addition, the players were required to shoot from behind a screen set up at the free-throw line and placed at a height that blocked their view of the hoop. The goggles and the screen required the athletes to change from detecting nonspecifying (less useful) to specifying (more useful) cues critical to accuracy. The players also increased the duration of the amount of time the goggles were open from a mean of 353 ms before training to 386 ms following training, a result similar to that found by Oudejans et al. (2002). Accuracy was determined relative to a control group that played in the same league.

Figure 5.13 shows the results for the jump shot. The attention-trained group improved their shooting percentages in games from a mean of 46.1% before training to 60.6% following, for a mean increase of 14.5%. The control group, who did not receive similar training, changed from 42.5% to 42.2%. Improvements in 3-point percentages were also determined for the attention-trained group, increasing from an average of 35.2% before training to 53.9% following, for an increase of 18.7%. This amount of improvement is far above what is normally found in basketball, but it is similar to the increase found by Harle

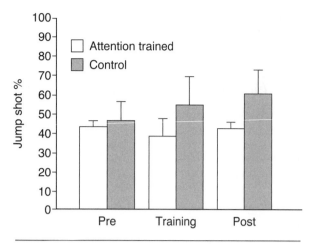

➤ **Figure 5.13** Improvement in percent jump-shot accuracy from the pretest, through the training of attention, to the posttest.

Derived from means in R.R.D. Oudejans et al., 2005.

and Vickers (2001). Both the Harle and Vickers (2001) and Oudejans et al. (2005) studies show that when athletes are trained to control their gaze and attention, improvements in shooting are found that are greater than those from physical or psychological training alone.

Gaze During Screen Training in the Jump Shot

Following the precedents of the Oudejans et al. (2005) study, Vickers, Panchuk, Morton, and Martell (in progress b) recorded the gaze of elite basketball players as they took shots from behind a screen while wearing an eye tracker. Both free throws and jump shots were taken from behind a screen that was located at the free-throw line and was raised to three heights. In the hoop condition, the players stood at the free-throw line and the screen was raised to a point where they could fixate only the top of the rim. In the line condition, the players fixated the line above the hoop; thus the hoop was visible if the athlete jumped. In the backboard condition, only the top of the backboard could be fixated; thus, it was impossible to see the hoop at any time. All shots were taken after a pass of the ball from a teammate.

The mean shooting percentage for the standing jump shot without the screen was 72% (SD = 13%); for the jump shot when the hoop could be seen, the mean was 68% (SD = 11%); when the line above the rim was visible, it was 61% (SD = 14%);

and when only the top of the screen was visible, it was 53% (SD =16%). Most shooters' accuracy levels were high, even in the condition when the hoop could not be seen at all, a result in agreement with Oudejans et al. (2005). The shooters who maintained the highest level of accuracy did not jump higher or change their fundamental technique; instead, before shooting they established an early quiet-eye fixation on cues in the background or on the floor that were aligned with the hoop. Some used a location on the middle of the top of the backboard or the middle of the line above the hoop. Others used a cue on the wall or cues on the floor aligned with the hoop. From these cues they deduced where the hoop was. It was clear that they were able to use novel locations within the perceptual-motor workspace other than just the hoop in order to shoot accurately. Specifically, they used an early quiet-eye fixation on the location that was in the center of their body relative to the backboard and the hoop.

Finally, those who failed to find a cognitive solution to the problem and instead used only a motor solution (e.g., jumping higher, changing their technique) soon became discouraged, especially in the line and top-of-board conditions, and shot at low levels of accuracy. This also probably explains why the Oudejans et al. (2002) study found low percentages in the screen condition where an athlete's view of the hoop was blocked. Occluding the goggles early in the shot removed any alignment cues the players might have used, forcing them to shoot largely using their memory of where the hoop was.

Quiet Eye and EEG in Rifle Shooting

In this section, we look at a second targeting task to a fixed target, that of rifle shooting. We delve deeper into what may be occurring in the brain during the quiet-eye period. Janelle et al. (2000) recorded both the quiet eye and **electroencephalography (EEG)** of elite and nonelite marksmen who took shots at simulated targets 50 m distant using the Noptel ST-2000 laser shooter-training system. EEG noninvasively records brain electrical activity through electrodes placed on the scalp. These electrodes summate postsynaptic potentials in the cerebral cortex and other areas of the brain (Davidson & Schwartz, 1976a; Davidson &

Schwartz, 1976b) and allow the patterns produced by electrical impulses across the surface of the brain to be plotted over split seconds of time.

EEG waves are defined by their frequency and are classified as alpha, beta, delta, and theta waves. Alpha waves occur at a rate of 7.5 and 13 waves each second. Alpha waves are the major rhythms seen in a normal relaxed adult, while beta activity occurs at a fast rate of 14-plus cycles each second. Beta activity occurs when we are alert or anxious with eyes open. Theta activity has a frequency of 3.5 to 7.5 cycles each second and is classed as a slow activity. Delta activity occurs at a rate of 3 cycles each second or lower and tends to be the highest in amplitude but the slowest. Delta waves occur during deep sleep.

Janelle et al. (2000) found progressive quieting of the left hemisphere of elite marksmen before the trigger pull. Similar quieting has been found in elite and intermediate-level shooters (Hatfield, Landers, & Ray, 1987; Haufler, Spalding, Santa Maria, & Hatfield, 2000) and in skilled golfers prior to the execution of a golf putt (Crews & Landers, 1993; Landers et al., 1994). The left hemisphere is involved in the serial processing of information, and the right hemisphere is specialized for visual–spatial processing (Davidson & Hughdahl, 1995). Janelle et al. also found that the quiet eye was significantly longer for the elite shooters (11 s) than for nonelite shooters (7 s). These quiet-eye durations are the longest reported to date and appear to be necessary in order to permit the exceptionally high levels of accuracy found in this task (95%-99%).

Quiet Eye in Biathlon Shooting Under Pressure

Why is it that some athletes are able to perform under high pressure, while others collapse under the combined weight of intense competition, high levels of physiological arousal, and psychological stress? Although researchers still do not have an answer to this question, examples abound of exceptional performances occurring under extreme pressure not only in sport, but in the military, fire fighting, police work, emergency medicine, and many other areas. In this section, we discuss a study that examined the gaze control of elite biathlon shooters as they took shots after incremental exercise in both low- and high-pressure settings. The objective of the study (Vickers & Williams, in press) was to determine why some athletes are able to handle the high stress of competition while others choke.

Since the classic studies of Setchenov (1903/1935), it has been known that the ability to perform high levels of physical work is not due to physiological factors alone. Setchenov found that more exercise could be performed after a complete state of exhaustion had been reached by diverting attention to an external mental activity. Several researchers have subsequently established that the ability to do more work is not due to circulatory, EMG, reflex, or other factors associated with the physiological system alone, but that a central nervous phenomenon plays a major role. (Assmussen & Mazin, 1978a, 1978b; Hoffman, 2000; Hoffman, Patterson & Carrougher, 2004; Kinomura, Larson, Gulyas, & Roland, 1996; Rotstein, Jablonowsky, Bar-Sela, Malamud, Tenebaum, & Inbar, 1999; Valet et al., 2004; Weber, 1914.).

Why Do We Choke?

Baumeister (1984, p. 610) defines **choking** as the "failure to perform up to whatever level of skill and ability the person has at the time." Competitive **pressure** often leads to choking and is composed of "any factor or combination of factors that increases the importance of performing well on a particular occasion" (p. 610). High-pressure environments are those where the performer perceives the stakes to be high and where poor performance may lead to a loss of position or stature. In contrast, low-pressure environments are those that contain few risks and the pressure to perform well is low, as is the tendency to choke.

Two types of models—self-focus and distraction—have been proposed to account for the phenomenon of choking. Self-focus models state that performance decrements occur when attention is directed inward to technical, physiological, or emotional aspects that are normally automated (Baumeister, 1984; Lewis & Linder, 1997; Masters, 1992; Masters & Maxwell, 2004). The skilled performer has developed implicit, highly automated routines that require little conscious effort. The need to explicitly attend to internal processes has been replaced by an implicit form of control characterized by a low level of conscious awareness and attention paid to controlling the skill. **Self-focus models of choking** predict that choking occurs in high-pressure settings when athletes redirect their attention to their physiological, technical, or emotional state or otherwise pay too much attention to internal processes that are normally automated and performed without thought.

In contrast, **distraction models of choking** (Bleilock & Carr, 2001; Eysenck, 1992; Eysenck & Carvello, 1982; Wine, 1971) state that choking occurs due to cognitive deficits that arise when the athlete's attention is diverted away from the primary task, causing a cognitive deficit that impairs performance. Sanders, Baron, and Moore (1978) define a distraction as any stimulus or response requirement that is irrelevant to the primary task. Distraction studies typically include a secondary task that draws attention away from the primary task, such as counting backward or other unusual tasks. Typically, performance on the primary task declines as memory load increases and the cognitive attention needed to perform well on the primary task becomes too low to maintain performance.

In addition to self-focus and distraction accounts of choking, it has also been shown that an external focus of attention leads to higher levels of performance than an internal focus (Wulf, McConnel, Gartner, & Schwarz, 2002; Wulf, McNevin, & Shea, 2001; Wulf, Shea, & Park, 2001). An **internal focus** is one that dwells on the techniques or emotions required in the activity, while an external focus is directed toward the outcome of the task or the goal being pursued. Wulf, McNevin, and Shea (2001) have further shown that when a motor skill is learned, attention shifts from an internal focus to an external focus. Athletes who remain immersed in internal thoughts are unable to attend to task-relevant cues, resulting in a deterioration of their performance, while an external focus is symptomatic of a lack of distraction that marshals the body's systems to better meet the task constraints. Given the three models of self-focus, distraction, and internal–external focus, it is clear that the ability to perform at a high level is due to the ability of athletes to control their attention in such a way that optimal physiological, psychological, or attentive states are reached and maintained.

Vickers and Williams (in press) selected biathlon shooting as their task because many of the conditions encountered during high-pressure competition can be simulated in the laboratory. In the biathlon, athletes race on cross-country skis, and at set intervals they take shots at targets that are at a distance of 50 m. As a race proceeds, the psychological pressure to shoot accurately increases because any missed targets result in penalty distances that normally lead to losing the race. Currently, the top 30 men and 30 women in the world hit an average of 86.7% of the targets (www.biathlonworld.com); therefore, they have found a way of maintaining a high level of visual focus and attention even under conditions of extreme physiological and competitive pressure.

In the study, elite biathlon skiers took standing shots at a target after exercising on a bike ergometer at individually prescribed power output *(PO)* levels of 55%, 70%, 85%, and 100% of their $\dot{V}O_2max$. The Noptel laser system was used to determine accuracy. With this system shots are taken to an optical target 10 mm in diameter located at a distance of 5 m that simulates the 50 m distance. Performance pressure was manipulated by testing the athletes in two counterbalanced conditions separated by 3 wk. In the low-pressure (LP) condition, they were told that the purpose of the testing was simply to give them information about their fixation on the target at the different *PO* levels, while in the high-pressure (HP) condition, the national team coach was present and they were told that their shooting percentages would be used in national team selections in 2 mo. Prizes were also made available to the most accurate shooters.

The main focus of the investigation was to assess how much each athlete changed from the LP to the HP condition and the effect this had on their ability to perform under pressure. Elite biathlon athletes typically spend 4-6 hrs per day in training. During this time, they develop habits that may be beneficial or harmful when performing under pressure. Vickers and Williams used established tests to determine the athletes' physiological arousal, anxiety, and gaze control on the target in the LP and HP conditions. For physiological arousal, they measured heart rate *(HR,* bpm) and rate of perceived exertion *(RPE)* (Borg, 1971, 1982a); for anxiety, they determined pre-competitive cognitive anxiety (Martens, Burton, Vealey, Bump, & Smith, 1990a, 1990b) and level of cognitive worry (Krane, 1994) before each set of shots. For gaze control, they measured the onset and duration of the final fixation on the target, or quiet eye *(QE)* (Vickers, 1996a). Before presenting the main results, let's look a bit closer at why cognitive anxiety, physiological arousal, and visual attention are critical factors in choking.

Cognitive Anxiety and Choking

Two components of anxiety have been defined in the literature: a mental component normally termed **cognitive anxiety** (or worry) and a physiological component normally termed **somatic anxiety** (Liebert & Morris, 1967; Martens et al., 1990a). An athlete who is cognitively anxious has "negative expectations and cognitive concerns about oneself, the situation at hand, and potential consequences" (Martens et al., 1990a, p. 541). Performers who experience high levels of cognitive anxiety are worried about their ability to perform and are fearful of the consequences of not performing well. Somatic anxiety is defined as "one's perception of the psychological affective elements of the anxiety experience, that is, indications of autonomic arousal and unpleasant feeling states such as nervousness and tension" (Morris, Davis, & Hutchings, 1981, p. 541). Somatic anxiety refers to the perception of one's physiological arousal symptoms, such as a rapid heart rate, shortness of breath, clammy hands, butterflies in the stomach, and tense muscles.

Of these two components, cognitive anxiety has been shown to have the greater and more controversial effect on sport performance (Hardy & Fazey, 1987; Hardy & Parfitt, 1991; Hardy, Parfitt, & Pates, 1994; Martens et al., 1990b). While Martens, Burton, Vealey, Bump, and Smith (1990) state that a high level of precompetitive cognitive anxiety is a detriment to performance, Hardy and Fazey (1987), Hardy and Parfitt (1991), and Hardy, Parfitt, and Pates (1994) state that, in the catastrophe model of performance, a high level of precompetitive anxiety only becomes a detriment when physical arousal becomes too high. Vickers and Williams (under review) therefore expected that if precompetitive anxiety *(CA)* increased from LP to HP (positive *d*-score), or if the level of worry *(CW)* increased from the LP to the HP condition (also a positive *d-CW* score), then the possibility of choking would increase, especially at the highest workload of HP *PO* 100%.

Physiological Arousal and Choking

Rate of perceived exertion (RPE) has played a decisive role in our understanding of the subjective sensation of the amount of physical work being performed. All humans have the ability to sense how hard they are working, and this is derived from the internal sensation of a high heart rate and rate of respiration, as well as the buildup of lactic acid in the muscles (Borg, 1982a; Noble et al., 1983). A vast amount of research has been conducted to find out what influences the experience of perceived effort (Borg, 1971, 1982a, 1982b; Noble, Borg, Jacobs, Ceci, & Kaiser, 1983; Whaley, Woodall, Kaminsky, & Emmett, 1997). The Borg scale has been developed to quantify the RPE (Borg, 1982a). A low value means that little or no work is perceived to have been done, while a high value means maximal effort is being expended and the work is perceived to be extremely hard.

In addition to *RPE*, the study also monitored *HR*. Biathletes develop the ability to decelerate their *HR* just before shooting. Their goal is to shoot when *HR* is no more than 80% of maximum because at this level they are able to control their breathing and body movements while taking the shots (Groslambert, Candau, Grappe, & Dugue, 2003; McArdle, Katch, & Katch, 2001). If *HR* exceeds 90% of maximum capacity, the athlete's respiration rate becomes rapid and the ability to shoot accurately is compromised. In this experiment, the athletes were required to shoot after exercising at a *PO* of 100% of their maximum *PO*. It was expected that those athletes who experienced an increase in *d-HR* or *d-RPE* from the LP to HP condition (positive *d*-score) would be more prone to choking than those who maintained their *d-HR* or *d-RPE* at the same or lower rate than what was found in the LP condition, especially at the highest workload of *PO* 100%.

Visual Attention, Quiet Eye, and Choking

In order to hit a target accurately, it is necessary to control the gaze so that the final fixation (quiet eye) is not only on the target, but is also of sufficient duration to ensure accuracy. This has been shown previously in this book in terms of pistol and rifle shooting to a set target (Janelle et al., 2000; Ripoll, Papin, Guezennec, & Verdy, 1985), as well as dart throwing (Vickers, Rodrigues, & Edworthy, 2001).

In later chapters, similar findings will be shown for the golf putt (Vickers, 1992), basketball shooting (Oudejans et al., 2002; Oudejans et al., 2005; Vickers, 1996a), and billiards (Williams, Singer, & Frehlich, 2002). In chapter 3, new literature was also presented showing a close relationship between control of the gaze and attention (Deubel & Schneider, 1996; Henderson, 2003; Kowler, Anderson, Dosher, & Blaser, 1995; Shepherd, Findlay, & Hockey, 1986; Zelinsky, Rao, Hayhoe, & Ballard, 1997). It was therefore expected that those athletes who maintained a longer quiet-eye duration on the target would not only shoot at a higher level, but also would be less prone to choking during the high-pressure condition.

Overall, it was also expected that the optimal state would have little change from LP to HP condition in the *d*-scores for *d-CA*, *d-CW*, *d-HR*, and *d-QE*. Those athletes who changed the least across the *PO* levels from the LP to the HP condition would be less prone to choking. Conversely, an increase in *d-CA*, *d-CW*, *d-HR*, or *d-RPE* or a decrease in *d-QE* would indicate that the athlete had changed from the LP to the HP condition in a way that would be more likely to contribute to choking, especially at the highest workload of HP *PO* 100%. It was also necessary to define

choking, and we did this relative to the conditions required to perform well in biathlon. Our definition of choking included three factors: first, it was based on performance in the HP condition only; second, choking took into account the total number of misses across the *PO* levels of the HP condition; and third, choking took into account the ability to perform at a high level when physiological arousal was at its highest during HP *PO* 100%. Athletes who did not choke were defined as those who missed the fewest targets during the HP condition and also maintained a percent accuracy ≥80% during HP *PO* 100%. Those who choked missed the most targets during the HP condition and had the lowest level of accuracy during HP *PO* 100% (>40%). Athletes who fell between these two performance levels were classified as neither.

The athlete's gaze was recorded using the vision-in-action system described in chapter 2. A frame of data recorded is shown in figure 5.14. Image A shows the athlete's eye, the x/y coordinates of the corneal reflection, and center of the pupil. Image B shows the visuomotor workspace of the athlete as recorded by the scene camera on the eye tracker. Visible is the 10 mm target (black dot) and the location of gaze on the target as

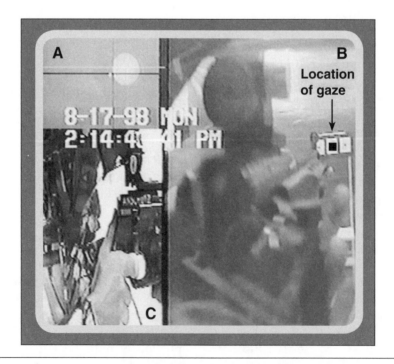

> **Figure 5.14**   A frame of vision-in-action data as collected in biathlon shooting.

Reprinted from J.N. Vickers and A.M. Williams, 2007, "Performing under pressure: The interactive effects of physiological arousal, cognitive anxiety, and gaze control in elite biathlon shooters," *Journal of Motor Behavior* (in press).

indicated by a white cursor (spatial accuracy ± 1° visual angle; precision of ± .5°). Only one target was used, the middle one as shown. Image C was recorded by an external camera that recorded the movement of the trigger finger and bolt of the rifle. Note that with this setup, it was not possible to record the gaze relative to the sights of the gun, but only relative to the target. The quiet eye was the final fixation that remained on any part of the target for a minimum of 100 ms prior to trigger pull. Quiet-eye offset occurred when fixation deviated off the target for longer than 100 ms; therefore, the quiet-eye period could carry through and beyond the trigger pull.

Analysis of the group's mean results for percent accuracy, *CA, CW, HR, RPE,* and *QE* were consistent with the literature for each of the variables. The level of *CA* was significantly higher in the HP condition than in LP. The level of *CW* increased across the workloads, but not significantly. Mean accuracy decreased over the *PO* levels and by *PO* 100% had declined to 50% or chance. Mean *HR* increased as planned experimentally, and mean *RPE* reflected the increased work being experienced at each *PO* level. Mean *QE* duration was significantly longer on hits than on misses. During *PO* 100%, *QE* duration had declined to half that found during the earlier workloads. These results were therefore as anticipated and predicted by the respective tests, with one exception. Although the athletes clearly were more anxious in the HP condition than in the LP, there were no significant effects that could be attributed to the level of pressure. This type of group analysis was unable to detect changes from LP to HP or to reveal possible reasons why some athletes choked while others did not. In order to examine this issue in greater detail, it was necessary to look at how each individual responded to the LP and HP conditions and determine the degree of change within *each* athlete across the HP workloads.

Given the criteria set for choking, it was found that 3 athletes (2 men, 1 woman) did not choke *(NC)* in that they missed the fewest targets during the HP condition as well as maintained a percent accuracy ≥ 80% at HP *PO* 100%. The remaining 7 were classified as choking *(C),* as they missed the most targets and had a percent accuracy ≥ 40% at HP *PO* 100%. None of the athletes fell between these 2 levels of performance. The accuracy of those who choked declined after *PO* 70% to a mean of 25.7% by *PO* 100%, while all those who

did not choke increased their accuracy to 80% by *PO* 100%. The results showed that *d-HR* did not differ significantly across the *PO* levels for either group, revealing that a cardiovascular limitation was not the cause of choking. The results also showed that *d-QE* differed significantly for the two groups across the *PO* levels; those who did not choke increased the duration of *d-QE* as the HP workloads increased, while *d-QE* remained the same or decreased for the group that choked.

Closer examination of the *d-QE* durations showed that with the onset of high-pressure competition, those who ultimately choked decreased their quiet-eye duration from what they had used in the LP condition, and also from what they used just prior to competing during HP. These results were contrary to previous studies on the quiet-eye period, albeit measured during nonexercise or low pressure conditions (Vickers, 1996; Janelle et al., 2001; Williams, Singer, & Frehlich, 2002; Oudejans et al., 2002, 2005), but were supportive of implicit model of choking (Baumeister, 1984; Lewis & Linder, 1997; Masters, 1992; Masters & Maxwell, 2004) where highly automated routines requiring little conscious effort or explicit attention are needed to control the skill. Although changing to a more rapid quiet-eye fixation worked very well at the lower workloads, this did not contribute to accuracy when the *PO* levels became very high. Instead, those who increased their *d-QE* during the higher workloads continued to shoot at a high level and did not choke. These results were supportive of past research on the quiet-eye period, as well as studies showing that an enhanced external focus of attention leads to higher levels of performance (Wulf, Shea, & Park, 2001; Wulf, McConnel, Gartner, & Schwarz, 2002). These results also supported models of choking that state that performance is enhanced when attention is maintained on aspects of a task that are central to success and not distracted by secondary tasks or concerns (Bleilock & Carr, 2001; Eysenck, 1982; Eysenck & Carvello, 1982; Wine, 1971). These results raise the question of why an increase in *d-QE* contributed to performing better under pressure. Three reasons are given in the sections to follow, with the first related to the role of automaticity in elite performance, the second to the Setchenov (1903/1935) phenomenon, and the third to the catastrophe model of cognitive anxiety and performance (Hardy & Fazey, 1987; Hardy, Parfitt, & Pates, 1994).

The Role of Automaticity in Elite Performance

Early models of skill acquisition, such as that proposed by Fitts and Posner (1967), state that athletes pass through three linear stages (cognitive, associative, and autonomous) as they become more highly skilled. During the cognitive and associative phases, conscious processing of information is required, while during the autonomous stage the ideal state is to perform without thought or apparent conscious control. Recall that this view of expert performance is similar to that of self-focus models presented earlier (Baumeister, 1984; Lewis & Linder, 1997; Masters, 1992, 2000). However, more recent models of skill acquisition identify a state beyond automaticity as being required before the highest levels of expertise can be achieved. Ericsson (2003) has studied experts in many fields (Ericsson, 1996; Ericsson, 2002; Ericsson, Krampe, & Tesch-Romer, 1993; Williams & Ericsson, 2005) and found that "expert performers counteract automaticity by developing increasingly complex mental representations so they can attain higher levels of control of their performance and therefore remain within the cognitive/associative phase" (p. 64). He goes on to state that when an athlete "gives up their commitment to seek excellence … they stop engaging in deliberate practice and focus only on maintaining their performance which results in premature automation (and 'arrested development')" (p. 65). Following this argument, the elite performer is one who is able to maintain cognitive control over all conditions encountered, no matter how difficult or unusual. In the biathlon study, the high-pressure condition forced the athletes to face a number of new and challenging conditions: the national coach was present, their scores were used in Olympic team selection, they were forced to exercise at a level that only occurs during intense competition, and prizes were awarded to the best shooters. Three of the 10 athletes were able to overcome all these pressures and in doing so increased their external quiet-eye focus to levels that differed significantly and appeared to insulate them from the causes of choking.

The Setchenov Phenomenon

A second explanation for why a longer duration of QE may prevent choking is provided by the Setchenov (1903/1935) phenomenon. Setchenov found that individuals who were fatigued to exhaustion could do more physiological work when a "diverting" activity was used to direct their attention to an external target or activity. Assmussen and Mazin (1978a, 1978b) subsequently found the phenomenon applied in a wide variety of tasks (both mental and physical) and that the amount of work that could be performed was greater with eyes open compared to eyes closed. Even when complete exhaustion was reached with the eyes closed, opening the eyes and focusing on an external target resulted in a 15-30% increase in the amount of exercise that could be performed. They explained that the input of afferent information acted to redirect attention away from the physiological demands of the task, resulting in an ability to perform at a higher level. The Setchenov phenomenon is therefore not related to an internal focus of attention, but instead to an external focus of attention mediated by vision. These results suggest that the ability to overcome the normally debilitating effects of maximum exercise can be aided through the use of an appropriate external focus of attention, as highlighted by the changes in d-QE found in the Vickers and Williams study.

Assmussen and Mazin (1978b) attributed the ability to do more work to the reticular formation, which they reported inhibits the ability to do work with the eyes closed; however, when the eyes are open, a release in inhibition occurs, resulting in the higher-level system exerting control over the lower systems. More recently Bear, Connors, and Paradiso (2007, p. 458) have further argued that the medullary rectinospinal tract of the reticular system "liberates antigravity muscles from reflex control … by descending signals from the cortex" leading to a state of heightened arousal. This explanation is also bolstered by PET studies (Kinomura et al., 1996), where participants were monitored as they went from a relaxed, awake state to an attention-demanding state. They found an activation of the midbrain reticular formation and thalamic intralaminar nuclei, confirming the role of these areas in increased attention and vigilance. In addition, fMRI studies of pain perception (Hoffman, 2000; Hoffman et al, 2004; Valet et al., 2004) have shown that there is greater tolerance for pain when an external distraction is present (using virtual reality and a Stroop task, respectively). Not only are participants able to tolerate more pain, but there is a reduced activation of the pain centers located within the reticular formation.

These studies, in combination, led Vickers and Williams (in press) to speculate that an increase in quiet-eye focus during intense high-pressure competition prevents the reticular formation from inhibiting the athlete's physiological response to work, thus leading to higher levels of performance. Translation of these results to the biathlon study suggests that those athletes who increased their external *QE* focus on the target at *PO* 100% may have prevented the reticular formation from inhibiting their physiological response to work, while those who did not increase their *QE* focus had to deal with a physiological system that was effectively being suppressed by the lateral pathways of the reticular formation. That this was a higher brain phenomenon was also bolstered by the fact that both groups had similar *d-HRs*, which did not change significantly from the LP to HP condition.

The Catastrophe Model of Anxiety and Performance

The catastrophe model of cognitive anxiety and performance (Hardy & Fazey, 1987; Hardy, Parfitt, & Pates, 1994) is one of the few that take into account the interactive effects of high levels of cognitive anxiety and physiological arousal on motor performance. This model states that a high level of precompetitive cognitive anxiety becomes a detriment only when physical arousal levels become too high (Hardy & Fazey, 1987; Hardy, Parfitt, & Pates, 1994). Vickers and Williams (under review) did not find that the combination of a high level of cognitive anxiety and a high level of physiological arousal always led to a catastrophe in performance during the HP condition. Instead, this occurred only for those athletes who had a negative *d-QE* focus on the target at the highest workload, while those who had a plus *d-QE* avoided the collapse and were still able to shoot accurately. These results therefore show that when physiological arousal is at maximum the beneficial interaction that leads to high levels of performance (and not choking) is an elevated level of cognitive anxiety, in combination with a heightened quiet-eye focus on relevant external information.

Quiet Eye in Action

Select a training partner or partners and develop a quiet-eye decision-training program for the free throw. Follow these steps:

1. List five quiet-eye characteristics that are needed to perform well in the free throw. When listing each characteristic, name the cognitive skill that is most important (anticipation, attention, focus and concentration, memory, pattern recognition, problem solving, or decision making).

2. Second, design a drill or progression of drills that will help you and your partner improve your accuracy in the free throw.

3. Practice the drills for 20 to 30 min per day. Your main goal is to develop the optimal focus as the free throw is prepared and executed.

Record your results. At the beginning of the first practice, record your pretraining accuracy for the first 10 shots before you do any quiet-eye training. Try to complete five training sessions. At the end of each practice session, record your percent accuracy on the final 10 trials on the blank graph provided on page 96.

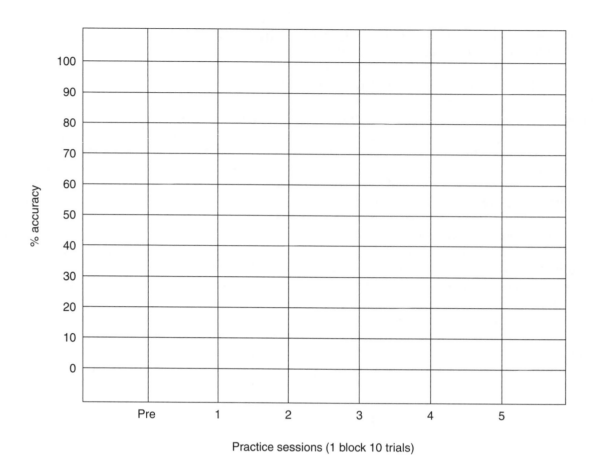

Practice sessions (1 block 10 trials)

From J.N. Vickers, 2007, *Perception, cognition, and decision training: The quiet eye in action* (Champaign, IL: Human Kinetics).

Prepare a short report in which you discuss the following topics:

1. List the five gaze control or quiet-eye characteristics that you selected to work on.

2. Provide a sketch of the drills used to train your quiet eye. Explain how each drill was used to improve your cognitive and quiet-eye focus.

3. What methods of practice did you use? (See chapters 9 through 12 for some ideas about how to vary your methods of training.)

4. Include the figure of results you generated from the blank graph and explain your percentage change over the five practices. Did you improve or get worse?

5. Using information from this chapter, discuss why your results occurred. In your opinion, what were the underlying reasons for your results?

CHAPTER 6

Gaze Control in Abstract-Target and Moving-Target Tasks

◄◄ *Where Have We Been?*

In the last chapter, research support for gaze control in fixed targeting tasks was presented. Elite performers define a single location on the target and direct their gaze to that location during the preparation of the aiming movement. The most important gaze is the final fixation, or quiet eye, which has an onset before the extension of the shooting arm. The duration of the quiet eye is longer during accurate shots; therefore, a spotlight of attention is needed before the final execution. The final aiming movements within this category of tasks are best performed quickly in an open-loop mode of control. When faced with high-pressure conditions, the ability to focus the gaze in an optimal quiet-eye period appears to insulate athletes from choking.

►► *Where Are We Going?*

In this chapter, gaze control research as found in abstract- and moving-target tasks is presented (see figure 4.1). Abstract targets, as the name implies, have hidden qualities that must be detected by the gaze and interpreted by higher cognitive processes in order to determine the correct motor solution; exemplars are golf putting and billiards. In most forms of abstract targeting, there are two or more visuomotor workspaces within which a number of targets exist. The performer has to determine which location is most important within each visual workspaces and also establish a sequence between target locations in order for higher levels of performance to be achieved. Gaze control to moving targets requires the performer to anticipate the speed and direction of the target and ultimately locate where a ball or other object must be aimed. One example is passing skills, such as those found in basketball, soccer, and American football.

Gaze Control in Golf Putting

Putting makes up between 42% and 45% of the game of golf and thus plays a major role in how well the game is played (Pelz, 2000; Wiren, 1991). However, it is not unusual for some individuals to be elite golfers in the drive and iron shots, yet have great difficulty in putting, or vice versa. Skill level in golf is determined, in part, by the **handicap** system. A handicap of 0 means that a golfer is able to play a complete round of golf in the number of strokes determined by the course designer. Normally a round of golf has 18 holes, each of which requires 3 to 5 strokes. The optimal number of strokes is around 72 on most 18-hole courses. A related system is called the *index,* which takes into account the type of course that the handicap is earned on. In this case, the handicap is adjusted to reflect the difficulty of the course. Professional golfers have handicaps of 0 or less, meaning that they are able to complete rounds of golf in fewer strokes than what was planned by course designers. The lowest score that has ever been recorded by a professional golfer in a regulation tournament is 59. The best golfers in the world average 1.8 or fewer putts each hole. In the sections to follow, gaze control while putting will be described. Putting on a sloped green is usually harder than on a flat surface, and because of this, it requires a different type of gaze control.

Gaze Control on a Sloped Green

In chapter 2, the gaze of high-skilled (mean handicap 6.2) and low-skilled (mean handicap 14.1) golfers was described as they performed 10 ft (3 m) putts on a flat surface (Vickers, 1991a, 1991b; Vickers, 1992). Most putts in golf, though, occur on greens with some degree of slope. Golfers who are good at putting are able to read the complexity inherent in the sloped green—they know how to read the different types of grasses, the many distances, the lie of the green, the slope, and the effect of weather and course maintenance on playing conditions. In order to perform well, the elite putter has the ability to read the abstract patterns in the green and determine in advance how the ball will roll or break to the hole.

Pelz (1994) identified four aim lines that golfers use when setting up a breaking putt. He first asked golfers to tell him where they were aiming; that is, he determined their initial read while they were standing behind the putt. This was followed by an objective assessment of the alignment on the clubhead prior to the stroke. Once over the ball, the golfers then described their final read. Finally, Pelz recorded the actual line taken by the ball as it traveled to the hole. He tested 1,500 golfers, of whom 50 were professionals (Pelz, 2000). He initially thought that the aim line was the best cue for teaching players how to play the sloping lie. But his results showed clearly that the final path of the ball to the hole did not correspond to the aim line or to most of the lines selected by the golfers before hitting. The majority of golfers tended to consistently estimate a point inside of the aim line, which Pelz called the visible break.

Pelz's studies (1994, 2000) provided a first insight into visual behavior during the putt, but he did not measure the gaze of the golfers while putting on a sloped surface. What do golfers actually see when they try to estimate the visible break? Do they run their eyes along the green and visually map out a curving line to the hole? Do they fixate the the hole using a **scan path** that can be linked to the roll of the ball? Most putts occur on greens where the slope causes the ball to roll in unpredictable ways as it approaches the hole. How do elite golfers read the abstract complexity of the green where they estimate the ball will begin its downward path to the hole? Being able to read where a putt is going to go before it is hit is the art of putting. The gaze plays a major role in how successful golfers are as they use their gaze and attention to estimate not only the aim line, but also the **breakpoint,** or the point on the green near the hole where the ball will begin to drop toward the hole. It is at this point that the force of gravity of the slope is greater than the forward speed of the ball. Both are affected by how hard the golfer hits the ball and the angle on the putter face. But even more important is the ability to select where the optimal breakpoint is on the green.

Two or More Visuomotor Workspaces

Whether a putt occurs on a flat or sloped green, the gaze and attention must be controlled precisely between two or more visumotor workspaces within which there is a spotlight for the gaze and attention. Figure 6.1 shows a frame of vision-in-action data. Image A shows the eye of the golfer with x- and y-coordinates, image B shows the scene in front of him with the location of gaze indicated by the black cursor, and image C shows his putting movements coupled in time. When a golfer sets up a putt, the first visuomotor workspace is located in front of the feet and includes the ball and club, as shown in image B. It is from this orientation that golfers determine the placement of the ball, the alignment of clubhead, the squaring of the stance, and other factors critical to success. During this time, most golfers have a line of gaze that drops in a straight line down to the ball.

Figure 6.2 shows the second visuomotor workspace, which includes the hole, the green about the hole, or a breakpoint near the hole. As mentioned, the breakpoint is the location on a sloped green where the golfer has determined that the ball will begin to break toward the hole. The selection of this location is dependent on a host of factors, especially the golfer's ability to perceive and interpret the curvature and elevation of the green, the texture of the grass, the firmness of the green, and the weight or pace on the club at contact.

Fixated information within each visuomotor workspace becomes a candidate for the spotlight of attention. The skilled golfer learns to control the gaze so that precise information is viewed

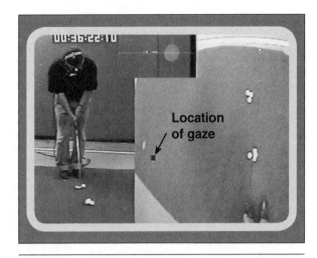

► **Figure 6.2** An elite golfer fixating the breakpoint while preparing the putt.

within the visuomotor workspaces. The ability to see fine detail and the salient features of the green and hole is crucial. Top golfers state that they do not fixate the hole or a spot on the green; instead, they select a single blade of grass, a small feature on the green, or the dimple or trademark on the ball to use as alignment aids. They use this information to fine tune their alignment on the putter head and execution of the stroke.

Scan Paths of Good and Poor Putters

Recall that a scan path combines the different types of gaze (fixations, saccades, pursuit tracking) into a map of what the athlete sees over time. Figure 6.3a shows the scan path of an elite golfer during five consecutive putts on a flat surface, while figure 6.3b shows the scan path of a near-elite golfer performing the same type of putts. Notice that the scan path of the elite golfer is precise. His gaze shifts from a location on the back of the ball to a precise location that he fixates on the hole. He defines a narrow focus within each target area, where he focuses his attention for an optimal period of time. The elite putter's scan path exhibits little uncertainty in where his target is. In contrast, the near-elite golfer does not define a single target on the hole, but lets his gaze roam over a wide area encompassing many degrees of visual angle. He is less precise in seeing a single location on the hole or the ball, and he does not seem to have a clear idea of where his target is.

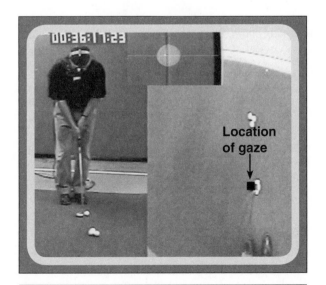

► **Figure 6.1** An elite putter fixating the back of the ball and club while preparing to putt.

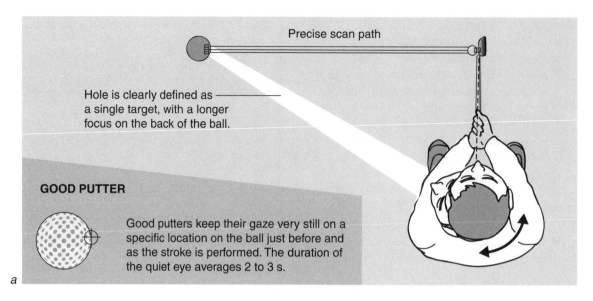

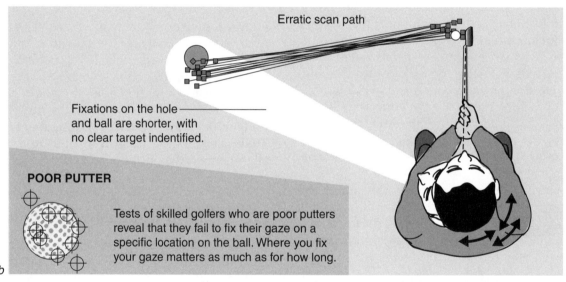

> ➤ **Figure 6.3**   Scan paths of *(a)* an elite golfer who is good at putting and *(b)* a golfer who has difficulty with putting.

Reprinted, by permission, from J.N. Vickers, 2004, "The quiet eye: it's the difference between a good putter and a poor one. Here's proof," *GolfDigest*, pp. 96-101.

Quiet Eye in Golf

Of all the gaze within the scan path in golf (fixations, saccades, pursuit tracking) to all locations (ball, club, hole, green), only one has emerged as an indicator of both higher levels of skill and accuracy, and that is the final fixation on the ball prior to the backswing (Vickers, 1992; Vickers, 2004; Vickers, Morton, & Panchuk, in progress). Figure 6.4 (top) shows that golfers with handicaps below 4 have a mean quiet-eye duration of 2 s, while those with handicaps above 14 average 1.5 s (Vickers, 1992). Figure 6.4 (bottom) shows

the quiet-eye duration of professional and novice members of the Ladies Professional Golf Association (LPGA) who performed putts of 3 m on a sloped green (Vickers & Crews, 2002). In both studies, the onset of the quiet eye occurred before the backswing, and it was located on either the back of the ball or the top.

Quiet-Eye Dwell Time

The **quiet-eye dwell time** refers to the portion of the quiet eye that occurs after the club contacts the ball. In putting, the quiet eye should remain on the green after contact for about 250 ms. But

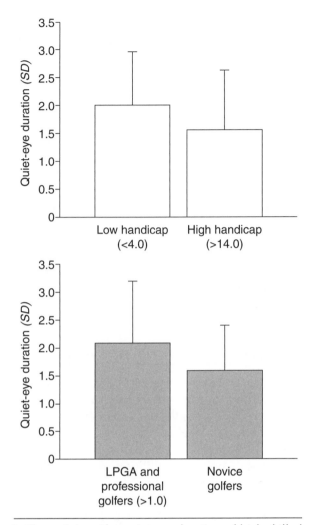

> **Figure 6.4**   The quiet-eye duration of high-skilled golfers compared with lower-skilled golfers. (Golfers with a low handicap are high skilled.)

it is very common for the gaze to move toward the hole before the ball is struck (Vickers, 1992). It takes 200 to 300 ms for a golfer to program a shift in gaze toward the hole, which means that any shift in gaze must be organized or programmed during the stroke. Pelz (2000) placed contact paper on the putter face that showed the impact points of elite and novice putters. Elite putters contacted the ball on the same narrow location of the putter face, while lower-skilled golfers recorded contact points over a wide area of the putter face. The ability to contact the ball with precision is dependent on having an early onset and long-duration quiet eye in which the quiet-eye dwell time is maintained until after the ball leaves the club face.

Optimal Location of the Quiet Eye

Golfers who are good at putting fixate one of the two locations shown in figure 6.5 (right-handed golfer). In the left of the figure, the quiet eye is located on the back of the ball where the putter head makes contact, while on the right the gaze is directed to the top of the ball. Which of these two locations contributes to greater accuracy? Both seem to be effective, but a weight of evidence favors the back of the ball. More elite golfers select the actual location where the putter face will contact the ball as the exact location of their quiet eye.

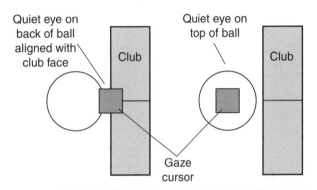

> **Figure 6.5**   The quiet-eye location on the left is the back of the ball where the putter face will make contact, while on the right the quiet eye is shown on the top of the ball.

By definition, the quiet eye in golf putting is the final fixation on the ball before the onset of the backswing. Most golfers establish a quiet eye on the ball as the stroke is executed. But an alternative is to establish a quiet eye on the hole or breakpoint as the stroke is performed (Alpenfels & Christina, 2005). In this style of putting, the golfer does not see the club or ball as the stroke is performed. Instead the gaze remains fixed on the target. Alpenfels and Christina (2005) report that golfers using this style are more successful in getting the ball close to the hole than in conventional putting, but they do not report if the golfers are more accurate overall. More research will be needed to see if this type of gaze control is as successful as the conventional style.

EEG and the Quiet Eye

Vickers and Crews (2002) studied the gaze and EEG recordings of elite and novice golfers. Recall that EEG recordings map the sequencing of mental operations in the brain. In the study, electrodes were placed on the scalp and electrical brain waves recorded. Typically, each waveform shows the average electrical activity recorded for 1 s. In skills such as golf putting (Crews & Landers, 1993) and rifle shooting (Hatfield, Landers, & Ray, 1987; Janelle et al., 2000), one of the most consistent findings with elite athletes is the relative quieting of the left hemisphere, with stable or subsequent increases in activation of the right hemisphere (as exhibited by decreasing alpha power). This activation pattern was matched with little or no change in the right hemisphere prior to task execution.

The brain maps in figure 6.6 represent the amount of activity during the final fixation, or quiet eye, in the golf putt. EEG activity from 10 sites was averaged over the final second before initiating the stroke. The two components of importance include the amount of activity (dark is high and light is low) and the degree of balance of activity in the two hemispheres. Of these components, the balance of neural activity is most important. The amount of activity may vary among golfers and with changes in arousal states, but overall when an optimal state is achieved, all areas of the brain fire synchronously, creating a coherent and relaxed state in the brain. Figure 6.6 shows that the poor putter (left) had more activity

in some parts of the brain than in others, while the elite golfer (right) had harmonized activity throughout the brain.

During the quiet-eye period, a coherent pattern of neural activity is created across both hemispheres and over the different locations, leading to neural harmony. Interestingly, Vickers and Crews (2002) found that the occipital area of the brain, the area that controls vision, shows a reverse pattern compared with the other brain regions. Elite golfers showed less activity at this location compared with novice golfers. This may be due to the presence of a more stable quiet gaze where the same information is fixated and processed continuously. Novice golfers who look repeatedly at the hole or target at a fast rate have diffuse brain activity and never seem to display the same focus and harmony.

Quiet-Eye Training in Golf

It is clear from the discussion thus far that the gaze control of elite golfers differs from that of golfers with lower skill levels. Elite putters have a lower frequency of gaze, and they direct fixations to specific locations on the ball and green, which is symptomatic of their ability to read the abstract patterns in the green. They also use a quiet eye located on the back of the ball for 2 to 3 s.

Vickers, Morton, and Panchuk (in progress) carried out a training study designed to determine if training a quiet eye (QE) would increase the accuracy of the golfers within the experimental setting. Fourteen golfers volunteered for the study and were randomly placed into two groups (QE trained and gaze trained). The two groups were matched by skill level based on their handicap before the pretest. Handicaps ranged from 0 to 29 strokes, with the mean of the gaze-trained group being 11.84 and of the QE-trained group 11.46. The quiet-eye trained group's handicaps ranged from 0 to 20, average 10.12, while the gaze-trained group's handicaps ranged from 2 to 19, average 11.84. The groups were also created with an equal number of low and high handicap golfers in each. Both performed putts in a pretest and posttest separated by 6 mo. All putts were taken on a sloped surface at randomized distances of 4 ft (122 cm) and 6 ft (183 cm). The tests took 30 min for the data collection and 30 min for the instruction that followed.

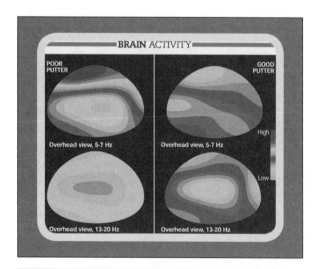

➤ **Figure 6.6**   Brain scans of a poor (left) and good putter (right) shown from overhead, with the forehead toward the top and occipital area at the bottom of each scan.

Reprinted, by permission, from J.N. Vickers, 2004, "The quiet eye: it's the difference between a good putter and a poor one. Here's proof," *GolfDigest*, pp. 96-101.

Before the pretest, the researchers found that it was not possible to select experienced golfers for a control group who had not already used the quiet eye in putting. Therefore, they provided the two groups with differing amounts of feedback about their gaze control and quiet eye. They also did not provide either group with instruction in technique as related to the stance or stroke.

After performing putts in the pretest, the gaze-trained golfers saw their vision-in-action data (as in figures 6.1 and 6.2) and received feedback on their gaze control, but they were given no precise instruction in terms of the quiet eye. The QE-trained group was instructed in a manner similar to the training given in the study on the basketball free throw, as presented in the last chapter (Harle & Vickers, 2001). First, the group viewed an elite prototype who exhibited the critical quiet eye as found in past gaze research (Vickers, 1992). The following points were stressed:

➤ Assume your stance and align the club so that the gaze is on the back of the ball.

➤ After setting up over the ball, fixate the hole and surrounding green and determine the breakpoint where the ball will begin to roll to the hole.

➤ Saccade from the hole to the ball and align the club so that the ball will travel to the breakpoint.

➤ Repeat this process no more than two or three times per putt. The final saccade should be from the breakpoint to the back of the ball and should be smooth and relaxed.

➤ The final fixation should be a quiet eye on the back of the ball. The onset of the quiet eye should occur before the stroke begins and last for 2 to 3 s.

➤ No gaze should be directed to the clubhead during the backswing or foreswing.

➤ The quiet eye should remain on the green for 200 to 300 ms of quiet-eye dwell time after the club contacts the ball.

Following instruction, the QE-trained golfers were shown their own gaze data and asked to identify how their gaze differed from that of the elite prototype. The instructor asked questions to elicit the golfers' understanding of their gaze relative to the expert. At the end of the session,

the golfers were then asked to identify one aspect of their gaze control that they would work on before the posttest. Most chose the quiet eye, in particular the quiet-eye dwell time, which is the amount of time the gaze remains fixated on the green after the club has contacted the ball. The posttest occurred 6 mo later and was similar to the pretest in that the putts were taken from 4 ft (122 cm) and 6 ft (183 cm). In addition, a transfer test was performed where the golfers had to perform a 6 ft (183 cm) putt from a new location with a novel break. Competitive pressure was added during the transfer by making a prize available to the golfer who made the most hits (out of 10) in the transfer condition.

Changes in Gaze Control

The QE-trained group significantly changed their quiet-eye duration from a mean of 3 s before training to 4 s after, compared with less than 2 s for the control group. The QE-trained golfers also increased their QE dwell time, as shown in figure 6.7, from shorter than 100 ms in the pretest to longer than 700 ms after training, while the gaze-trained group maintained durations of approximately 100 ms. The QE group also increased the amount of time spent in the preparation phase in a manner similar to that found

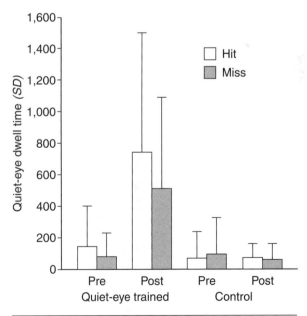

➤ **Figure 6.7** Mean quiet-eye dwell time on hits and misses while performing breaking putts, pretest to posttest.

in basketball, while the gaze-trained group did not make a similar change. With a change in gaze control, there appeared to be a self-organization of the stroke without overt coaching.

Changes in Accuracy

Figure 6.8 shows the percentage of putts made during the pretest, posttest, and transfer test by the low- and high-skilled groups. The dotted line illustrates the percent of putts (50%) made from 6 ft (183 cm) by professional golfers in competition (Pelz, 2000). In the pretest, the high-skilled gaze-trained group made 42% of their putts compared with 50% for the QE-trained, even though the two groups had similar mean handicaps at the outset, while the low-skilled groups had similar and lower levels of accuracy (32%). During the posttest, the high-skilled gaze-trained group increased its accuracy to 46% and the QE-trained group to 51%. During the transfer test, the high-skilled gaze-trained group made 70% of their putts and the QE-trained group made 77%. These values compared to 59% and 60%, respectively, for the low-skilled golfers in the QE-trained and gaze-trained groups. Overall, there was a significant improvement in accuracy by both training groups from pretest to posttest to transfer. Although

the QE-trained golfers had the highest accuracy overall, they did not improve significantly more than the gaze-trained golfers. It would appear that being aware of the quiet eye and being able to view their personal gaze data after the pretest had almost the same effect as receiving quiet-eye training. Overall, the increases by both training groups were impressive, but especially for the high-skilled golfers, as improvements at this skill level are often more difficult to achieve than when at lower skill levels.

Quiet Eye in Billiards

Our next exemplar in the subcategory of abstract targeting skills is billiards. In order to be successful in billiards, pinpoint aiming is required. Figure 6.9 shows a typical billiards table with a white cue ball, an object ball, a target ball, and pockets. The objective of the game is to aim the cue ball at one of the object balls so that it ultimately goes into one of the pockets. The target ball comes into play on complex shots where a number of balls collide before one goes in the pocket. Players have to aim precisely on the contact point of the object ball, and it takes total concentration to maintain the gaze on that location (Kurz & Stergiou, 2004).

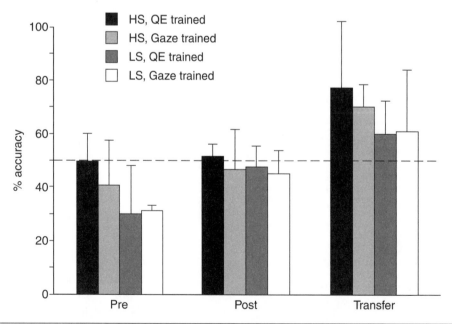

➤ **Figure 6.8**   Changes in accuracy from pretest to posttest to transfer test on 6 ft (183 cm) breaking putts of the QE-trained and gaze-trained groups. The dotted line indicates the percent of putts made by professional players from a similar distance during competition, as reported by Pelz (2000).

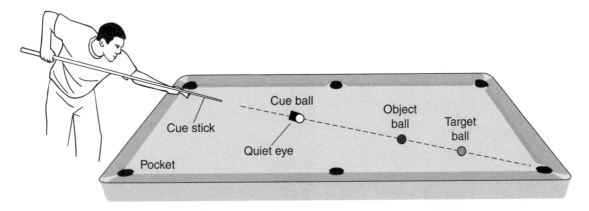

➤ **Figure 6.9** A billiard table showing the cue ball, object ball, target ball, and pocket. The contact point of the object ball is the location of the quiet eye.

Williams, Singer, and Frehlich (2002) recorded the gaze of highly skilled and novice players as they performed shots of varying complexity. The highly skilled players were known for having a solid stroke and an exceptional sense of aim, while the novices had limited experience with the game. In two experiments, researchers manipulated the quiet-eye duration during easy, intermediate, and difficult shots. For the easy shots, the object ball lay near a corner and hitting it into the pocket was easily done. The intermediate shots required the players to strike the cue ball and hit the cushion before hitting the object ball. The hard shot required the cue ball to be struck so that it caromed off the object ball into another target ball located near the corner pocket. Since more complex motor responses require longer preprogramming times (e.g., Henry, 1980; Henry & Rogers, 1960; Klapp, 1977), it was expected that the quiet-eye duration was related to cognitive programming, and therefore the more complex shots would require a longer quiet-eye period.

In experiment 1, the players took continuous shots until they made 10 hits and 10 misses for each of the easy, intermediate, and hard shots. The results showed that, regardless of complexity, more accurate shots were characterized by longer durations of quiet eye, with successful shots taking approximately 210 ms longer to complete than unsuccessful ones. There were no increases in the duration of the backswing and foreswing; however, the preparation phase took longer on the more complex shots. The skilled players spent more time preparing the stroke for each level of complexity than the novice players.

In terms of gaze behaviors, the skilled players' visual-search behaviors were more economical, and they fixated the cue and object balls longer. The less skilled players used more fixations of shorter duration, particularly to the cue and object balls. They allocated their quiet-eye duration equally to the cue ball, object ball, and target ball, and they did not appear to know how to discriminate among these objects or locations. The quiet-eye period was significantly longer for the highly skilled players than for the novices in all levels of shots, and it was also longer on hits compared with misses.

In experiment 2, the validity of the quiet-eye period as a measure of cognitive programming was examined by manipulating how long the players could prepare the shot. Each player's mean preparation time was reduced by 25% and 50% of what they had used in the first experiment. Regardless of the skill level of the player or complexity of the shot, when the amount of preparation time was constrained, shorter quiet-eye periods accrued, resulting in poorer performance as shown in figure 6.10. Williams, Singer, and Frehlich (2002) interpreted the quiet-eye duration as the critical period when cognitive processing was carried out.

Gaze Control in Moving-Target Tasks

The final category of targeting skills occurs when the target is in motion and the gaze and attention system are used to anticipate the target's

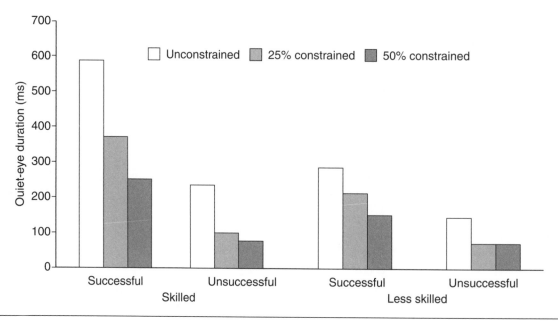

➤ **Figure 6.10**   Mean quiet-eye duration (ms) for successful and unsuccessful shots for skilled and less skilled groups by each level of constraint.

Journal of Motor Behavior, 34, 2, 197-207, 2002. Reprinted with permission of the Helen Dwight Reid Educational Foundation. Published by Heldref Publications, 1319 Eighteenth St., NW, Washington, DC 20036-1802. Copyright © 2002.

movement prior to a pass or kick. Examples of tasks in this category are passing to a receiver in football, basketball, soccer, ice hockey, or similar sports, as well as attempting to hit an elusive target as in boxing and martial arts. Williams and Elliott (1999) investigated the effect of competitive pressure on the gaze of elite karate athletes. During a simulated karate match, the athletes were found to protect themselves from fast actions of the opponent's feet and hands by centering their gaze on the upper chest. From this central location, they could monitor any attack of the opponent. The study also found that the athletes changed their gaze control under conditions of high anxiety, using more saccades and fixations to peripheral areas than when nonanxious, resulting in less effective performance. There have been surprisingly few visual-search or vision-in-action studies done in this subcategory of targeting skills.

Interpreting the Quiet-Eye Period in Targeting Tasks

Although the quiet-eye period has been identified as a characteristic of skill and accuracy in targeting skills (as well as in interceptive and

tactical tactics, as will be shown in the next chapters), interpreting what it means has provided a number of different perspectives. In the following section, four interpretations of the quiet-eye period are provided, first from **cognitive neuroscience**, second from **ecological psychology** and dynamic systems, third from sport psychology, and lastly from the beneficial combination of cognition and physiological arousal as found in the **Setchenov phenomenon**.

Cognitive Neuroscience

Researchers from a cognitive neuroscience perspective have speculated that during the quiet eye, the neural networks that control the skill are being organized and that an optimal period of time is needed to accomplish the skill. The different mean durations found in the basketball free throw, basketball jump shot, rifle shooting, golf putting, and billiards suggest that the complexity and precision of each task require a task-dependent optimal quiet-eye period.

Posner and Raichle (1994) have identified three attention networks that may be central to this organization. The **posterior orienting network** is responsible for controlling the gaze and attention in space. This network, which is located in the parietal region, directs the gaze to specific locations of importance in a task. It is also responsible for preventing the disengagement of the gaze to other locations. Free-throw shooters, golfers, rifle shooters, and cricket players may use the posterior network to align their gaze to specific locations in space and maintain the gaze at a single location. The second network, the **anterior executive network,** is responsible for bringing into consciousness critical aspects of what is being fixated. This network interprets what is being viewed and imposes a higher-order understanding on the task based on past experience and knowledge. Skilled players bring a richer knowledge base and more refined rules than less skilled performers, who are often unsure of what they need to see as they perform. The **vigilance network** is responsible for coordinating the posterior and anterior networks and preventing unwanted or distracting information from gaining access to the other networks during periods of sustained focus. The vigilance network is responsible for the sustained concentration seen in elite players, especially during pressure-filled games of long duration.

Ecological Psychology and Dynamic Systems

Researchers from an ecological or dynamic systems perspective argue that the spatial-temporal information is a central aspect of the "education of attention," a concept first proposed by Gibson (1966, p. 51). Newell and McDonald (1994) and Williams, Janelle, and Davids (2004) describe the perceptual-motor workspace as the location where perception and action are specified; the quiet eye is a more specific location within this space. Oudejans, Koedijker, Bleijendaal, and Bakker (2005) and Oudejans, van de Langenberg, and Hutter (2002) have suggested that quiet-eye information is central to the intrinsic dynamics of skilled actions. Quiet-eye analyses reveal the nature of the intrinsic dynamics between perception and action and the outcome of the skill.

The quiet eye also facilitates orientation of the body and arm movements in space and allows for the execution of movement that is attuned to the affordances and other constraints that are present. In the next chapter a quiet eye will be shown to optimize optic flow and permit a better orientation of the performer relative to targets and objects

in space. The orientation of the body in space is not carried out by an internal feedback system but through the generation of dynamical relationships between the position of the athlete's body and gaze in space relative to a target or object. The training study of Oudejans et al. (2005) presented in the previous chapter lends credence to this view. The shooting ability of basketball players increased significantly over that of a control group through the use of a screen that occluded the basket, enabling a longer quiet-eye period.

Another equally plausible view within the ecological and dynamic systems perspective is that the quiet eye may act as a visual pivot (Ripoll, 1991; Williams, Davids, & Williams, 1999) that improves the egocentric orientation of the basketball player's body and aiming arms to the target. In a recent attempt to replicate Oudejans et al.'s (2005) result, Vickers, Panchuk, Morton, and Martell (in progress b) found that some players maintained a high level of accuracy when the hoop was screened completely so that only the top of the backboard could be seen. These players preserved their accuracy by selecting a unique quiet-eye location that was aligned with the hoop, such as the marks on the floor, letters in a sign above the hoop, or lines in the wall behind the hoop. As long as they refreshed this unusual but egocentric quiet-eye location, they were able to shoot accurately.

Sport Psychology

Yet still another perspective is offered from sport psychologists, who argue that the quiet-eye period is an index of focus and concentration. The biathlon study (Vickers & Williams, under review) lends credence to this view in that only those shooters who increased their quiet-eye duration above that used in practice were able to overcome the normally debilitating effects of the high physiological workload, competitive pressure, and anxiety. Using a quiet eye may facilitate being **in the zone,** which many elite athletes report during optimal performance. It may be that when the same target location is fixated for a long duration of time, the stable quiet eye creates a feeling of emptiness because there is no change in external visual information. The gaze is stable and when the correct information is fixated, processing can occur without as much change as when the gaze is constantly shifting to new locations.

Cognitive-Physiological Facilitation: Setchenov Phenomenon

A final reason why the quiet-eye period may be beneficial was presented in the biathlon study (Vickers & Williams, in press), which showed that athletes who employed a longer quiet-eye duration continued to perform well even after exercising at a *PO* level of 100% of their individual maximum. Athletes who had a lower duration choked under the combined weight of high pressure, high anxiety, and physiological arousal. Setchenov showed that individuals who were fatigued to exhaustion could do more physiological work when a diverting activity was used to direct attention to an external target or activity and away from internal processes. Subsequent studies have shown that directing attention externally to relevant task information improves performance in a wide variety of tasks, creates a greater effect with the eyes open compared to the eyes closed, and appears to be related to the reticular formations regulating physiological arousal and the perception of pain (Assmussen & Mazin, 1978a, 1978b; Bear et al., 2007; Hoffman, 2004; Kinomura et al., 1996; Valet et al., 2004; Wulf, McNevin, & Shea, 2001; Wulf, Shea, & Park, 2001; Wulf et al., 2002). In combination, these studies suggest that maintaining a quiet-eye focus that is optimal may insulate the athlete from the normally delimitating effects of extreme exercise, anxiety, and pain and allow athletes to maintain or even increase their level of performance.

Regardless of the theoretical perspective taken, there is considerable research evidence showing that the quiet-eye period is a characteristic of higher levels of skill and accuracy in a wide range of targeting tasks. The quiet eye is the last good look that an athlete gets before performing the final movement in a task. Elite athletes find a way to get the information they need at just the right time, and this is a factor in why they perform so well. Finally, although it is now possible to describe the location, onset, offset, and duration of the quiet eye in many targeting tasks, considerable research still needs to be done to provide a complete understanding of this intriguing phenomenon. In the next chapter, we look at the quiet eye and gaze control in the second major category of skills, that of interceptive timing tasks.

Quiet Eye in Action

Select a training partner or partners and develop a quiet-eye decision-training program for the golf putt. Follow these steps:

1. List five quiet-eye characteristics that are needed to perform well in the golf putt. When listing each characteristic, name the cognitive skill that is most important (anticipation, attention, focus and concentration, memory, pattern recognition, problem solving, or decision making).

2. Second, design a drill or progression of drills that will help you and your partner improve your accuracy in the putt.

3. Practice the drills for 20 to 30 min per day. Your main goal is to develop the optimal focus as the golf putt is prepared and executed.

Record your results. At the beginning of the first practice, record your pretraining accuracy for the first 10 putts before you do any quiet-eye training. Try to complete five training sessions. At the end of each practice session, record your percent accuracy on the final 10 trials on the blank graph provided on page 109.

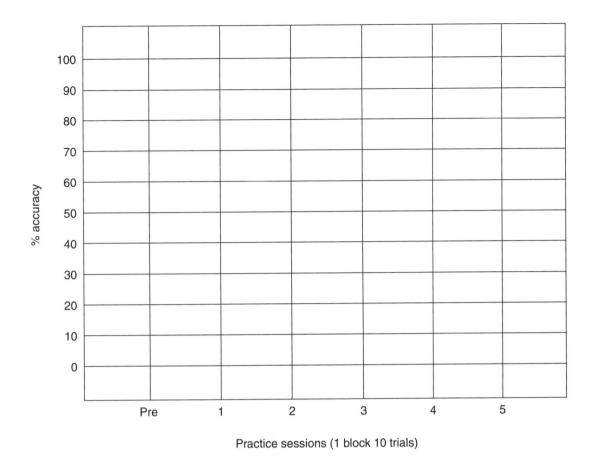

Practice sessions (1 block 10 trials)

From J.N. Vickers, 2007, *Perception, cognition, and decision training: The quiet eye in action* (Champaign, IL: Human Kinetics).

Prepare a short report in which you discuss the following topics:

1. List the five gaze control or quiet-eye characteristics that you selected to work on.
2. Provide a sketch of the drills used to train your quiet eye. Explain how each drill was used to improve your cognitive and quiet-eye focus.
3. What methods of practice did you use? (See chapters 9 through 12 for some ideas about how to vary your methods of training.)
4. Include the figure of results you generated from the blank graph and explain your percentage change over the five practices. Did you improve or get worse?
5. Using information from this chapter, discuss why your results occurred. In your opinion, what were the underlying reasons for your results?

Gaze Control in Interceptive Timing Tasks

◀◀ *Where Have We Been?*

Chapters 5 and 6 presented gaze control in targeting tasks where an object was propelled toward a fixed target in space (as in basketball), toward targets fixed in space with abstract qualities (as in golf or billiards), or toward moving targets (as in passing to a receiver). We saw that the goal in these tasks is to place an object, such as a ball, in or on the target with a high degree of accuracy. To achieve this, the gaze must be controlled in an optimal manner in order to acquire the visual information needed to perform well. The quiet eye was introduced as a gaze that provides this information. For each targeting task, the quiet eye has a specific location, onset, offset, and duration. Perhaps most importantly, its onset begins before the final impulse phase of the aiming movement. Performance is lower in targeting skills when the athlete is too early or too late in acquiring the information needed to organize and control the aiming skill.

▶▶ *Where Are We Going?*

In this chapter, we now look at interceptive timing tasks where the gaze is used to track an object that moves toward the athlete and that has to be controlled in a specific way. Examples of tasks in this category include catching a ball, hitting a baseball or cricket ball, receiving a serve in volleyball, hitting a tennis ball, and goaltending. An important quality of interceptive tasks is whether performers have developed gaze control strategies that allow them to predict the flight of the object. All objects can be propelled so that the flight is easy or difficult to predict. Elite performers have developed two gaze control strategies—one that they use when the flight of the object is relatively constant, and a second that they use when the object spins, slides, curves, or moves erratically as it approaches.

Interceptive Timing Tasks Defined

Davids, Savelsbergh, Bennet, and van der Kamp (2002, p. 2) define interceptive actions as those that require the

> coordination between the performer's body or a held implement, and an object, surface, gap or target area in the environment. That is, they typically involve two types of coordination processes. First, like many complex actions, interceptions involve a high level of coordination between body parts, joints or limb segments. The second coordination process involved is between key limbs (or even with respect to the whole body) and a target object or surface in the environment. With respect to the latter type of coordination process, interceptive movements typically require a limb segment or held implement to be in the right place at the right time, often with an additional constraint of imparting a controlled amount of force into an intentional collision with an object or surface.

It is clear that this definition by Davids et al. (2002) concentrates on the motor control systems needed to perform interceptive timing actions. In this chapter, a different perspective is used as we concentrate on describing how the gaze is used to fixate, track, and anticipate the speed, direction, and other characteristics of an object that moves toward the performer and is controlled in a specific way.

Motor Control During Interceptive Timing Tasks

A central characteristic of interceptive timing actions is the ability to control both the speed and direction of the limb so that the object is contacted with optimal timing. The motor timing variables normally assessed are the onset, offset, and duration of movement time, as well as velocity at contact. These variables identify, in order, when the athlete initiates the action, how long the movement takes, when the movement ends, and how hard the object is hit.

Extensive research has been carried out on the timing of interceptive actions, and one of the most intriguing results is the invariant nature of some aspects of motor control (Davids et al., 2002; Schmidt & Lee, 2005). A feature is said to be invariant if it does not change much from trial to trial. One aspect that does not vary much is the sequence, or order, of events in a motor task. Another is the relative timing of these events, or the temporal structure. For example, in table tennis, Bootsma (1991), Bootsma and van Wieringen (1988), and Rodrigues, Vickers, and Williams (2002) determined that movement onset, movement-time duration, and arm velocity at contact do not differ significantly for high-, intermediate-, and low-skilled players.

Bootsma and van Wieringen (1988) have also found that the precision of the timing at contact and variability at contact ranged from only 2.0 to 4.7 ms. Rodrigues et al. (2002) found that arm velocity did not differ between high-skilled (91.59 cm/s, $SD = 33.68$) and low-skilled players (89.75 cm/s, $SD = 36.68$) at contact. Among normal adult subjects, the available evidence shows that movement-time onset, movement-time duration, movement-time offset, and velocity at contact are far more similar than different across skill and accuracy levels.

Predictable and Unpredictable Object Movement

There are two subcategories of gaze control in interceptive timing tasks (see figure 4.1), and these depend on whether the flight of the object is easily predicted or not. All objects have the capacity for predictable or unpredictable flight, so the skilled athlete has to develop a gaze control strategy to use in each case. During predictable object motion the flight of the object is determined using fixations or pursuit tracking as it is delivered and during early flight. When the flight of the object is unpredictable, then both early and late tracking of the object is needed, often interconnected by a quick saccade. Often the complexity of object flight depends on the task and the skill of the person pitching, hitting, serving, kicking, or throwing the object. In baseball, for example, certain pitchers are able to deliver the ball so that it is much harder to hit. The same is true in tennis and volleyball as well as in all forms of shooting on a goaltender. Perhaps the most difficult object to track is one that bounces in front of the athlete as occurs in cricket bowling, leaving little time to respond.

Three Gaze Control Phases of Interceptive Timing Tasks

Whether object motion is easy or hard to predict, all interceptive timing tasks have in common three gaze control phases: object recognition, object tracking, and object control. During the **object-recognition phase,** fixations and pursuit tracking are used to study the movements of the object and the individual propelling the object as it is pitched, bowled, kicked, shot, or otherwise propelled toward the athlete. Some controversy currently exists over what occurs during this phase in successful and unsuccessful performances. Visual-search studies (e.g., Salmela & Fiorito, 1979; Williams & Burwitz, 1993) have found that advanced cues from the body of the person propelling the object (head, hip, arm, leg action) underlie high levels of skill, but vision-in-action studies have found that fixations or tracking gazes on the object being propelled play a critical role when the speed of the object is moderate (Bard & Fleury, 1976; Land & McLeod, 2000; Panchuk & Vickers, 2006; Vickers & Adolphe, 1997).

During the **object-tracking phase**, smooth pursuit-tracking gazes are used to maintain the image of the object on the fovea in order to detect if it spins, accelerates, or decreases in speed; changes direction; or is affected by wind, sun, or a host of other factors that can occur. There are inherent limits in human pursuit tracking. If the speed of the object exceeds 150°/s, then the pursuit-tracking system is unable to maintain the image on the retina (Bahill & LaRitz, 1984; Pola & Wyatt, 1991). Saccades, which are ballistic eye movements that can reach speeds in excess of 900°/s, are also used to regain tracking of the object when it moves unpredictably. Therefore saccades are used to race ahead of the object so that pursuit tracking can occur once more before contact (Land & McLeod, 2000). During saccades information is suppressed, so the athlete is not aware of the blurring and displacement of the image that occurs during this rapid eye movement.

During the **object-control phase**, fixation and tracking gaze are used to stabilize the eyes and head as the object is caught with the hand, kicked to a teammate, hit as in baseball or cricket, passed to a teammate as in volleyball, and so on. Each task places specific demands on the gaze control system that must be met during this phase, but the central one is that a goal is achieved. The performer has to integrate all the necessary information across the three phases in order to realize a successful performance. In baseball this may be hitting to a specific field, in volleyball it may be passing to the setter, and in ice hockey or soccer goaltending it may be preventing a rebound. In the following sections we now look at each of the three phases in selected tasks where research has been completed.

Object Recognition: Anticipating Object Flight

It is currently unclear which cues are most useful in terms of anticipating the flight of the object during the object-recognition phase. Studies carried out using the visual-search paradigm (Salmela & Fiorito, 1979; Singer, Cauraugh, Chen, Steinberg, & Frehlich, 1996; Williams & Burwitz, 1993; Williams, Ward, Knowles, & Smeeton, 2002) have found that the most important cues come from the person's head, shoulder, kicking leg, and hips. In contrast, vision-in-action studies in which the subjects performed the action show that fixations and tracking gazes are restricted primarily to the object before and during flight (Bard & Fleury, 1976; Land & McLeod, 2000; Panchuk & Vickers, 2006; Vickers & Adolphe, 1997).

Visual Occlusion Studies

A valuable experimental technique used in the visual-search paradigm is film occlusion, where sections of a video are masked in order to limit the amount of information available. The occluded video is then shown on computer monitors or on life-size displays and the participant responses are recorded. Reaction time, decision time, and movement time are assessed under various constraints. Jones and Miles (1978) used film occlusion to determine anticipation of the tennis serve. Video clips of the serve were occluded so that 336 ms and 126 ms of ball flight were observable after the server hit the ball, as well as a third condition that showed the serve until 42 ms before ball–racket contact. Elite players could predict the direction of the serve from the 42 clips, indicating they could extract more meaning than the novices from the brief movements of the server.

Salmela and Fiorito (1979) used a similar technique to determine how ice hockey goaltenders read the flight of the puck. Film sequences of shots to the four corners of the net were shown using either a wrist shot or a slap shot. The film sequences were then occluded 83.33 ms, 166.67 ms, and 333.33 ms before the shooter's stick contacted the puck. The goaltenders had to predict which corner of the net the puck was directed toward. The goaltenders were least successful in predicting the location of the shot when the films were occluded 333.33 ms before contact; they were also better at detecting the horizontal direction of the shot than the height, or vertical dimension. The type of shot also played an important role; success rates were higher for the wrist shot than for the slap shot, which is normally taken with greater speed.

Using a similar approach, Williams and Burwitz (1993) identified the cues used by goaltenders in the soccer penalty shot. Their results also showed that highly skilled goalkeepers were better at predicting the direction of the shot than the height. These differences were attributed to the lack of experience some goaltenders may have in facing left-footed shooters, who are fewer in number.

Although these studies show that goaltenders are able to use early cues from the shooter to anticipate the direction of the puck or ball, and they provide some indication of the minimum amount of information required for success, they fail to show the origin of the information. Gaze data represent an important advancement in the study of high-speed games because they allow researchers to better understand the dynamic organization of visual behavior and provide an understanding of the mental processes and general principles of semantic visual function (Ripoll, 1991).

Reading Baseball Pitches

Shank and Haywood (1987) used the visual-search paradigm to study the eye movements of elite and novice baseball players reading pitches. They selected pitches performed by highly skilled pitchers and presented them to elite and novice players on a monitor. The complete windup and delivery of the pitcher were included in each video sequence, as well as the first 200 ms of the ball's flight. The subjects' eye movements were recorded as they viewed each pitch, and verbally they were required to indicate the type of pitch being delivered (fastball or curve).

The elite athletes correctly identified 89% of all pitches, while the novices were correct in identifying only 60%. Clearly the elite athletes were better at detecting aspects of the pitcher's delivery of the ball, thus allowing them to better predict the type of incoming pitch. From the windup until the release of the ball, the elite athletes fixated the release point of the ball and did not look at the ball or the pitcher's head, arm, or any other part of the body. In contrast, the novices fixated the head of the pitcher, or they alternated fixations from the head to the ball. The two groups also differed on when they initiated pursuit tracking on the ball after it was released from the pitcher's hand. The novices tended to saccade before the release of the ball from the pitcher's hand, while the elites waited until after the release of the ball and then made a rapid saccade to initiate tracking. The elites and novices did not differ in how long it took to saccade to the ball and initiate tracking; the elites averaged 148.32 ms $(SD = 43.63$ ms) and the novices averaged 150.98 ms $(SD = 35.43)$. These time intervals represent the amount of time typically needed to transition from a fixated gaze to one that tracks an object; we therefore see that for both groups a considerable amount of time was required. Since the ball's flight in baseball lasts only 450 to 500 ms, the ball would be well on its way to the plate before tracking began.

A final aspect of this study concerned the players' verbal reports. The elite hitters reported that they looked for the ball rotation, some of the pitcher's delivery, and the path of the ball, and they made these reports even as they fixated their gaze on only one location—the ball. It is clear that they were able to see much more than what was indicated just by the location of their gaze. The player's verbal reports showed that, even as they fixated one location (the ball at release), they were aware of the ball during the delivery. Perhaps this was due to their use of the ambient system, or to their memory or extensive experience in the game. Although the novices actually fixated more locations while the pitches were being delivered, they "simply had more difficulty naming any kind of pitch from any type of motion, responding slightly better than chance" (Shank & Haywood, 1987, p. 1195). Elite batters therefore anchor their gaze at the release point.

Reading Soccer Penalty Shots

Savelsbergh, Williams, van der Kamp, and Ward (2002) recorded the eye movements of elite and novice soccer goaltenders as they responded to videotapes of penalty kicks presented on a life-size screen. A joystick was used to predict the direction of the shot. Savelsbergh et al. found that elite goaltenders initiated their responses later (closer to ball contact) than novices. Elites and novices did not differ significantly in their ability to predict the location of the penalty shot (36% for elites and 26% for novices), and both groups demonstrated greater ability to predict the horizontal direction (77%) of the shots than the vertical (38%). Novices spent more time fixating the trunk, arm, and hip regions, while elites spent more time fixating the head early in the trial and then the kicking leg, nonkicking leg, and ball region as the shot was taken. The elite goaltenders used fewer fixations than novices (2.9 versus 4.0), and these were of longer duration (585 ms versus 430 ms).

Williams, Ward, Knowles, and Smeeton (2002) determined the anticipation of low- and high-skilled tennis players who responded to life-size video images of strokes being performed toward them. They were required to "return" the ball using an appropriate tennis stroke. The elites were superior in anticipating the direction of the strokes and spent more time fixating central areas of the video player's head–shoulders and trunk–hip regions, while the lower-skilled players looked at the racket and the ball to guide their responses. A second experiment then trained a new group of tennis players to use the cues used by the skilled players to better anticipate the return of strokes. A field test on court was also used to determine transfer to the court. Those who received perceptual training improved their performance in tests of anticipation in the lab and also on court compared with placebo and control groups who did not receive the same training, but these improvements did not translate to actual improvements in tennis performance. No significant improvements were found for any of the groups in returning the ball to specific locations on the court.

Object Tracking: Reading a Moving Object

In this section we look at object tracking, or the ability to maintain the gaze on an object as it moves toward you. Imagine being in a room where the lights are turned off as a ball travels toward you. In experiments by Sharp and Whiting (1974, 1975), participants had to catch a ball with one hand when the lights in the room turned off, which occurred early in flight, late in flight, or at different times in between. Not surprisingly, performers were affected by the duration of viewing time. When viewing times of the approaching ball were shorter than 200 ms, performance was worse than when the ball could be seen for a longer period of time.

Sharp and Whiting also found that the ball was viewed with two systems, which they called the **image–retina system** and the **eye-in-head system.** If the duration of ball-viewing time was shorter than 245 ms, the eyes and head remained motionless and the image–retina system was used to read the image of the ball as it washed across the retina. During this amount of time, there was simply not enough time to move the eyes to track the object, and only a fleeting glimpse of the ball was perceived. When the duration of light was longer than 365 ms, tracking of the object was initiated using both head and eye movements and the image was maintained on the fovea longer using the eye-in-head system. This system allowed a more sustained view of the ball and contributed to higher levels of catching. The study also found that there was a transition period between 245 ms and 365 ms where participants shifted from using the image–retina system to the eye-in-head system. The results showed that both systems are available to provide information about objects in flight, but the time required to transition between the two is quite long, about 120 ms or more. Tracking the object earlier with the eye-in-head system is therefore preferable to the image–retina system alone.

Can We Track an Object and Attend to Another Location at the Same Time?

Another vital question regarding the tracking phase is whether it is possible to track an object and focus on something else at the same time. Researchers have shown that it is very difficult to successfully track and catch a ball while attending to another stimulus in the background. For example, imagine that you are the catcher in baseball and the ball is being thrown to you from third base. A runner is also coming toward you, trying to score at home plate. Is it possible for you to see the player running toward you and the ball being thrown toward you at the same time, or should you concentrate on tracking the ball alone?

Montagne, Laurent, and Ripoll (1993) had participants attempt to track an approaching ball and also anchor their gaze on one of two locations at the same time—at 0° (i.e., directly in line with the ball's flight) and at 33° (i.e., to the right or left of the ball). They found that when the gaze was anchored at either location, thereby affording use of the image–retina system instead of the eye-in-head tracking system, the percentage of successful catches was lower than when tracking occurred. Accuracy was lowest when the gaze was anchored on location at 33°, indicating the ambient system was not capable of providing the information required for successful catching. These results also reveal that it is best for a catcher to concentrate on catching the ball first and then worry about seeing the runner coming from third base.

These results, along with those from Sharp and Whiting (1974, 1975) and Haywood (1984), reveal three important things about how the gaze and attention systems function during object tracking. First, it is important to keep the gaze on the object, and nowhere else, for a sustained period of time. The ambient system is limited compared with the foveal system in the extent to which it can handle useful information in interceptive timing tasks. Second, the pursuit-tracking system takes quite a while to get up to speed to track an object (longer than 120 ms). Therefore it is important to anticipate when an object has to be tracked as it comes toward you. Third, performing at a high level requires the use of attention. Kowler, Anderson, Dosher, and Blaser (1995) explored the relationship between attention and pursuit tracking in a study where an object was tracked even as the background moved. Smooth pursuit eye movements maintained an accurate line of sight on the object even in the presence of distracting background stimuli moving at a different velocity, and the success of this high degree of selectivity was due to attention (Murphy, Kowler, & Steinman, 1975). A weight of evidence therefore shows that the gaze and attention need to be focused on the object as it approaches; it is very difficult to pay attention to another object or location at the same time.

When to Track a Moving Object

Is it important to keep the gaze on the object during its entire flight, or are certain time periods more important than others? Hubbard and Seng (1954) described the problem of batting as one "of tracking a moving object, predicting its course and, at the right point in its flight, deciding to swing or not" (p. 42). They wanted to know how long a baseball batter kept his eyes on the baseball and if keeping his eyes on the ball was necessary to contact the bat with the ball. They used an intricate set of mirrors and cameras to record the eye, head, and batting movements of professional players as they hit pitches on a regulation diamond.

Although they were not able to record the gaze of the players, they did find that there was less head movement when a swing was made than when the player made no attempt to hit the ball (let it go by). A second finding was that the ball did not appear to be tracked late in its flight, therefore defying the long-standing advice of coaches to maintain tracking on the ball until ball–bat contact. Hubbard and Seng suggested that two factors might account for the absence of late tracking. First, as the pitch approached the plate it reached very high angular velocities (above 1,000°/s for a 90 mph [145 kph] pitch). This rate exceeds the capacity of the human pursuit-tracking system. Second, batters have the ability to anticipate the ball's flight during the object-delivery and early flight phase, so there is little need for them to track the ball later in its approach.

Object Tracking: Unpredictable Object Flight

In this section, we look at studies that included the final two phases of interceptive timing tasks: object tracking and object control in tasks where the flight of an object is typically unpredictable. Land and McLeod (2000) recorded the gaze of three cricket batsmen as they viewed balls delivered via a ball-projection machine and hit them as they would in a game setting. One was a highly skilled player, another was an intermediate-level player, and the third was a weak but keen amateur. Cricket differs from the previous interceptive tasks we have looked at so far (ball catching and tracking a baseball) in that the ball bounces just before it is hit, as shown in figure 7.1. The bowler also places different spins on the ball so that when it bounces, the late flight is erratic and difficult to hit. The flight phase of the ball averages between 600 and 650 ms, which is similar to the duration of a 90 mph (145 kph) baseball.

The portion of time after the bounce is between 150 and 200 ms.

Figure 7.1 shows the pursuit tracking of the elite player (dark circles) versus a lower-skilled one (open circles) during a good pitch. Both tracked the ball immediately for 100 to 200 ms and then used an anticipatory saccade that raced ahead of the ball to the point where the ball bounced on the ground, where the fovea "lay in wait" (Land & McLeod, 2000, p. 1341). Following the bounce, the ball was tracked for about 150 ms during the final part of its flight by the high-skilled player but not by the low-skilled player. The main difference between the players was in the speed and variability of the saccade to the bounce. The elite player timed his saccade so that he could maintain a longer period of tracking both before and after the bounce, while the low-skilled player lost sight of the ball and then had greater difficulty getting the gaze back on it during the final approach.

Object Tracking and Object Control: Hitting Targets in Table Tennis

Land and McLeod's (2000) study provided new insights into tracking objects at high speeds during interceptive timing tasks, especially when the object's movement is unpredictable. But their results do not explain how athletes respond to an incoming object and then hit it successfully to another target area on the field of play. This happens often in games such as tennis, table tennis, and volleyball, where the object must not only be tracked and received but also batted, hit, kicked, or controlled to a precise location. How is the gaze controlled in these instances where there is temporal, spatial, and competitive

pressure? Does the gaze have to be controlled in a specific way in order for performance to be high during the control phase? These were the questions asked by Rodrigues et al. (2002) in a table tennis study where high- and low-skilled athletes made returns to cued target locations across the table.

Figure 7.2 shows a regulation table surrounded by six motion analysis cameras that recorded the movement of the ball during its flight, as well as the movement of the hitting arm. Two target areas (one left and one right) were located on the opposite side of the table, within which the ball was to be hit as hard as possible. The participants also wore an eye tracker with a magnetic head tracker. The configuration of equipment in figure 7.2 made it possible to record the ball in flight, the gaze relative to the ball, and the movements of the arm as the forehand action was completed. The ball was served by an experienced player, who delivered it so that the second bounce landed in the circular area on the forehand side of the participant. Ball flight durations did not differ due to skill, accuracy, or the experimental conditions, and they ranged between 760 and 810 ms (*SD* range 49-70 ms). High- and low-skilled players were required to hit the ball as hard as they could with a forehand action while still maintaining a high level of accuracy.

Three temporal cues were used to signal which target to hit. During the precue condition, the cue light came on 3 s before the server began to deliver the ball, and in the early-cue condition, the cue light came on 500 ms after the serve and before the ball was contacted by the participant. In the late-cue condition, the light came on only 300 ms before contact with the ball; therefore, the ball was very close to the participant when the cue light indicated which of the two targets to hit toward.

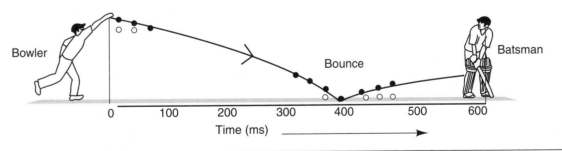

➤ **Figure 7.1**   A cricket bowler delivering the ball to a batsman, with pursuit-tracking gaze of an elite player (●) and lower-skilled player (O). The solid line represents the flight of ball.

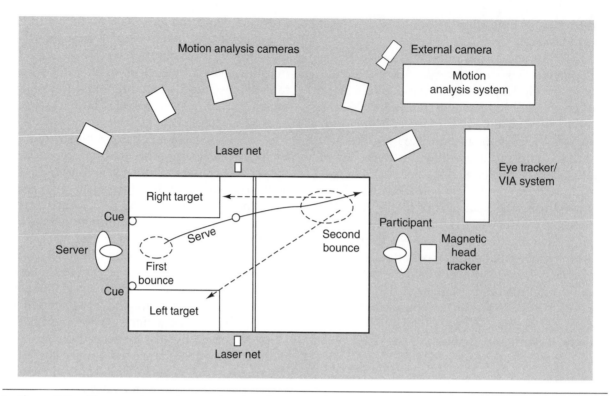

> **Figure 7.2**   The experimental setup showing the server, the participant, the flight of the ball during the serve, and the two target areas. The eye tracker, magnetic head tracker, motion analysis system with six cameras, external camera, laser timing device, and right and left cue lights are illustrated.

Reprinted, by permission, from J.N. Vickers, S.T. Rodrigues and L.N. Brown, 2002, "Gaze pursuit and arm control of adolescent males diagnosed with Attention Deficit Hyperactivity Disorder (ADHD) as compared to normal controls: Evidence of dissociation in processing short and long-duration visual information," *Journal of Sport Sciences* 20(3): 201-216. http://www.informaworld.com

Vision-in-action data were recorded concurrently, as shown in figure 7.3, in order to ensure the accuracy of calibration and also to serve as a second source of data used to verify that data collected using the motion analysis and eye–head tracking systems were accurate. Image A shows the eye of the participant, and image B shows the field of view of the participant, including the server, the two target areas, and the cue lights. The white cursor shows the location of the gaze relative to the ball and targets. An external camera (C) recorded the player's movements and that of the ball. Visible on his arm are the motion analysis markers used to determine the forward movement of the arm to contact. Gaze data were recorded at a rate of 30 Hz for the vision-in-action data and at 60 Hz relative to the eye–head integration system.

Hitting Targets Under Time Constraints

As expected, the low-skilled players were significantly less accurate, making 31% of their returns compared with 50% for the high-skilled group.

The most important differences were caused by the cueing of the lights. Both groups were relatively accurate when the cue light came on 3 s before the serve, as well as when 500 ms were available, but both had low accuracy when they had only 300 ms (late cue) to select the target and make the hit. There was clearly a critical period of time between 500 ms and 300 ms when performance was negatively affected irrespective of the athlete's skill level.

An additional question that Rodrigues et al. (2002) explored was whether the difference in accuracy was due to deficiencies in the control of the arm, control of the gaze, or both. Onset, offset, and duration of arm movement did not differ significantly due to skill level, accuracy, or cueing condition. The results were therefore consistent with those of other researchers displaying an invariant motor timing (Bootsma & van Wieringen, 1990; Schmidt & Lee, 1999). Both high- and low-skill players had higher velocity values on misses than on hits, but overall the movement-time results did not shed any light on why performance was so much lower in the late-

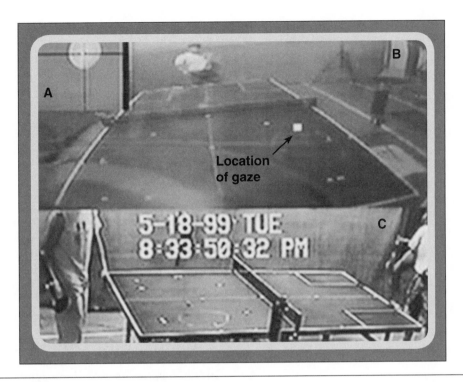

➤ **Figure 7.3**   A frame of vision-in-action data collected in table tennis.

cue condition. The more important variables were those related to tracking the ball prior to hitting.

The duration of tracking on the ball was determined across the ball flight duration to see if the same type of gaze control, as reported by Land and McLeod (2000), was also found in this task, where the ball bounced close to the athlete before being returned. Figure 7.4 shows the mean pursuit tracking in the pre-, early- and late-cue conditions as determined from the eye–head analysis. The x-axis shows the percentage of ball flight from 0% to 100%, with 0% occurring as the ball left the server's bat and 100% when the participant hit the ball. The y-axis shows the gaze location relative to the ball in degrees of visual angle. A value of 0 visual angle (degrees) meant the gaze was on the ball, and above 3° (the horizontal dotted line) indicated the gaze was no longer being tracked by the focal system. The vertical dotted lines in the bottom two plots show when the cue light came on in the early and late conditions. The quiet-eye duration was defined as the duration of tracking time within 3° of visual angle before the onset of the final forward movement of the arm in the foreswing. Figure 7.4 (top) shows that a quiet eye was present in 95% of all trials when the cue light came on early. The quiet-eye duration extended from an early onset at 8% and offset at 60% of total ball flight duration. The middle plot shows

the quiet-eye duration when the cue light came on 500 ms before contact. Here we see that the gaze was on the ball from 3% to 37%. The bottom plot shows the quiet-eye duration in the late-cue condition occurring only briefly, from 3% to 23%.

Quiet-Eye Duration in Table Tennis

Quiet-eye durations differed significantly, as shown in figure 7.5. Mean quiet-eye duration was 410 ms in the precue condition and 272 ms in the early-cue condition, indicating that there still was sufficient time to read the flight of the ball, but when the quiet-eye duration was only 176 ms, as occurred in the late-cue condition, there was not enough time to read the ball's flight, detect the target, and make the hit accurately. These results differ from those of Land and McLeod (2000) in two ways. First, there was no late tracking of the ball after the bounce, even in the early condition, probably due to the presence of the cue lights, which drew the gaze and attention to the target. The participants had no choice but to take their eye off the ball in order to determine which target to hit toward. Second, even the highly skilled performer needed 272 ms or more ball-tracking time in order to perform well. Once tracking on the ball averaged 176 ms, performance declined regardless of skill level.

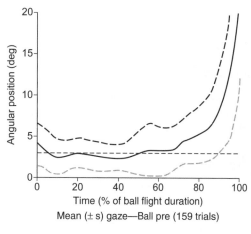

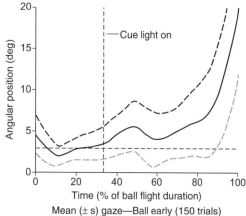

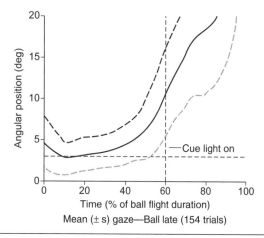

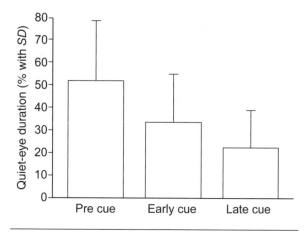

Figure 7.5 Quiet-eye duration during the three cue conditions (pre, early, and late).

Figure 7.4 Percent of trial spent in quiet-eye tracking on the ball (with standard deviation) in the pre-, early-, and late-cue conditions. The horizontal axis shows the percent of ball flight duration, and the vertical axis shows the gaze relative to the ball in degrees of visual angle. The horizontal dotted line shows the 3° threshold for quiet eye; vertical dotted lines show cue onset in the early and late conditions.

Reprinted, by permission, from S.T. Rodrigues, J.N. Vickers and A.M. Williams, 2002, "Head, eye and arm coordination in table tennis," *Journal of Sport Sciences* 20(3): 171-186. http://www.informaworld.com

Object Recognition, Object Tracking, and Object Control

In this section, we now look at studies in volleyball and ice hockey that have investigated all three phases (object recognition, object tracking, and object control) at once in the live sport setting. The goal was to understand how the gaze is controlled over all three phases and the type of gaze control that contributes to higher levels of performance. Many of the same perceptual problems faced by players of table tennis are also faced by receivers in volleyball, who have to study the movement of the server in order to anticipate the ball's flight, track the ball, and then control it using a pass to the setter. Previous studies presented in this chapter (e.g., Shank & Haywood, 1987) have shown that reading the delivery of the ball is critical, as is the ability to track the object once it is in flight. But these studies concentrated on separate phases of the task and did not provide a complete picture across all three phases of object recognition, object tracking, and object control.

In this section, we look at the gaze and motor behavior of elite Team Canada male volleyball athletes who received serves and passed to the setter area on a regulation court (Vickers & Adolphe, 1997). The goal was to determine if elite and near-elite players differed in gaze in the three phases of object detection—object recognition, object tracking, and object control—and the extent to which differences in gaze control accounted for their differences in being able to pass to the setter accurately.

Although all the players performed at the Olympic and world level, their game statistics showed that half were elite players and the other half near-elite players who were just beginning their international careers. Pass accuracy was determined using the system of the International Volleyball Association (IVA), shown in figure 7.6. The target is where the setter typically stands during competition. The elite receivers averaged 63% of their passes to area 4, while the near-elite receivers averaged less than 50%. Figure 7.6 also shows the setup of the experiment, including the server, the flight path of the ball, the athlete receiving the serve while his gaze was recorded by the eye tracker, and a teammate standing behind to keep the cable from interfering with the athlete's actions.

Figure 7.7 shows two frames of vision-in-action data collected in the study. The gaze images (A) were recorded by the scene camera on the eye tracker worn by the athlete, and the motor images (B) were recorded by an external camera placed in front to record his physical movements as he received the ball and passed to the setter area. Figure 7.7 (left) occurred as the serve was delivered, and shows the athlete's gaze (the black cursor) on a point where the ball was tossed and then struck by the server's hand. Figure 7.7 (right) occurred during the flight of the ball and shows the player's gaze on the edge of the ball while it traveled toward him. A time-code generator (not shown) recorded time simultaneously in the two images at a rate of 30 frames/s (each frame = 33.33 ms), making it possible to determine the temporal characteristics of the gaze during the object-recognition, object-tracking, and object-control phases.

Effect of Age, Physiology, Technical, and Training Characteristics

Since all the athletes were on a national team, a wealth of data was available about their height, weight, percent body fat, $\dot{V}O_2$, blood pressure, anaerobic power, 20 m sprint, vertical reach, spike jump, block jump, and hip flexion. No significant differences were found between the elite and near-elite athletes on any of these variables. These results were therefore consistent with other studies that show that athletes at the upper levels of sport tend to be similar in terms of cardiac function, anaerobic power, muscular strength, power, and body composition (Komi, 1992; McArdle, Katch, & Katch, 2001; Titel & Wutscherk, 1992). The elite and near-elite groups did, however, differ in years of formal training in volleyball, with the elite athletes averaging 12 y of training and the near-elite athletes averaging 7 y.

Consecutive serves were delivered until 10 hits and 10 misses were completed. In addition, percent accuracy was determined over all the serves and was 64% for the elites and 60% for the near-elites, a difference that neared significance ($p < .06$). The near-elites were more accurate in

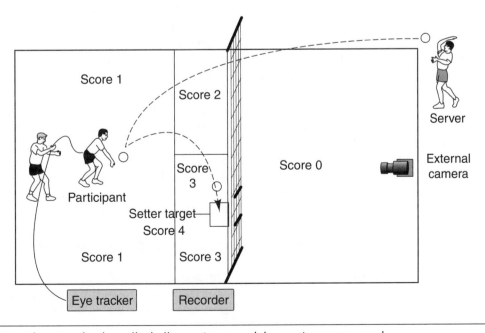

▶ **Figure 7.6**   The setup for the volleyball experiment and the scoring system used.

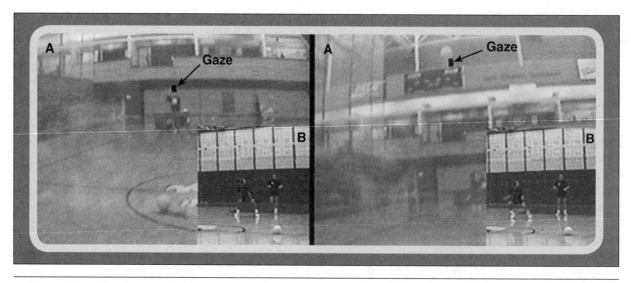

➤ **Figure 7.7**   Two frames of vision-in-action data during the volleyball serve reception.

Reprinted, by permission, from S. McPherson and J.N. Vickers, 2004, "Cognitive control in motor expertise," *International Journal of Sport and Exercise Psychology* 2(3): 274-300.

the experiment than in competition (64% versus 56%), and this was attributed to the floater serves being delivered at a relatively slower speed than what might occur in competition. Duration of the serves was similar for elites (1,465 ms; SD = 88 ms) and near-elites (1,478 ms; SD = 94 ms).

Gaze Control

The duration of the serve was similar for elites and near-elites and averaged 801 ms (SD = 22 ms). During this time, both groups directed their gaze primarily to the ball. In less than 4% of serves there were tracking or fixated gazes to the server's head, hitting arm and hand, or other body locations. The near-elites were more likely to track the ball upward as it was tossed in the serve, and this gaze was associated with lower levels of accuracy. In contrast, the elites fixated the area where the ball was struck by the server's hand (see figure 7.7). This gaze was a characteristic of successful trials and agreed with those reported by Shank and Haywood (1987) in baseball, but ran contrary to those reported in visual-search studies (Salmela & Fiorito, 1979; Williams, Davids, Burwitz, & Williams, 1994; Williams, Ward, Knowles, & Smeeton, 2002).

The athletes tracked the ball on average one time each serve as it approached, but they differed on tracking onset, tracking offset, and duration. The elites tracked the ball significantly longer, (*mean* [M] = 1,400 ms (SD = 709 ms), while the near-elites averaged 768 ms (SD = 726). Five of the six elites initiated tracking as the ball was being served and started to accelerate their gaze in a tracking movement in advance of the ball even before it was struck. Five of the six near-elites initiated tracking late, as the ball approached the far side of the net. The elites continued tracking the ball until it was 109 ms before contact, which was about 2 to 3 m in front, compared with 144 ms for the near-elites or 3 to 4 m in front.

It was clear that the elites were able to seamlessly transition from the fixation that occurred during the serve into a tracking gaze on the ball that continued during the early flight phase—in other words, they anticipated the onset of flight better than the near-elites did. The near-elites lost sight of the ball in the transition from the serve to the flight phase and were only able to regain tracking as the ball approached the middle of the court. Consequently, the near-elites had higher levels of saccades to the ball (elites 28%; near-elites 42%) and more tracking off the ball (elites 6%; near-elites 27%), as well as more gaze that were out of the range of the eye-tracker system (elites 9%; near-elites 25%).

Quiet-Eye Duration in Volleyball

Quiet-eye duration was defined as the portion of tracking on the ball that occurred before the first step to play the ball. The elites had a quiet eye that lasted 432 ms, while the near-elites did not have a quiet eye. That is, they did not have a period of tracking before they began stepping to play the ball. The elite players delayed their stepping movements until they had a clear picture of where the ball was going. In contrast, the near-elites did not stand quietly as the ball was served and approached but instead often began to step even before the server hit the ball, thus making it difficult to maintain the gaze on the ball.

It is not unusual to hear volleyball coaches tell their athletes to track the ball right into their arms. Athletes with this style of gaze control have a distinctive head and shoulder scrunch that occurs at contact. But do skilled performers use this type of head and gaze control at contact? Elites used this style in only 7% of trials, and near-elites in 8%. Instead, the most prevalent gaze at contact, occurring in 73% of elite trials and 49% of near-elites trials, was to leave, or park, the gaze in front as the ball was contacted. This gaze behavior created a period of **eye–head stabilization** at contact that was similar to that reported by Ripoll and Fleurance (1988) and by Rodrigues et al. (2002) in table tennis. During this time the gaze was maintained in front and in the spatial area where the ball traveled after it left the receiver's forearm. This meant that the receiver easily regained visual control over the ball immediately after contact. The near-elites were more prone to look toward the setter target before the ball contacted their arms, which they did in 20% of all trials (versus less than 5% for the elites).

Motor Control

Vision-in-action data also provide valuable insight into the motor control. The total number of steps to play the ball and the number of step corrections made before each reception were derived from the motor image (B of figure 7.7). The mean number of steps to play the ball was similar for elite and near-elite groups, but the near-elites had significantly more step corrections. This meant that they changed course more often as the ball was coming toward them.

The location where the ball was received was coded from the motor image in figure 7.7. The near-elites received the ball at more difficult locations (low below the knees and high at the shoulders), while the elites tended to receive the ball at the optimal location (waist height). The elites also aligned themselves so that they received the ball down the midline of the body, while the near-elites made more receptions to one side or another.

The combined results for gaze control, step correction, and ball-reception locations suggested that the elites read the serves better than the near-elites, thereby enabling better anticipation of the ball's flight. The near-elites often stepped in the wrong direction and then had to recover using step corrections that culminated in a reception that was not at the optimal location.

In summary, we see that elite athletes in volleyball are adept at controlling the gaze within and across the three phases of the task. In the object-recognition phase, they fixate the ball at the location where the ball is struck by the server's hand, and they begin tracking even before the server hits the ball. It appears that they anticipate the ball's flight and avoid the saccade that occurs when the gaze must transition from a fixed location to one of tracking. Second, during object tracking they track the ball to within 2 to 3 m of contact. Third, during object control, their gaze remains parked in front and lies in wait until the ball passes through the visual field on the way to the setter target. This gaze sequence facilitates the elite players' ability to physically play the ball—they use fewer step corrections and receive the ball at more optimal locations. In contrast, the near-elites are late in initiating tracking on the ball, track the ball for shorter durations, and find it difficult to sustain tracking near to contact. Prior to contact, many also look to the setter target. These gaze behaviors appeared to contribute to a greater number of corrective steps, reception of the ball at more difficult locations, and overall lower levels of performance.

Quiet-Eye Training in Volleyball

The Team Canada athletes from the study by Vickers and Adolphe (1997) were invited to participate in a 6 wk quiet-eye training program where the goal was to improve their ball tracking and pass to the setter (Adolphe, Vickers, & LaPlante, 1997). A quiet-eye training program was designed in which athletes received video feedback of their gaze behavior, followed by five quiet-eye training sessions on court. The training sessions consisted of video feedback of their vision-in-action data and participation in a progression of exercises on the volleyball court that were designed to improve quiet-eye tracking and performance in both the experimental and game setting.

The athletes were first shown the gaze control of an elite prototype. Four gaze behaviors were emphasized, as follows:

➤ During the serve, the ball should be detected using a fixation that is located at the coincident point of the toss and where the server's hand makes contact. Athletes should avoid tracking the ball upward since this may cause their gaze to lag behind the ball after contact.

➤ As the ball is struck by the server's hand, continuous tracking on the ball should be maintained throughout the early flight phase.

➤ Tracking offset should occur when the ball is 2 to 3 m in front and well before the pass is received.

➤ The gaze should be held, or parked, in front as the pass occurs (eye–head stabilization).

The athletes were then shown their own vision-in-action data on dual monitors and asked to determine the difference between their gaze control and that of the prototype. A questioning approach was used, where the athletes were given time to view both their own vision-in-action data and that of the prototype in order to be able to see, understand, and better internalize their focus of attention and control of gaze as well as that of the elite performer. The athletes were then asked to make a decision about how they could improve their gaze and attention control in practices.

All training sessions were conducted during the regular practice times on a regulation volleyball court and were 30 min in length. Four quiet-eye exercises were designed to facilitate the early detection and improved tracking of the ball. These exercises were based on an event from the life of the baseball player Ted Williams, who commented that he could see the seams on the baseball as he hit it. Some reporters

challenged him to actually do this and placed numbers and letters on baseballs and had him attempt to identify these as he hit the ball. He indeed could call them out before or as the ball was struck. The quiet-eye training exercises were as follows:

➤ *Track and pass a tennis ball.* The receiver stood about 3 m from the wall. A partner tossed a tennis ball over the receiver's head so that it rebounded off the wall. The receiver had to track the ball and pass continually against the wall, progressing from tracking and catching to passing the ball using the forearm action. The speed of the toss was increased.

➤ *Track and detect drill.* Numbers between 1 and 20 were placed on the volleyball, as shown in figure 7.8. When the ball was served and in flight, the receiver called out the number as soon as he could see it. Variations included using letters instead of numbers and placing both a letter and a number on the ball with the receiver calling both. Requiring the athlete to call the number acts as a cognitive trigger that tells the athlete and the coach whether the athlete could indeed see the number before passing the ball. When the athlete mastered one symbol, the complexity of the exercise was increased by placing more than one symbol on the ball.

➤ *Track and detect drill with a barrier.* The ball was served from behind a barrier (blackboard) situated so as to block the view of the server. The receiver tracked the ball in flight and called out numbers, letters, or both.

➤ *Track and detect drill after a full-body turn.* The receiver stood on the baseline with his back to the court. The coach called "Go" after the server tossed the ball. On the signal, the player turned 180°, detected and tracked the ball, and called out the letter, number, or both. This drill progressed to full serves of varying types and speeds.

One month after the quiet-eye training sessions were completed, the athletes' gazes were recorded on court once again using the vision-in-action system. The results showed that after quiet-eye training, all the athletes had an earlier tracking onset and had improved their tracking duration, and most displayed the ability to hold their gaze parked in a moment of eye–head

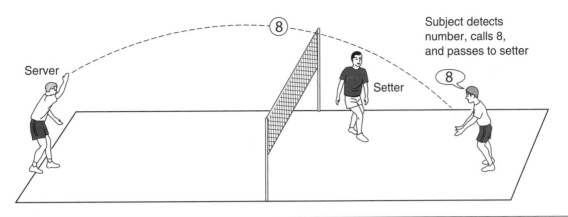

> **Figure 7.8** Volleyball track and detect drill with a barrier.

stabilization as the ball was passed. In addition to improving their quiet-eye tracking and gaze control, the athletes also improved in a number of skills that were not overtly trained. Their step corrections decreased, as did the location where they received the ball. Overall, they moved into position quicker and took the ball in the midline of the body better, which improved their performance in the task. These results suggest that knowing how to improve gaze and attention aids the self-organization of the skill without direct coaching of the motor behavior.

All of the athletes played internationally, so it was possible to compare their serve-pass statistics with those of athletes from other countries playing at the same level. The players were followed for 3 y, and figure 7.9 shows that those athletes who received quiet-eye training steadily improved their pass accuracy (means 65%, 69%, 72%), while the pass accuracy of those athletes who did not receive the same training remained relatively constant over the three seasons, as would be expected (means 65%, 68%, 61%).

Relationship Between Gaze Control and Verbal Reports

A number of studies have examined the verbal reports of athletes in response to questions about their performance (see Ericsson & Simon, 1993; McPherson, 1993), but few have also looked at the relationship between control of the gaze and the performers' response to questions about how they focus when they perform.

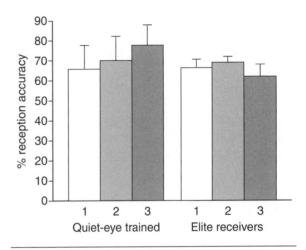

> **Figure 7.9** Percent improvement of the quiet eye–trained group and players in serve-pass receptions over three seasons of international volleyball competition.

In a study on the volleyball reception and pass similar to that found in Vickers and Adolphe (1997), McPherson and Vickers (2004) examined the relationship between volleyball players' verbal reports and their gaze behaviors while receiving serves and passing to the setter area. The goal was to determine the extent to which athletes' verbal reports were also reflected in their gaze control. That is, when volleyball athletes provide a verbal report of what they are seeing during the performance of a trial, to what extent is their verbal information reflected in the actual gaze behavior recorded when performing the skill?

Five male volleyball players volunteered to be participants. Two athletes (E1, E5) were junior members of Team Canada and played internationally, while three (E2, E3, E4) were trying out for the team during the summer training camp where the data were collected. The goal of the task was to complete the pass to the setter area for accuracy on a regulation volleyball court, as in Vickers and Adolphe's 1997 study. Questions were posed to the athletes and verbal reports collected both before data collection (in pretask interviews) and on court at regular intervals.

Figure 7.10 shows the relationship between passing accurately to the setter and the number of verbal statements the athletes made about how they tracked the ball (e.g., "watch the ball, focus on the ball, look at the ball, see the ball"). The four athletes who had the highest accuracy in passing (E1, E2, E3, E5) made the fewest comments about their ball tracking, while E4, who had the greatest difficulty passing, had the highest number of verbal reports.

McPherson and Vickers also wondered if there was a relationship between passing accuracy and the relative duration of tracking the ball. Figure 7.11 shows that the athletes with the

highest accuracy (E1, E2, E3, E5) were uniform in having an early onset of tracking on the ball, followed by a period of early tracking (quiet eye) and a period of eye–head stabilization (the parked gaze) prior to ball contact. In contrast, although E4 spent 75% of total ball flight time in tracking compared with 40% to 50% for the other athletes, his tracking occurred too late, thus not giving him enough time to have the stable head and parked gaze that are required to ensure accuracy. Overall, the results showed that E4's overemphasis on one aspect of the skill (ball tracking) worked to his detriment in a skill that requires the use of a number of gaze behaviors that are intricately timed and sequenced. The study suggests that quiet-eye training where athletes are able to see their gaze control and are asked to verbally describe the nature of tracking relative to an expert prototype may lead to improvement in this aspect of the skill. And since elite gaze control is understood in this skill, training programs can be used to guide performers to better sequencing of their gaze over time (Adolphe et al., 1997).

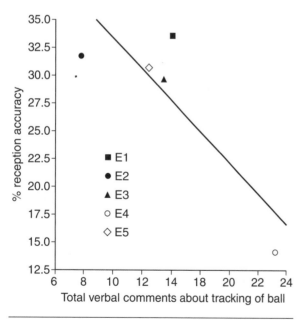

➤ **Figure 7.10** Bivariate regression plot showing the relationship between the accuracy of the passes to the setter and the number of statements made about tracking the ball.

Reprinted, by permission, from S. McPherson and J.N. Vickers, 2004, "Cognitive control in motor expertise," *International Journal of Sport and Exercise Psychology* 2: 274-300.

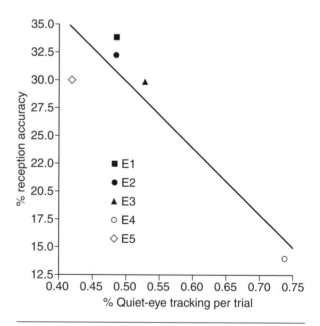

➤ **Figure 7.11** Bivariate regression plot showing the relationship between accuracy in passing to the setter and the relative percent of time spent tracking the ball each trial.

Reprinted, by permission, from S. McPherson and J.N. Vickers, 2004, "Cognitive control in motor expertise," *International Journal of Sport and Exercise Psychology* 2: 274-300.

Gaze Control in Ice Hockey Goaltending

The final interceptive timing task presented in the gaze framework in figure 4.1 is ice hockey goaltending (Panchuk & Vickers, 2006). In this task the gaze of elite ice hockey goaltenders was determined while they either stopped shots from an elite shooter or were scored on. The gaze of the goaltenders was analyzed during all three phases (object recognition, object tracking, and object control). In this task, the flight duration of the puck averaged only 115 ms during 5 m shots and 179 ms for shots taken from 10 m. Recall that in the table tennis study described earlier, even elite players were unable to return the ball to targets when they could track the ball for only 272 ms. How is it, then, that ice hockey goaltenders can stop pucks with such short flight times?

High-speed sports such as ice hockey goaltending are characterized by perceptual uncertainty and time constraints that require a performer to process visual information and perform within a limited time frame (Ripoll, 1991). During a hockey game, goaltenders face shots that travel upward of 160 kph (Hache, 2002). These shots are often taken from point-blank distances and at speeds that reach angular velocities in excess of 500°/s (Bahill & LaRitz, 1984; Pola & Wyatt, 1991). When an object reaches velocities that great, the functional capacity of the human visual system is exceeded and a performer can no longer accurately track the object to contact using pursuit eye movements. Despite these limitations in pursuit tracking, goaltenders in ice hockey stop an average of 90% of all shots they face (www.nhl.com).

The majority of our knowledge about how goaltenders respond to shots comes from studies where goaltenders respond to videotape simulations of soccer shots presented under different spatial–temporal constraints (McMorris, Copeman, Corcoran, Saunders & Potter, 1993; Salmela & Fiorito, 1979; Williams & Burwitz, 1993). By occluding portions of information at various times during the preparation and execution of the shot, researchers assessed the extent to which goaltenders are able to make the right decision relative to the availability of information. Earlier in this chapter, a visual occlusion study by Salmela and Fiorito (1979) also showed that ice

hockey goaltenders can make saves if they can see the final 83 ms of the shot as it is delivered but have much greater difficulty if 300 ms of the shot are occluded.

Savelsbergh, van der Kamp, Williams, and Ward (2005) investigated the visual-search behaviors of 16 expert soccer goaltenders classified as successful or unsuccessful in making saves during simulated penalty kicks. Their study sought to resolve the "somewhat contradictory" (p. 1687) findings within the literature on soccer goaltending regarding the main source of predictive information during the penalty kick. Tyldesley, Bootsma, and Bomhoff (1982) and Williams and Burwitz (1993) showed that the hips, kicking leg, and trunk were fixated just before and during ball–foot contact, while Franks and Harvey (1997) identified the nonkicking foot. The goaltenders were divided into two groups (successful and nonsuccessful) based on their performance in a goaltending simulation where they viewed 30 penalty kicks and predicted the direction of the shot by moving a joystick as if to intercept the ball. The videotaped shots were performed by elite youth players (aged 18.9 y) who directed the ball to one of six target locations using deceptive moves whenever possible. The clips included the players' approach to the ball, their actions before and during ball contact, and the first portion of ball flight. Average ball flight time was 648 ms and mean ball velocity was 16.84 m/s; no measures of the approach or kicking action were provided and only a small portion of the ball flight was permitted.

The successful goaltenders saved 47.8% of penalties faced, while the nonsuccessful saved only 21.1%. When the two groups were compared with the group of novices from Savelsbergh et al. (2002), it was found that the novices saved 25.9% of shots; therefore the unsuccessful expert goaltenders performed no better than novices. The successful players stopped more penalties and were more accurate at predicting the side and height of the shots. They also initiated their response closer to foot–ball contact (230 ms prior) compared with the unsuccessful players (359 ms) and the novices (479 ms). These differences were not reflected in a general reaction-time test (done during the pretest), which found the three groups to have similar reaction times (ranging from

238-262 ms). The successful players therefore delayed their response, allowing more information to be gained during the run-up to the kick. Interestingly, there were no differences in fixation duration for the successful and unsuccessful goaltenders (average 501 and 529 ms, respectively), or number of fixations (average 3.0 and 2.9 ms), but differences were found in fixation location. The successful goaltenders fixated the nonkicking foot, which was planted about 350 ms before ball–foot contact, while the unsuccessful goaltenders fixated the head and kicking leg.

Overall, studies in soccer goaltending (Franks & Harvey, 1997; Savelsbergh et al., 2002, 2005; Tyldesley et al., 1982; Williams & Burwitz, 1993) have consistently shown that fixations to the body of the shooter underlie higher levels of performance. Although a controversy exists in terms of the final source of that information (e.g., the nonkicking leg or the head and kicking leg), these studies are universal in showing that body-based cues from the shooter are most important, not those related to the flight of the ball.

There has been only one attempt to examine the eye movements of ice hockey goaltenders as they face shots in a live ice hockey setting. In chapter 2, a study by Bard and Fleury (1981) was presented that showed that both novice and expert goaltenders focused the majority of their fixations on the puck and stick, and not the body of the shooter.

In order to determine how goaltenders stop shots with such short flight times, as well as the critical cues underlying saves, Panchuk and Vickers (2006) recorded the gaze and motor behavior of elite goaltenders on ice as they attempted to stop wrist shots taken from 5 m and 10 m by the best shooters on their teams (as selected by their coaches). The setup is as shown in figure 7.12. Eight elite goaltenders were included who played competitively for an average of 15 y (range was 12-19 y). The mean save percentage for the goaltenders from the most recently completed competitive season was .88 (range was .77-.92), which compares to 92% for the National Hockey League.

Vision-in-action data were collected, as shown in figure 7.13. The gaze image (B) was recorded by the scene camera on the eye tracker and shows

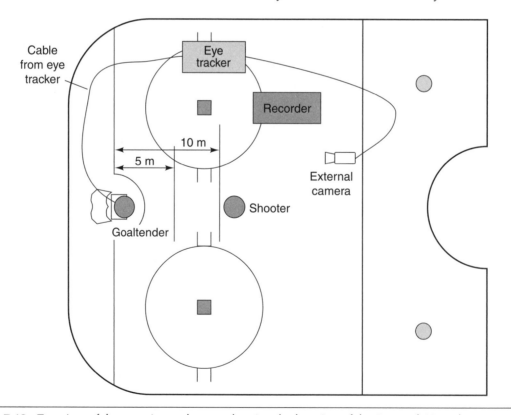

> **Figure 7.12**　Top view of the experimental setup, showing the location of the 5 m and 10 m shots.

Reprinted from Human Movement Science, Vol. 25, D. Panchuk and J.N. Vickers, Gaze behaviors of goaltenders under spatial-temporal constraints, pp. 733-752, Copyright 2006, with permission from Elsevier.

the scene in front of the goaltender as the shots were taken. Shown on image B is the gaze cursor, which indicated the participants' point of gaze with an accuracy of 2° of visual angle (width of the cursor). The motor image (C) was recorded by an external camera that recorded the movements of the goaltender, shooter, and puck as the shots were taken. The eye image (A) was recorded by the eye camera on the eye tracker and contains horizontal and vertical axes for the pupil and corneal reflex, which were produced through a helmet-mounted infrared light source reflected off the visor into the eye, allowing measurement of the eye line of gaze with respect to the helmet. Images A, B, and C were originally collected at a rate of 30 Hz (or 33.3 ms/frame). This data was subsequently deinterlaced at a rate of 60 fields each s (1 field = 16.67 ms).

Percent saves made by the goaltenders were lower than what had been recorded in games. The goaltenders saved 71% of shots from 5 m and 77% from 10 m, compared with a game average of 88% (range was 77%-92%). This might have been due to the experimental task being more difficult because the shots were taken close to the net and there was nothing obstructing the shooter's sight. During the course of a game, a goaltender faces approximately 30 shots from a variety of distances, speeds, and angles, and not all would be considered quality opportunities. The lower save percentage may also be a reflection of the high skill level of the shooters, who were among the very best on their teams, whereas in games shots are taken by a greater variety of low- and high-skilled shooters.

Phases of the Action

Five phases were identified, the first three belonging to the shooter and the final two to the goaltender. The beginning of the preparation time (PT) was preset at 1 s back from the release of the puck off the shooter's stick, which was an ample amount of time given the elite level of the shooters. The onset of body movement (BM) occurred when any part of the shooter's body moved as the shot was initiated. The shooting movement (SM) occurred with the first observable motion of the shooter's stick and ended when the puck left the stick. Reaction time (RT) was the period of time from release of the puck from the stick until the first observable movement of any part of the goaltender's body to initiate a save. The movement time (MT) followed the offset of the RT and included the goaltender's stopping movements with a foot, hand, or stick. The temporal order

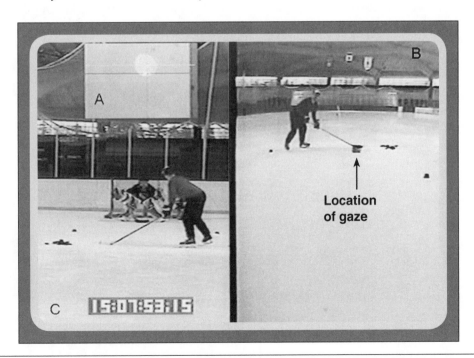

➤ **Figure 7.13** A frame of vision-in-action data showing (A) the eye of the goaltender in the eye image, (B) the location of his gaze in the gaze image, and (C) the movements of shooter and goaltender in the motor image as taken by an external camera.

of these phases did not differ between shooters or across trials. Figure 7.14 shows the duration (%) of the phases during the 5 m and 10 m shots. The durations of the phases differed significantly for the 5 m and 10 m shots. In the 5 m shot, the shooters used longer preparation time, whereas during the 10 m shots, the shooters employed a shorter preparation time. The first movement of the body and the initiation of the shooting movements occurred later in the 5 m shots, providing the goaltenders with a reduced window of time when information could be picked up, while in the 10 m shots they had more time to read the cues available. Yet none of these differences affected the goaltenders' ability to make saves.

The goaltenders' *RT* phase was the period of time from the release of the puck until their first movement to stop the puck. Mean *RT* was very brief (20 ms to 46 ms), well under the threshold of visual reaction time at both distances, which we saw in chapter 3 averages 180 to 200 ms for novel tasks but can be as low as 100 ms on well-learned ones (Carlton, 1981a; 1981b). The short *RT* results provide evidence that the goaltenders used information from earlier in the shot to anticipate the shots. These *RT* results are similar to those previously found in ice hockey goaltending (Salmela & Fiorito, 1979) and in soccer goaltending (McMorris et al. 1993; McMorris & Colenso, 1996; McMorris &

Hauxwell, 1997; Savelsbergh et al., 2005; 2002; van der Kamp, 2006; Williams & Burwitz, 1993). Only one saving movement was observed for each trial, and the *MTs* were very fast, averaging between 115 and 178.54 ms. Although the goaltenders faced two significantly different shots in terms of the temporal duration of the shooters' actions, overall the *MT* employed to stop the shots from both distances did not significantly affect the goaltenders' performance (saves versus goals).

Gaze Locations

Eight fixation or tracking locations were used by the goaltenders—the shooter's head, the shooter's upper body, the shooter's lower body, the puck, the shooter's stick, the puck–stick combination, the ice in front of the release point of the puck, and the ice in front of the goal. Figure 7.15 shows the percentage of fixations to each location. The greatest concentrations of locations were on the stick and puck as the wrist shot was prepared and executed (70.53%), followed by the ice in front of the stick (25.68%). Very few fixations were allocated to the head (0.42%), upper body (0.63%), lower body (0.42%), puck (0.42%), or ice nearer to the net (0.63%). The goaltenders were similar in selecting just one focus for their gaze and attention as the shots were prepared and executed. These

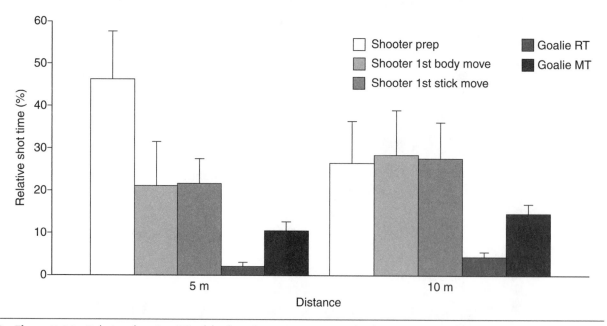

> **Figure 7.14**   Relative duration (%) of the five phases (preparation, body movement, stick movement, reaction time, and movement time) during the 5 m and 10 m shots.

Reprinted from Human Movement Science, Vol. 25, D. Panchuk and J.N. Vickers, Gaze behaviors of goaltenders under spatial-temporal constraints, pp. 733-752, Copyright 2006, with permission from Elsevier.

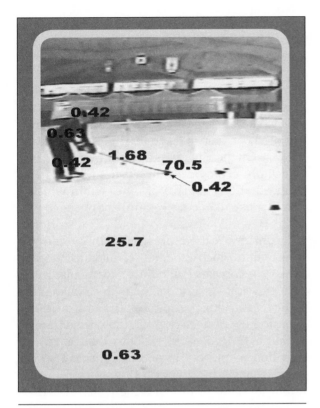

➤ **Figure 7.15** Percentage (%) of fixation and tracking by location.

Reprinted from Human Movement Science, Vol. 25, D. Panchuk and J.N. Vickers, Gaze behaviors of goaltenders under spatial-temporal constraints, pp. 733-752, Copyright 2006, with permission from Elsevier.

results therefore agree with Bard and Fleury (1981), who found that experts and novice goaltenders focused the majority of their fixations on the puck and stick; however, they differ from those found in soccer, where body-based cues, especially directed to the nonkicking leg, have been reported to underlie higher levels of performance (Franks & Harvey, 1997; Savelsbergh et al., 2005).

The results in both soccer and ice hockey suggest that the primary focus for elite goaltenders is the one that first gives away the shooter's intentions. For wrist shots in ice hockey, the focus is on how the shooter manipulates the movement of the puck on the stick as the shot is taken. Shooters develop a number of deceptive techniques where they lag the stick, delay the wrist snap, roll the puck, and perform other maneuvers to hide the true direction of the shot, making close attention to these aspects a necessary skill. Salmela and Fiorito (1979) suggested that the orientation of the stick on the wrist shot provides critical cues for the goaltender, a claim supported by the results from this study. Because goaltenders focus on

the stick–puck interface, they are able to read the orientation of the stick during the shooting action and thus anticipate the direction of the shot. Awareness of this would give the goaltender the opportunity to make a prediction about the direction, height, and speed of the puck. Taken together, these factors create a situation where the gaze control strategy used by the performers zeroes in on the area of the task that contains the most pertinent visual information. This would also suggest that the most critical cue required for initiating the stop occurred during the final *SM* phase of the shot, but as will be shown in the next section, saves occurred when the final fixation, or quiet-eye onset, was much earlier than this.

Quiet-Eye Onset, Duration, and Offset

Quiet-eye *(QE)* duration was significantly longer on saves than on goals for both distances. Figure 7.16 shows the duration of *QE* on saves and goals superimposed over the durations of the five phases of the 5 m and 10 m shots. *QE* onset occurred during the first 300 ms of all shots, before either the first movement of the shooter's body or first movement of the stick. The *QE* period extended over the *BM, SM,* and *RT* phases and had an offset within two frames (66.6 ms) of the puck leaving the stick.

QE duration was longer on saves than goals at both the 5 m (saves 935.83 ms; goals 774.17 ms) and 10 m (saves 968.75 ms; goals 878.13 ms). The mean *QE* duration ranged from a low of 61.1% of total trial time to a high of 84.7 %. More importantly, figure 7.17 shows that all eight goaltenders had a longer *QE* duration on saves than on goals at both distances, in terms of both absolute (ms) and relative time (%). Note also the relatively small standard deviation, indicating most of the goaltenders had similar durations.

If the critical cue to stop the puck appeared in the final 240 to 335 ms when the wrist shot was executed, why did the goaltenders fixate the stick and puck for such a long duration beforehand? A plausible explanation for the long quiet eye comes from studies by Morya, Ranvaud, and Pinheiro (2003) and van der Kamp (2006), who investigated the effect of keeper-dependent and keeper-independent strategies on the shooter's ability to make penalty shots in soccer. When a keeper-dependent strategy is used, the shooters

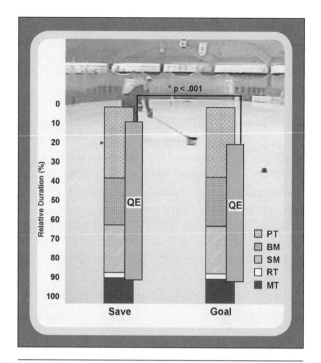

> ➤ **Figure 7.16** Coupled relative durations (%, *SD*) on saves and goals of mean phase durations (%, *SD*) and mean *QE* (%, *SD*).

change their shot in response to the goaltender's actions. When a keeper-independent strategy is used, any action by the goaltender is ignored and the shot is taken according to a preset plan. In a computer-based simulation of the penalty kick, Morya et al. (2003) found that soccer shooters are able to successfully change their response if they are cued between 400 and 500 ms before the ball contact. On the other hand, van der Kamp (2006), in a more ecologically based field simulation, found that the interval of time within which a penalty taker could successfully be changed was large, ranging between 174 and 773 ms prior to ball contact. We therefore see that the window of time within which a shooter can make a change in the shot is very large, and thus a goaltender has to be prepared to respond to a shooter's changes in tactics over a long time period. The long quiet-eye duration fits perfectly within these time frames.

Successful goaltenders focus their gaze and attention on only one location in order to respond to any changes in strategy by the shooters during a long interval of time. Hache (2002) describes more about why a singular long-duration focus on the puck is critical in a game like ice hockey: "Along with anticipating a shot, concentration is

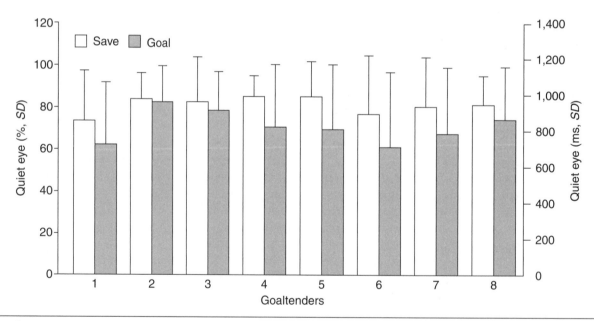

> ➤ **Figure 7.17** Relative (%) and absolute (ms) duration of quiet eye (*M* ± *s*) for the goaltenders.

also very important in stopping pucks. A quick reaction time is useless unless it is backed up by a relentless focus on the puck. Just a blink of the eye or a moment of distraction, and the next thing you will notice is the other team celebrating a goal. This is why NHL goaltenders try to focus on the puck itself rather than the puck carrier or other players. Sure, knowing where potential puck receivers are is helpful (peripheral vision is useful for this purpose), but the small black dot is what the goalie is interested in" (p. 135). Finally, given that this study was done on ice under realistic conditions and that a high-speed, ballistic movement was required in order to make a save, it is plausible that the long quiet eye also facilitated a degree of physiological readiness in which the goaltenders prepared their body to react to the velocity of the puck, although this explanation warrants further exploration.

The ability to make saves in ice hockey is therefore not significantly affected by differences in the duration of the shooters' actions, the ability to track the puck in flight, or the distance from which the shot was taken; instead, it is dependent on the goaltender's ability to maintain a prolonged quiet-eye fixation on the puck and stick within 3° of visual angle from early in the preparation of the shot until a short period after release of the puck. It is during this time that any changes in the shooter's strategy must be detected and responded to. Virtually no fixations are directed toward the actions of the shooter's body, and in this sense Panchuk and Vickers' (2006) results differ from those found in soccer, where the most critical cues appear to come from the nonkicking foot (Franks & Harvey, 1997; Savelsbergh et al., 2005). This is not to negate the importance of body-based cues in ice hockey goaltending, but these cues had to have been detected using the ambient system since fixation and tracking on the puck and stick or on the area of ice just in front of the release point of the puck accounted for 96.20% of all fixation and tracking gazes in the current study.

From a theoretical approach, these differences would fit within a **constraints-led perspective** (Newell & McDonald, 1994), which states that task constraints (organism, environment, and task) affect how a skill is performed and how the gaze is controlled (Williams, Janelle, & Davids, 2004). It is also important to stress that all of the goaltenders were more successful when they had a longer quiet eye at both distances. Since a shooter can successfully change the direction of a shot up to 773 ms before release and in as little time as 174 ms (van der Kamp, 2006), the long duration of quiet eye was necessary to permit the detection of a wide range of changes that could occur within this time period. Finally, the percent of tracking gaze on the puck as it traveled to the goal was negligible, as was the percent of gaze in the crease area.

Gaze Control in Action

Select a training partner or partners and develop a quiet-eye decision-training program for goaltending (select either soccer, ice hockey, or field hockey). Follow these steps:

1. List five quiet-eye characteristics that are needed to perform well in goaltending. When listing each characteristic, name the cognitive skill that is most important (anticipation, attention, focus and concentration, memory, pattern recognition, problem solving, or decision making).

2. Second, design a drill or progression of drills that will help you and your partner make more saves in goaltending.

3. Practice the drills for 20 to 30 min per day. Your main goal is to develop the optimal focus as the shot is prepared and executed.

Record your results. At the beginning of the first practice, record your pretraining accuracy for the first 10 shots before you do any quiet-eye training. Try to complete five training sessions. At the end of each practice session, record your percent accuracy on the final 10 trials on the blank graph provided on page 134.

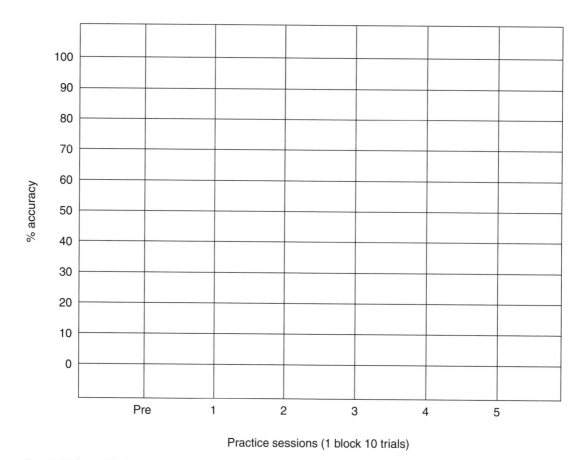

Practice sessions (1 block 10 trials)

From J.N. Vickers, 2007, *Perception, cognition, and decision training: The quiet eye in action* (Champaign, IL: Human Kinetics).

Prepare a short report in which you discuss the following topics:

1. List the five gaze control or quiet-eye characteristics that you selected to work on.
2. Provide a sketch of the drills used to train your quiet eye. Explain how each drill was used to improve your cognitive and quiet-eye focus.
3. What methods of practice did you use? (See chapters 9 through 12 for some ideas about how to vary your methods of training.)
4. Include the figure of results you generated from the blank graph and explain your percentage change over the five practices. Did you improve or get worse?
5. Using information from this chapter, discuss why your results occurred. In your opinion, what were the underlying reasons for your results?

Gaze Control in Tactical Tasks

◄◄ *Where Have We Been?*

In chapter 7, gaze control during interceptive timing tasks was described. Two major subcategories were presented, gaze when object flight is predictable and when it is unpredictable. Since objects can be propelled with either characteristic, the elite performer is one who has developed two gaze control strategies, one for when the flight of the object is relatively constant and a second for when the object moves erratically. In addition, all interceptive timing tasks have three gaze control phases: object recognition, object tracking, and object control. The gaze has to be controlled optimally within and across these three phases in order to achieve a high level of success.

➤➤ *Where Are We Going?*

In this chapter, gaze control during tactical tasks is described. Gaze control in tactical tasks often subsumes the first two categories of gaze control (targeting and interceptive timing), but it also adds a third quality—pattern recognition. Athletes must learn to read meaningful patterns during two subcategories: locomotion over and around objects and locations, and during offensive and defensive plays. All team sports have developed sophisticated offensive and defensive set plays that must be instantly recognized and the appropriate actions taken under severe time pressure. In addition, elite players are able to recognize and exploit novel patterns of play.

What Are Tactical Tasks?

Tactics can be defined as the science of organizing and maneuvering forces in games, battles, or other endeavors to achieve a limited or immediate aim. Most tactical situations require the planning of maneuvers as they will occur during actual contact with a competitor or an enemy. A word used synonymously with tactics is strategy, which is the science and art of planning and conducting a contest, sport, or military campaign. Strategy is also described as the carefully devised plan of action to achieve a goal, or the art of developing or carrying out such a plan.

Tactical tasks in sport require control of the gaze and attention over multiple visuomotor workspaces, within which one or more spotlights of attention may be found that enable the performer to be successful. The gaze framework presented in figure 4.1 shows two subcategories of tactical tactics: (1) locomotion and (2) offensive and defensive plays. Both subsume the gaze control and attention found in targeting and interceptive timing tasks and add a third dimension, the ability to read and extract meaning from dynamic patterns of action.

Virtually all tactical tasks require **locomotion,** which is "the movement of one's body around an environment, coordinated specifically to the local or proximal surrounds—the environment that is directly accessible to our sensory and motor systems at a given movement (or, at most, within a few moments). When we locomote, we solve behavioral problems such as identifying surfaces to stand on, avoiding obstacles and barriers, directing our movements toward perceptible landmarks, and going through openings without bumping into various things" (Montello, 2005, p. 258-259). Both object and travel fixations are used during locomotion. **Object fixations** are directed toward objects in space, thus allowing the momentary detection of information. During object fixations the gaze is stationary on an object, even as the feet continue walking or running. **Travel fixations** are carried along by the feet, and there is a continuous flow of information at the speed of locomotion.

This chapter describes the gaze of people walking over and around obstacles, as well as when learning to perform in a task where the solution to success is difficult to discern (a trap task). The gaze of elite speed skaters is also described as they skate at full speed on an Olympic oval. In all cases, performers must control their gaze over multiple visuomotor workspaces that may include spotlights for their attention. Next, gaze control during tactical tasks is described. Tactical tasks differ from locomotor tasks in that they are more complex due to the presence of an opponent whose intention is to make the tactical workspace difficult to discern. The penalty shot against a goaltender in ice hockey is presented, and finally, gaze during soccer and ice hockey offensive and defensive plays is described. Extensive knowledge often has to be acquired in order to understand the many set and novel plays that characterize modern sport. All of these tasks have one thing in common: It is not enough to fixate a target (as in the targeting category of tasks) or intercept a moving object (as in the interceptive timing category of tasks); it is necessary to extract the meaning from patterns of dynamical action and get into positions where these tasks can be performed successfully. To do this requires visual-spatial intelligence, which is described in the next section.

Visual-Spatial Intelligence

Visual-spatial intelligence is "the ability to navigate across town, comprehend an animated display of the functioning human heart, view complex multivariate data on a company's website, or read an architectural blueprint and form a three-dimensional mental picture of a house" (Shah & Miyake, 2005, p. i). Visual-spatial intelligence is central to sport performance and requires an ability to read complex patterns of movements, resulting in actions that lead to a goal being attained. The ability to comprehend the often abstract nature of the spatial organization of moving athletes and objects is a special skill required in sport. Within sport there exist well-known set plays (e.g., give and go; the screen; the fast break; zone defense; person-to-person defense), as well as novel tactical situations that arise.

Team games are not the only sports that require visual-spatial intelligence; virtually all sports involve some form of tactics. Consider that in many forms of racing, athletes have to read the configuration of ever-changing packs of racers; drafting is a tactic used in cycling and speed skating that requires the ability to gauge the position of oneself to others at high speed; and triathlon athletes must develop the ability to find their way while swimming in open water and while riding and racing within large groups of competitors. Visual-spatial intelligence is also needed to determine the best route down a ski race course, a kayak course, or when sailing.

Often athletes may be good at performing a specific skill (e.g., shooting on goal), but they may have trouble reading complex patterns of moving players and making the best decisions under extreme temporal pressure. Terms such as *game sense, court sense,* and *court intelligence* have been used to describe people who have a high level of visual-spatial intelligence. These individuals know how to read complex tactical plays and position themselves at just the right spot at the right time to receive a pass, stop an opponent, or set up a teammate.

Tversky (2005, p. 2) has suggested that human spatial thinking is made up of four components: "the space of the body, the space surrounding the body, the space of navigation, and the space of external representations." These four spaces can also be related to the four principles underlying gaze control that were presented in chapter 4. Recall that the number and type of locations and objects that need to be fixated are important, as is the number of visuomotor workspaces over which the gaze must be controlled. Within each visuomotor workspace exists a spotlight of attention that must be attended to in order for optimal gaze–action coupling to occur. It is through the use of these gaze characteristics that athletes develop a fine sense for the space of their body, the space surrounding the body, the space of navigation, and the space of external representations.

When learning a motor skill, we first have to become aware of and master the spaces within which we perform. To do this, fixations and tracking gazes are directed to the objects and locations that are of greatest use. These may be arrayed over one visuomotor workspace or over many. Part of being spatially intelligent is an ability to access this information as efficiently as possible. Within each visuomotor workspace there may be a spotlight of attention that is key in determining how the space will be navigated. Over time and with practice, skilled motor performers develop internal representations of all the visuomotor workspaces that exist in their sport, thus allowing them to move with ease and effectiveness under all conditions of play. An integral part of spatial

intelligence is the ability to couple the gaze with the appropriate motor behaviors in a wide variety of both expected and unexpected environments.

Context and Target Gaze Control

Neisser (1967, 1976) and more recently Tenenbaum (2003) haved proposed a model in which performers control their gaze in different ways. Tenenbaum (2003) explains that in tactical settings, athletes have to know "where to direct the gaze to capture the most important features in the environmental display" (p. 194). Figure 8.1 presents the two types of gaze control he proposes for expert (left) and novice (right) athletes. When elite athletes face a complex tactical problem, they maintain a fixation in the center of the display from which peripheral cues are perceived as part of larger chunks of information. **Chunking** occurs in memory when diverse pieces of information are consolidated into meaningful concepts, ideas, or sequences of thought or actions. Because elite athletes have richer knowledge structures, they are able to orient their gaze to the center of the display and use their peripheral vision to control and monitor the action. Others have referred to this location as a **visual pivot** (Ripoll, 1991; Williams, Davids, & Williams, 1999). It is suggested that elite performers are able to perceive complex perceptual workspaces by looking at a central location that activates large chunks of information in memory. Novice or nonexpert athletes differ from experts in directing their gaze to discrete targets located throughout the display. In this case, the athletes are described as target controlled and do not have the depth of chunked knowledge to understand what is in the periphery using the ambient system. Therefore, they have to look directly at the objects and locations in the display. This type of gaze control is considered to be less effective.

The bottom of figure 8.1 shows two different long-term working memory (LTWM) systems, taken from the work of Ericsson and Kintsch (1995). The expert (on the left) has a richer store of knowledge from which to retrieve information and solutions, whereas the novice (on the right) has less knowledge to draw upon. As a consequence, Tenenbaum (2003, p. 196) argues the elite athlete is able to perceive the overall pattern

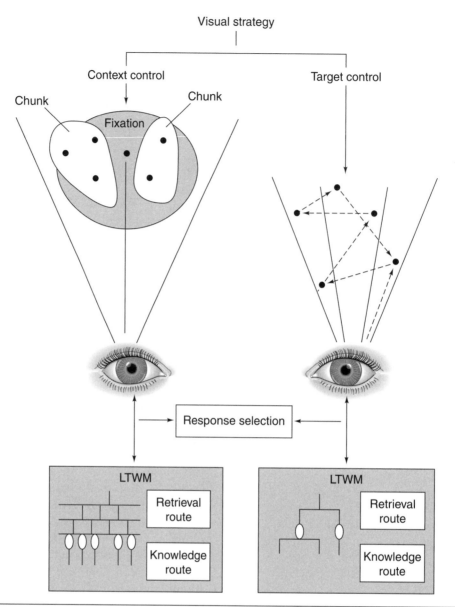

➤ **Figure 8.1**   Tenenbaum's model showing the visual strategies of expert (left) and nonexpert (right) sport performers.

Reprinted, by permission, from G. Tenenbaum, 2003, Expert athletes: An integrated approach to decision making. In *Expert performance in sports: Advances in research*, edited by J.L. Starkes and K.A. Ericsson (Champaign, IL: Human Kinetics), 200.

of play, while the novice is more target or object dependent. Tenenbaum (2003, p. 197) explains further using two strategies originally proposed by Neisser (1967, 1976):

the target control strategy consists of detecting targets within the display until a target is detected, which is compatible with the mental representations in long-term memory. The context control strategy consists of a visual search carried out under the control of memory representations,

which are not necessarily sensitive to individual objects, but rather to the number of items in the display. Under such a strategy the observer is under a situational control when the stimulus is compatible with the representational memory of the context. We posit that with practice, as the number of representations and their logical connections increase, the players who apply mental operations in an open environment will shift from target control to context control so that they may a) reduce the information-processing load (i.e., complexity); b) increase the efficiency of the visual scan; and c) simplify the long-term working memory elaborations for response selection.

Tenenbaum's model is based on visual-search studies where participants viewed video displays presented in two dimensions. In these types of studies the tactical information displayed often lacks all of the information found in real visuomotor workspaces. The spaces that athletes perform in are often large and the gaze must be controlled over the full width, height, and depth of the space. The pressure to perceptually and physically perform with full awareness is so great that a centralized gaze or visual pivot is often unable to detect the many changes that occur in the movement of objects over time (e.g., the spin of a ball, the dip of a puck). This was shown in chapter 4 (see tables 4.1 and 4.2) where the gaze of athletes was reported in a number of tasks using vision-in-action methods. It was found that athletes do centralize the gaze and look into spaces, but this does not constitute a high percent of gaze. Instead, both elite and near-elite performers direct their gaze to specific cues found within the visuomotor workspace. This is the thesis of Klein's **recognition-primed model of decision making,** which is presented in the following section.

Klein's Recognition-Primed Model of Decision Making

Klein's (1999) recognition-primed decision model (RPD) of decision making describes many of the qualities that expert decision makers exhibit in high-stress environments. Klein developed the RPD model from extensive study of experts who work in firefighting, medical emergency rooms, the military, and police work. Although these environments are often ill defined and ill structured, experts consistently solve the problems found there in efficient and effective ways. Klein states that

> during the past twenty-five years, the field of decision-making has concentrated on showing the limitations of decision makers—that is, that they are not very rational or competent. Books have been written documenting human limitations and suggesting remedies: training methods to help

us think clearly, decision support systems to monitor and guide us, and expert systems that enable computers to make decisions and avoid altogether fallible humans . . . . This book was written to balance the others and takes a different perspective. Here I document human strengths and capabilities that typically have been downplayed or even ignored. (p. 1)

He found that experts' decisions are based on critical cues in the environments that are often missed by others. He explains that "experts see the things the rest of us cannot, [and] often experts do not realize that the rest of us are unable to detect what seems obvious to them" (1999, p. 147). In the RPD model, experts are separated from nonexperts by their ability to detect the most important cues without hesitation and in a way that leads to decisive and appropriate actions. Many of the characteristics Klein lists describe expert decision making in sport.

➤ *Experienced decision makers who offer solutions are present.* Expert firefighters, pilots, soldiers, doctors, nurses, athletes, and coaches routinely solve complex problems and develop methods for making effective decisions on a consistent basis.

➤ *There is time pressure.* Decisions have to be made in minutes, seconds, or milliseconds. There is often time for only one decision. The correct decision results in success, but the incorrect decision means defeat. In sport, the clock often dictates what will occur, and we all know of exceptional performances in the dying seconds of contests or in brief periods of time.

➤ *Decisions are made in the face of inadequate information.* In all action environments, uncertainty must be dealt with on a routine basis. In sport, uncertainty rules the day and comes from opponents, teammates, weather, officials, fans, parents, media, and many other sources.

➤ *Procedures are both well defined and poorly defined.* Protocols that aid treatment are planned, but even the best plans are unable to deal with everything that happens. Despite the many rules that govern sport, there are many gray areas that require unique problem-solving and decision-making abilities. Many times coaches and athletes function at what they feel are instinctual levels. Later in this chapter we will see that what is often called *instinct* or *intuition* is scientifically measurable and therefore understandable.

➤ *Cue learning is required and is the basis of good decision making.* Experts in all domains have learned what is important and what is of no consequence. The gaze research presented in this book shows that we can now measure what cues athletes actually use and how the cues underlie their decision making. Learning how to detect the most important cues in high-pressure settings is critical. We also know that learning how to ignore many cues is just as important.

➤ *The context of decision making changes constantly.* A solution in one situation is not automatically the solution in the next. The ability to respond to emergency situations is dependent on perceiving each context. Sport, by nature, is fluid, dynamic, and unpredictable. Even relatively common things, like changes in playing venues, can have a great effect on how an athlete performs and therefore should never be underestimated.

➤ *The context of decision making is dynamic in that there is no one right solution all the time.* Quick detection, adaptability, and exploitation are the norm rather than the exception in terms of expert decision making in high-pressure settings. In order to train effective decision-making skills in sport, a variety of methods or tools must be used (a topic covered in detail in chapters 9-12).

Klein's RPD model consists of three variations that function according to the complexity of the decisions that have to be made. Together these three variations permit an analysis of different types of decision making found in sport. Each variation begins with the detection of cues using one or more of the senses (vision, audition, kinesthesia, taste, olfaction). In the following sections, the different variations are presented and applied to sport and other settings. Linkages are also made to the three categories of gaze control (targeting, interceptive timing, and tactical tasks) as found in the gaze control framework.

RPD Model: Variation 1

Figure 8.2 presents variation 1 of the RPD model, which occurs when there is a simple match between a familiar event and a well-known action. Variation 1 (if . . . then) is found in situations where typical cues are present and where the task is one of recognition followed by a known

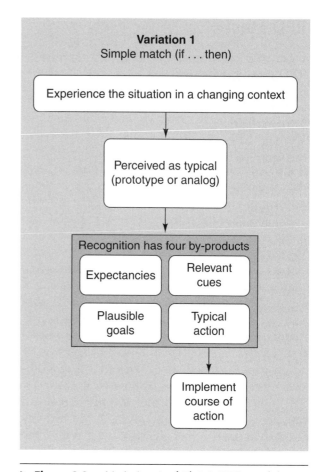

➤ **Figure 8.2**   Variation 1 of Klein's RPD model.

Klein, Gary, *Sources of Power: How People Make Decisions*, figure 3.1. © Massachusetts Institute of Technology. Published by The MIT Press.

action. Within sport environments, this if–then simple match scenario is very common due to the repetitive nature of the skills and tactics performed in most sports.

Variation 1 thus aptly describes what happens in sport a good deal of the time. Indeed, the purpose of extensive training is to make much of the unpredictable world of sport predictable, and therefore something that can be controlled more easily. Many if–then visual cues were defined in chapters 5 to 7, where the gaze was described in targeting and interceptive timing tasks. Through training, athletes learn how to detect an effective cue, such as the front hoop in the basketball jump shot, as shown in fixed targeting tasks in chapter 5. The detection of the hoop is then matched with an action consistent with basketball shooting. When a simple match occurs, the performer's expectancies, relevant cues, plausible goals, and typical actions occur in a largely predictable if–then matching scenario.

RPD Model: Variation 2

Figure 8.3 presents the second variation of the RPD model, where more complex information is introduced at an early stage but the action performed is well known. In variation 2, new information must be processed that is often atypical or unusual, but the action is largely the same as that performed many times before. A situation that is atypical or unusual requires the recognition of new information that must be interpreted in terms of expectancies, goals, and actions. Once the new information is clarified and anomalies resolved, the action is performed the same as countless times before.

Variation 2 (if ??? . . . then) occurs in sport when performers have to acquire new or unusual information but still make familiar movements. In this variation, the situations are unfamiliar and contain elements that must be figured out or diagnosed each time. An example occurs in **abstract targeting tasks** such as golf

putting as presented in chapter 6. The putting stroke is similar from putt to putt, but to be successful the golfer has to figure out the unique characteristics of each green. Variation 2 is also needed when, for example, the opposition uses a new play, when an official makes an unusual call, when the weather becomes challenging, and where the same skills and tactics are routinely adapted to handle the new information. In these types of cases, performers have to assess each situation, interpret the available information, and then perform a well-known action.

RPD Model: Variation 3

Figure 8.4 presents the third variation of the RPD model (if then . . . ???), which requires taking in familiar information that is then used to produce a novel action. Here the information that is available is familiar and adequate; however, the action taken is atypical.

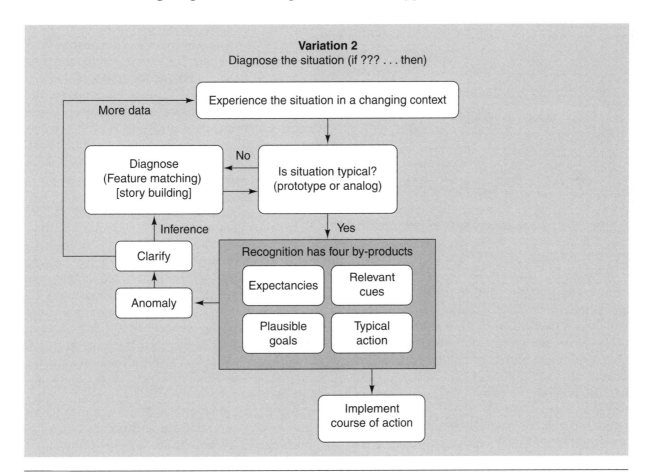

➤ **Figure 8.3** Variation 2 of Klein's RPD model.

Klein, Gary, *Sources of Power: How People Make Decisions*, figure 3.1. © Massachusetts Institute of Technology. Published by The MIT Press.

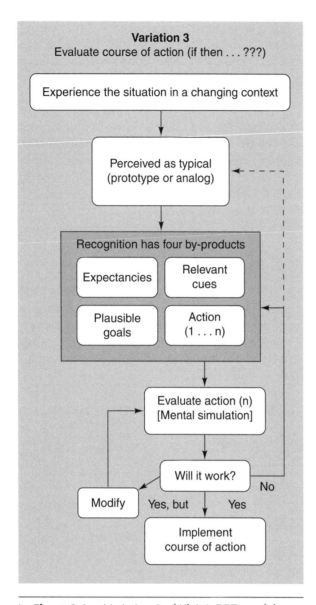

Variation 3
Evaluate course of action (if then . . . ???)

Experience the situation in a changing context

Perceived as typical
(prototype or analog)

Recognition has four by-products

Expectancies

Relevant
cues

Plausible
goals

Action
(1 . . . n)

Evaluate action (n)
[Mental simulation]

Will it work?

Modify   Yes, but   Yes

No

Implement
course of action

> **Figure 8.4**   Variation 3 of Klein's RPD model.

Klein, Gary, *Sources of Power: How People Make Decisions*, figure 3.1. ©
Massachusetts Institute of Technology. Published by The MIT Press.

An example of variation 3 comes from an incident in sail racing involving Isabel Autissier, who was a participant in the 1998-1999 Vendee Globe, a solo sailing race in the Southern Ocean. This is the most grueling of all races, taking the sailors into the Southern Ocean below the 50th parallel where they essentially circumnavigate Antarctica over 40 to 50 days. The waves are huge, and gale force winds blow for weeks. The boats in the 1998-1999 race were broad beamed, almost like Windsurfers with immense sails. They had an unknown weakness that only became apparent once the racers reached the worst of the seas—they could not right themselves once capsized. All sailboats must have the ability to turn right side up should they capsize, but these boats could not, therefore putting the solo sailors in a situation where they could not self-rescue and continue sailing.

Autissier's boat was dismasted and then overturned. The two closest racers were 200 km ahead and tied for the lead. As is the convention in sailing races, they were both asked to turn back and give assistance without penalty to their own times. Autissier's location was known because a signaling device on her boat was functioning. Therefore, in terms of the first part of variation 3 of the RPD model, there was no uncertainty regarding where she was. However, the first sailor refused to turn back, citing the impossibility of sailing back into the huge wind and waves. The second sailor, Italian racer Giovanni Soldini, turned back immediately into the mountainous seas. A day and a half later he found the overturned boat, but no sight of Autissier. Two times he circled the boat shouting into the wind and received no response. As a solo sailor in 10 m seas, it was impossible to board the boat for fear of collision or worse. Instead, he circled the boat again and used a novel action to see if she was still aboard: He threw a heavy hammer on the overturned hull. Autissier, who was barely clinging to life, heard the sound and was able to exit onto the hull and make her way to Soldini's boat. Throwing hammers on boats is not normally what sailors do, but it was a new action that worked very well that day.

How this story ended is also interesting. The first sailor compounded his bad manners and brought charges against Soldini, claiming that with Autissier aboard he was no longer a solo sailor. The international outcry was immediate and swift. Not only was Soldini reinstated, he was also awarded the normal makeup time under the rules of racing. He went on to win and, most important of all, reinforced the time-honored tradition of sailors on the high seas who make high-stakes decisions and help one another without hesitation.

Variation 3 (if then . . . ???) is the most complex of all the variations and occurs when the information present is known and understood but a completely new action has to be taken due to unusual circumstances. An example that occurs in sport is when key players are injured or fouled out, or when a team has to perform actions unique to the context and time. Such a situation arose during the gold medal game of the 2002 Winter Olympics, when the Canadian women's ice hockey team was called for a large number of penalties and so had to play virtually the entire game with up to three players fewer than the opposition. Normally teams are scored on when this occurs, but the players adjusted their actions and handled the opposition in a way that is rarely seen in ice hockey. Normally even one penalty can cause a goal in championship ice hockey games, but the opposite occurred in this case. Indeed, the imposition of so many penalties seemed to improve the focus and decision-making skills of the players as the game went on.

A final example, which could be considered variation 4 although not identified as such by Klein, occurs when both the information available and the action taken are novel. Consider the true story of an elite gymnast who had to withdraw at nationals because the beam was oriented so that she had to face a large crowd. She could not find her normal spotting cues and therefore could not adjust her actions, which negatively affected her expectancies, goals, and ultimately her course of action. Even though she was performing a self-paced routine, the information available had a huge effect on her and caused her to take an unusual action. Variation 4 occurs in sport quite often. For example, figure 8.5 shows Tiger Woods performing an unusual golf stroke from an unusual lie. Here he is hitting the ball using a technique variation that he probably employed only on this shot. Both the information that was available to him and the stroke he had to make were somewhat novel.

Consciousness and Decision Making

Athletes make decisions all the time when they perform in sport, but are they conscious of the decision-making processes they use? Many teachers, coaches, and psychologists recommend acting without thought, advice reflected in slogans such as "Just do it" and "Act, don't think,"

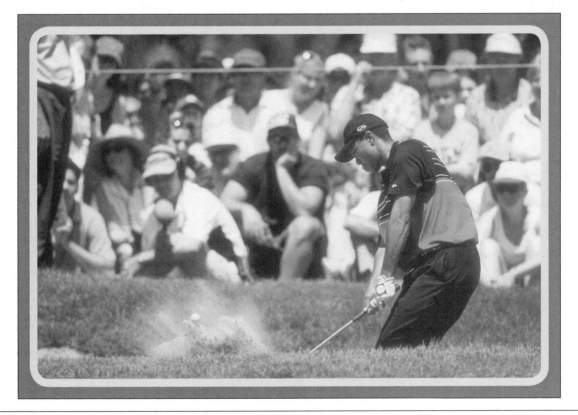

▶ **Figure 8.5**   Tiger Woods illustrating variation 4, performing an unusual golf stroke from an unusual lie. The caption from *How I Play Golf* (Woods, 2001) is, "The game has brought me to my knees many times, from which there is definitely a different view" (p. 208).

as well as popular books such as *Blink* (Gladwell, 2005) that ask us to trust our subconscious selves in all situations. Often we do not know how we arrive at decisions, but this does not mean that the science of decision making in complex action environments cannot be understood.

To illustrate how the conscious and unconscious aspects of decision making can be understood scientifically, Klein (1999) tells the story of an incident that occurred on a British naval ship during the closing hours of the 1991 Gulf War. The warship was a few miles off the coast and a blip on the radar screen indicated that an object, possibly a missile, was coming right at the destroyer. It would reach the ship in a few seconds; therefore a decision had to be made in seconds whether to shoot it down. At the last moment, the gunnery captain ordered the object shot down. How he correctly identified the blip as hostile was a mystery to everyone, including himself, as there were no obvious cues to reveal that the incoming object was unfriendly. Indeed, two hours after firing, it was still not known if he had shot down an Allied plane or an enemy missile. Did he make the decision to save himself and his crew, or was there objective evidence to support his decision making?

Klein was called in to investigate. Through interviews, he found that much was typical that day—the gunnery captain and his crew knew there was a high probability of missile attack due to the critical stage of the war. They also knew that the enemy had a store of missiles and only a short time in which to use them since they would soon be overrun by Allied forces. His crew was ready and well trained and had situational information specific to the context that indicated a greatly increased probability of attack. The captain and his crew had acquired expectancy information and were prepared to act. The captain also knew that if a missile was fired, he had very little time in which to respond. He and his crew were therefore primed to attack quickly and decisively. But none of these expectancies explained how he knew the blip on the screen was a missile and not an Allied aircraft.

The key emerged from Klein's analysis of the radar data and how the captain had visually perceived the blips on the screen. The captain and his crew knew that Allied aircraft always flew at 3,000 ft (914 m) and that blips from these aircraft were always continuously visible on the radar screen. The captain also knew that a missile coming from land had to accelerate from ground zero and therefore was not visible on radar until it reached an altitude above 1,000 ft (305 m) due to ground interference. This was the key cue. Allied aircraft were constantly visible since they never flew below 3,000 ft (914 m), whereas a missile became visible only above 1,000 ft (305 m). What the captain had detected was the absence of the missile on the radar screen during its first few moments of flight and then its sudden appearance. He was not consciously aware that this was why he made the decision he did, but objective analysis of the data later confirmed that this was the case.

This story shows that a seemingly unconscious perception can have an objective basis that can be identified and understood scientifically. Klein refers to this as decision making based on expert intuition. He defines *expert intuition* as intuition based on events that has its roots in visual, auditory, kinesthetic, and other forms of information that are acquired through extensive training and can be identified and measured. Because everything happens so quickly in dynamic sport environments, expert performers are often unaware of how they make the decisions they do. But this does not mean we cannot understand scientifically how they make decisions. Finally, Klein explains that the ability to make good decisions under all conditions is a source of power, one that separates the expert performer from the near expert and novice. In the next section, we explore this idea further through an analysis of the gaze control and attention in simple and complex locomotion tasks, followed by the gaze control and attention of elite speed skaters skating at speed on an Olympic oval.

Gaze Control During Locomotion

Tactical situations in sport require that athletes use locomotion to walk, run, skate, ski around, or jump over both stationary and moving objects at varying speeds. During locomotion, the visual field in front changes constantly, and within each visual field there are a number of visual targets and locations that must be attended to in order to navigate safely.

Making Our Way Around and Over Obstacles

Patla and Vickers (1997) recorded the gaze of participants as they approached and stepped over obstacles of varying height (no obstacle, 5 cm, 10 cm, 30 cm), as shown in figure 8.6. When people walk at a normal speed, they let their gaze travel along the pathway in front and use travel fixations to monitor where they are going. These fixations are anchored about 1 to 2 m in front of the feet and are carried along at the rate of locomotion.

Travel fixations monitor optic flow (Gibson, 1979); therefore, both the focal and ambient systems function to orient the person within the environment. Gibson (1979, p. 229) explains that during optic flow humans "see where they are going without having to look where they are going." When people walk, the changing **optic array** and the changes in angular position

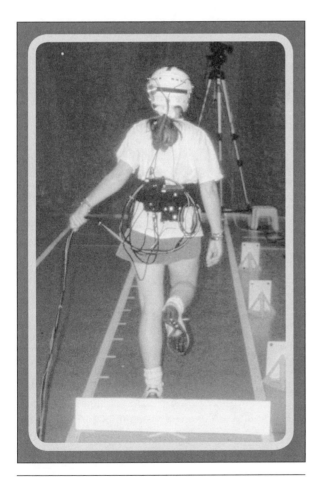

➤ **Figure 8.6** A participant stepping over an obstacle while wearing a mobile eye tracker.

of locations in the environment are registered continuously on the retina. As the size, orientation, and rate of expansion of the object change, the locomotor system adjusts automatically without conscious effort or awareness. Travel fixations have the qualities shown for the expert performers described in Tenenbaum's model in that the gaze is often positioned in the center of the visual field and is used to subconsciously monitor events. During a travel fixation, the gaze is maintained in frontal space and acts as a visual pivot that aids ongoing locomotion.

Object fixations are the second type of gaze used during locomotion. These fixations are used to attend to objects, even as the feet continue walking or running. In order for the body to move effectively, the gaze dwells on specific objects even as the feet continue to move. Object fixations must be of sufficient duration to allow people to navigate safely and solve tactical problems even when moving at a high rate of speed. Patla and Vickers (1997) found that when participants approached obstacles of different heights, they fixated the obstacle well in advance before reaching it. The height of the obstacle affected both the frequency and duration of object fixations. Frequency of fixations increased as a function of obstacle height, with more fixations allocated to higher obstacles than to lower ones. Fixations were directed to the top of the obstacle during the approach and to the area on the floor where the takeoff foot landed. These gazes were used in a **feed-forward** or top-down manner and provided the locomotor system with the advance information needed to step correctly. During top-down feed-forward control, information is sent ahead from the higher neural centers and incorporated with incoming sensory information for use in motor planning.

How much time is needed to step over obstacles of different height? During normal locomotion, an object is identified at least two steps, or about 300 ms, before reaching the obstacle (Hollands, Patla, & Vickers, 2002; Patla & Vickers, 1997). If an obstacle is higher or more complex, then more object fixation time is needed. Well before the step is taken over the obstacle, the gaze is directed down the travel path and toward the next locations where stepping will occur. Since information gathered 300 ms in advance is needed to navigate an obstacle while walking, imagine the additional time needed by an athlete who is running, skating, speed skating, cycling, or skiing at high speeds. It is vital that athletes learn to look ahead and detect critical obstacles in the environment so that they can plan their steps well ahead of time.

Patla and Vickers (1997) found that travel fixations were the most dominant gaze behavior, accounting for 60% of all fixations during loco-motion. Later studies investigated the gaze of participants who walked toward one of five cued target lights (Hollands, Patla, & Vickers, 2002). The same result emerged even when specific information had to be fixated and walked toward or over. The most dominant gaze behavior was travel fixation, and object fixations were used only when a complex problem had to be solved. Other researchers have found similar gaze behaviors, even in cats avoiding small objects (Fowler & Sherk, 2003; Wilkinson & Sherk, 2005).

Locomotion: Learning to Avoid the Trap

In simple locomotion tasks like the ones just presented, a mixture of 60% travel fixations and 40% object fixations appears to be sufficient to ensure safe and effective walking. But is this ratio of object to travel fixations adequate when the task is more complex? In order to better under-stand how people use object and travel fixations to solve complex motor problems, we now look at a complex tactical problem called the *trap task*, as used in a study by Vickers and Patla (1999). Figure 8.7 shows the trap task, which consists of eight blocks organized in two sections (approach and trap) on the floor. In the study, participants were required to walk along the set of raised blocks without touching the floor, stepping awk-wardly, or losing their balance. Unbeknownst to the participants, the blocks were arranged in such a way that stepping on the first block with the wrong foot forced them to use an awkward crossover step and subsequently lose balance (see figure 8.8). The participants were not allowed to see the trap task before beginning their first attempt. The researchers wanted to know how many participants would fail on the first attempt, how long it would take the individuals who failed the first trial to solve the task, and what

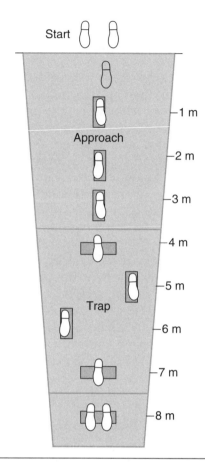

> **Figure 8.7** The trap task, with approach and trap sections.

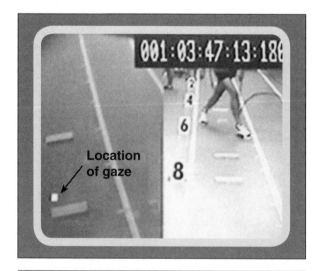

> **Figure 8.8** A frame of vision-in-action data show-ing a person who has become trapped (right); his gaze is shown at the same time on the left side of the image.

type of gaze control was used during successful and unsuccessful navigation. Figure 8.8 shows a frame of vision-in-action data and a participant who has fallen into the trap. The right image shows him using an awkward crossover step, while the frame on the left shows the location of his gaze (white cursor) near one of the blocks at the same time.

On the first trial, two of the participants navigated the trap without error, and the other six failed. The successful participants were removed because they may have stepped on the first block with the correct foot by chance. Of the remaining six, four learned to avoid the trap by the third trial and performed perfectly thereafter, and two failed to solve the task over the total of five trials permitted. Figure 8.9 shows the percent of object and travel fixations of the four participants who learned the task. On trial 1 (when all participants failed), 50% were travel fixations and 35% were object fixations directed to the blocks in the approach (20%) or trap (15%)

areas. These participants held their gaze in front and stepped using optic flow in a manner similar to what was reported in earlier studies (Patla & Vickers, 1997). During trials 2 and 3, they then changed their gaze so there was an increase in object fixations to the blocks in the approach (0 to B3) and a decrease in both travel and object fixations to the trap area. In order to discover the secret of the trap task, they changed their gaze and their lead foot on block 1, thus enabling the correct stepping sequence. During trials 4 and 5, the percentage of travel fixations then returned quickly to its original level.

Figure 8.10 presents the results of the two participants who failed to solve the trap task during the 5 trials. During trial 1, they used an equal percentage of travel and object fixations to the near blocks, but they had fewer fixations than the group that succeeded due to their using a high percentage of other gazes (saccades, blinks, head movement). During trials 1 through 4, they increased the percentage of travel fixations and decreased object fixations to the blocks, a gaze strategy opposite

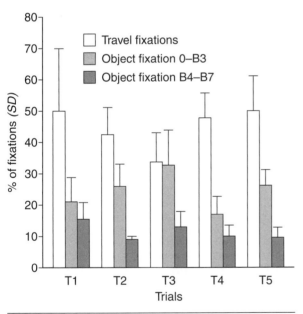

> **Figure 8.9** Percent of gaze (travel and object fixations) used by participants who failed on trial 1, solved the problem by trial 3, and then maintained successful performance through trial 5. The percentages do not equal 100% because the remaining percentage in each trial was for saccades, blinks, and data that were uncodeable due to excessive head movement.

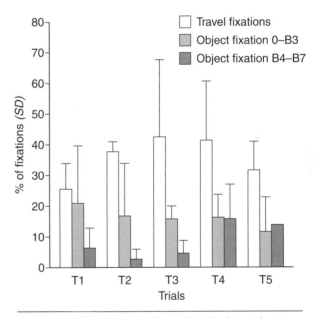

> **Figure 8.10** Percent of travel and object fixations used by the participants who failed on trial 1 and did not solve the problem thereafter. The percentages do not equal 100% because the remaining percentage of gaze was uncodeable due to excessive movement of the head.

of those who solved the trap problem. They never seemed to be aware of the importance of using a high percentage of object fixations to the blocks in the approach area where the secret to the trap task lay, thus allowing the correct step to be taken on block 1.

Overall, these results show that when a complex locomotion problem is faced, the first tendency is to use travel fixations, but these are inadequate in terms of solving complex loco-motor problems. In order to be successful, the percentage of object fixations to relevant objects and locations in the task environment has to be increased until the task is learned. When these results are considered in light of Tenenbaum's (2003) study, we see that a centralized gaze (travel fixations) was not enough to solve the problem but was preferred once the task was learned, when the participants quickly reverted to travel fixations and were effective thereafter.

Gaze Control in Speed Skating

Speed skaters travel the same 400 m of ice, which often leads observers to assume they have to make few decisions given the sameness of their environment and the need to simply go fast around an unobstructed path of ice. In truth, speed skaters have to make a great number of tactical decisions most often under extreme time pressure. There is the need to start without a fault and to gain milliseconds that often affect the outcome of the race. Then while maintaining speeds greater than 40 kph, the speed skater must enter two turns on each lap, skate the apex, and exit while maintaining a precise position and track path over the skates. Since speed skaters always skate with or against another skater, they also must exit from the turn in a way that permits a smooth lane transition or crossover. In addition, speed skaters must learn to monitor their speed by developing an internal clock that is often accurate within milliseconds of their actual times. To enter two turns at precisely the right spot and exit from those two turns in exactly the correct location, and to do so lap after lap at high speed, requires anticipation, focus and attention to cues, concentration, and good decision-making skills. Even in a sport where the environment is relatively predictable, there is tremendous variability in how elite and near-elite athletes see the same environment.

The gaze behaviors of five elite speed skaters were recorded just before the 2006 Turin Olympics (Vickers, 2006). Three of the five went on to win medals. A theory of attention that may explain how skaters control their gaze at speed is the attentional narrowing theory of Easterbrook (1959). As performance conditions become more complex and more challenging, which occurs at high speeds, performance typically deteriorates unless the optimal cues are fixated at the appropriate times. Skaters must optimize the position of their body over their skates such that in a 3,000 m event, for example, the process of entering the corner, building through the apex, and exiting at full speed is repeated more than 14 times; therefore, focus over an extended period of time is required in order to link the required movements at full speed.

Many of the conditions encountered by speed skaters are also found in auto driving. The inherent demands of auto racing have made it an ideal task for investigation of attentional mechanisms and the eye-movement parameters that underlie those mechanisms. Janelle et al. (1999) assessed the effect of a central driving task and a peripheral light-detection task on driving performance over three driving sessions. Driving performance decreased when distracting peripheral lights were present; distracters in the periphery tend to reduce performance quality due to a reduction in attentional resources. Reaction time to peripheral stimuli increases as the pressure of racing builds and situational demands increase. An Olympic oval is a very large space where teammates, rivals, coaches, and members of the public are in close proximity and where coaches often call out or show race times and provide feedback. Even in the midst of all these distractions, it is critical that the gaze be oriented in an optimal way.

Parallels may also be drawn between the requirements of gaze control and visual attention found in car driving and those found in speed skating in terms of navigating turns. Riemersma (1981) found that car drivers depend on edge-line motion to maintain the alignment of the car on the road, with the greatest effect found during night driving. Land and Lee (1995) and Mestre and Durand (2001) showed that when negotiating a curve, a critical cue fixated at high speed is the tangent or reversal point. This is shown in figure 8.11 from a study by Mestre, Mars, Durand, Vienne, and Espie

(2005). This singular point is located midway on the inside of the curve. In speed skating, it is often called the *apex* of the turn and is recognized by coaches and athletes alike to be the location where the body must be positioned over the skates such that the exit from the turn can be made under control. Otherwise, the athlete cannot prevent skating into the far lane and thus loses valuable time. Mestre & Durand (2001) stated that the tangent point attracts the gaze and is therefore critical in providing the information needed to travel safely at high speeds. If the tangent point is also a critical cue used by elite speed skaters, then orienting the gaze inside to this location should contribute to faster skating speeds.

The data were collected on an Olympic oval with three lanes, each 4 to 5 m wide. The inner lane was the practice lane, and the two outer lanes were used for competition. A frame of vision-in-action data is shown in figure 8.12, as recorded by a mobile eye tracker worn by the skaters. The right image shows the athlete's gaze as recorded by the scene camera. Superimposed on the image is a circle, which indicates the skater's location of gaze. The left image was recorded by two external video cameras (one at each end of the oval) that recorded the skater as the laps were performed. Lap speeds were recorded using a timer integral to the eye tracker.

Travel fixations were carried along by the skating strides and were held relatively stable on or between four lines on the track. The athletes directed their gaze to the inside practice lane, directly in front in lane 1 or lane 2, or outside toward the bumper pads. They also directed their inside to the tangent on the turn. Object

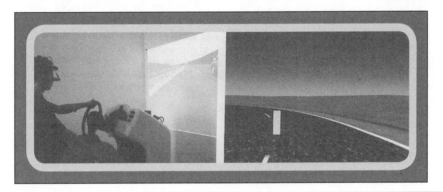

➤ **Figure 8.11** On the left, a driver executes a corner while wearing an eye tracker. On the right, the tangent of the turn is indicated by the vertical bar. When the drivers were told to fixate the bar as they drove the turn, they sustained higher speeds and spun out on fewer occasions.

Reprinted, by permission, from D.R. Mestre, et al., 2005, "Gaze behavior during simulated driving: Elements for a visual driving aid," *Driving Assessment 2005 Proceedings Paper*. Available: http://ppc.uiowa.edu/driving-assessment/2005/final/papers/45_mestreformat.pdf.

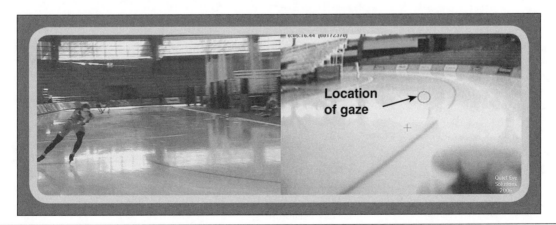

➤ **Figure 8.12** A frame of vision-in-action data collected in speed skating, showing the athlete's skating movements on the left and his gaze at the same time on the right as he enters the turn.

Reprinted, by permission, from J.N. Vickers, 2006, "Gaze of Olympic speed skaters while skating at full speed in regulation oval: Perception-action coupling in a dynamic performance environment," *Cognitive Processing* 7(5): S102-S105.

fixations were directed to people, cones, signs on the bumper pads, and other objects in the field of view. Saccades were rapid shifts of the gaze from one location to another. Figure 8.13 shows how the elite and near-elite skaters differed in the orientation of their gaze. The elite skaters directed a total of 86% of their gaze to the inside line or to the tangent point, whereas the near-elite skaters directed 60% of their gaze to these locations. The near-elite skaters also tended to look ahead and toward the outside lane more than the elite skaters did.

Figure 8.14 presents a bivariate regression plot of lap speed on the *y*-axis and the duration of the gaze orientations on the *x*-axis. Shown is the amount of lap speed variance accounted for by type of gaze used. The regression lines reveal that increasing the duration of the gaze to the inside tangent, the inside lane, or in front increased the skaters' lap time, while orienting the gaze to the outside line or lane contributed to slower skating times. The greatest aid to speed was orienting the gaze to the tangent point. The longer the athletes

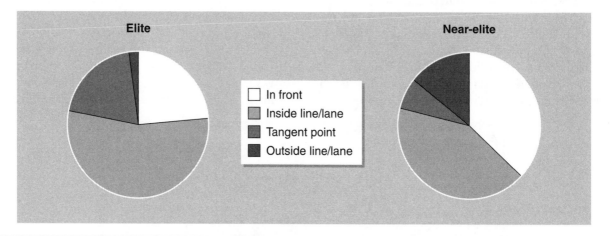

> **Figure 8.13**   Percentage of fixation or tracking to different locations on the ice of elite and near-elite speed skaters skating at training speeds on an Olympic oval.

Reprinted, by permission, from J.N. Vickers, 2006, "Gaze of Olympic speed skaters while skating at full speed in regulation oval: Perception-action coupling in a dynamic performance environment," *Cognitive Processing* 7(5): S102-S105.

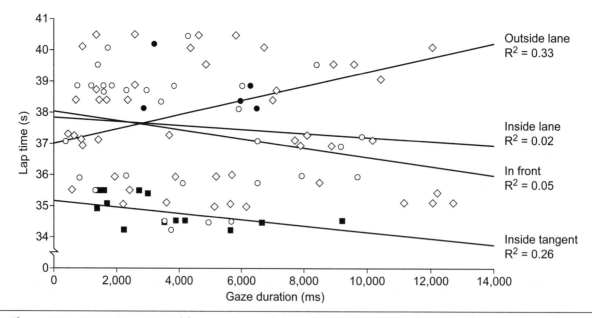

> **Figure 8.14**   Four orientations of the gaze in speed skating (outside lane, inside lane, in front, inside tangent) and the relationship of the duration of each gaze to skating lap times (s).

Reprinted, by permission, from J.N. Vickers, 2006, "Gaze of Olympic speed skaters while skating at full speed in regulation oval: Perception-action coupling in a dynamic performance environment," *Cognitive Processing* 7(5): S102-S105.

were able to maintain their gaze at this location, the better they were at maintaining or increasing their speed. During this time it is normal that speed skaters build speed out of the turn, so this result is not unexpected.

Elite speed skaters appear to use this gaze to counter the forces of gravity that act to pull them off the track. In addition, some of the athletes established their gaze on the tangent point earlier than others. Further investigation of the onset and duration of the gaze relative to the tangent point will be needed to determine how this affects the athlete's speed.

Shooting to Score on a Goaltender

In this section, gaze control during the penalty shot in ice hockey is described. This task is categorized as a tactical task because of the presence of the goaltender. Shooting on goal without a goaltender would be classified as a targeting task because the target is fixed and there is an unobstructed view of the net. But the presence of a goaltender makes a problem for the gaze tactical in nature. During the penalty shot there are multiple visual fields, within which there may be one or more spotlights for the gaze and attention.

The penalty shot is awarded when there is a flagrant foul on a player who has a clear opportunity to score. It is also used during shoot-outs to determine a winner in tied games. Unlike penalty kicks in soccer or penalty strokes in field hockey, ice hockey players are allowed to skate with the puck before shooting. The penalty shot begins with the puck on the center face-off spot and the goaltender standing in the goal. The player taking the shot skates with the puck and has one attempt

to score. As the shooter skates toward the net, the goaltender is free to move in any direction. Recent rule changes in ice hockey have led to the penalty shot playing a major role in the outcome of games. During the 2006 National Hockey League (NHL) season, a total of 103 penalty shots were taken and 35 goals were scored (34%) (see NHL.com). The advantage is clearly with the goaltenders, who are successful in stopping 66% of all shots.

Some shooters have great difficulty in scoring during the penalty shot, whereas others are more successful. In an effort to determine whether control of the gaze is a factor in scoring, male ice hockey players aged 16 to 18 y were selected from the top teams for their age group in the City of Calgary (Vickers, in progress). All were the top shooters on their teams and among the best in the high-level league in which they played. The players skated against a professional goaltender until 10 goals and 10 saves were made. The percentage of goals scored by each athlete was determined, and from this the players were classified as high scoring (31%) or as lower scoring (21%). A frame of vision-in-action data is shown in figure 8.15, similar to that collected in the study. Image A shows a shooter wearing an eye tracker about to take the shot, while image B shows his gaze (circle) at the same time located to the goaltender's left, near his glove hand.

Each shot was divided into three motor phases (i.e., preparation, preshot, shot). The high- and low-scoring players did not differ in the duration of these phases. During the preparation phase, the players skated toward the puck. During this time, the high-scoring players fixated the puck (50%) and the net (22%),

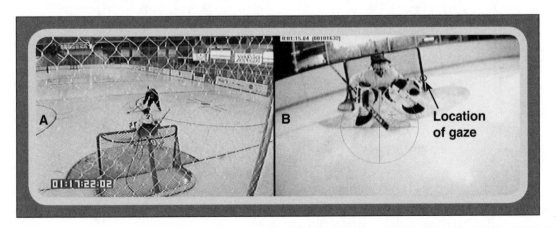

> **Figure 8.15** Vision-in-action data of a head-up shooter performing the ice hockey penalty shot.

whereas the low-skilled fixated the puck (31%), the ice (29%), and the net (25%). During the preshot phase, the skaters picked up the puck and skated toward the goaltender. During this time, the high- and low-scoring shooters were similar in fixating the ice (47%) and different locations on the net (23%).

Figure 8.16 shows the percentage of fixations during the shot phase, which was held constant at seven frames (or 233.33 ms before the release of the puck from the stick). The high-skilled shooters (left) used a head-down style where they directed their fixations to the ice in the vicinity of the puck (62%), the puck (2%), the blade of the stick (2%), or the upper left side of the net (22%). In contrast, the low-skilled shooters (right) used a head-up style where they fixated the upper left side of the goal (52%), followed by fixations on the ice (27%), the goaltender (17%), and the puck (3%). Given that the head-down shooters were more successful, it may be that this style of shooting is harder for goaltenders to read because the shooter provides fewer clues about where the puck is going. In contrast, the low-scoring shooters used the head-up style, which may have given the goaltenders more opportunities to pick up clues as to where the shooter intended to shoot.

Alternatively, in the previous chapter, Morya, Ranvaud, and Pinheiro (2003) and van der Kamp

(2006) identified two styles of shooting in soccer penalty taking—keeper dependent and keeper independent. When a keeper-dependent strategy is used, shooters are prepared to change their shot in response to the goaltender's actions, and during the keeper-independent strategy the actions of the goaltender are ignored and the shot executed as planned earlier. Both Morya et al. and van der Kamp found that the keeper-independent strategy was more successful. It might be that the head-down style facilitates the use of a keeper-independent strategy and is more effective, as it prevents the shooter from being affected by the goaltender and changing the shot at the last moment.

Gaze Control During Offensive and Defensive Plays

The second subcategory of tactical tasks describes the gaze control during offensive and defensive plays. Tactical plays are well known in a sport and are most often trained in a deliberate way. Examples would be the fast break, zone defense, the throw-in, and so on. Novel plays emerge spontaneously during play and arise as a result of unusual playing conditions or **creativity** on the part of one or more players. Gaze control research relative to tactical plays is now presented in soccer and ice hockey.

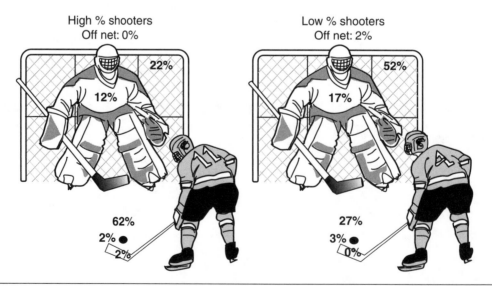

> **Figure 8.16** Percentage of fixation or tracking gaze of high-scoring (left) and low-scoring (right) players during the shot phase of the ice hockey penalty shot.

Gaze Control in Soccer Tactics

We now look at studies that have investigated the control of gaze and attention during team tactical situations in soccer where set plays such as 1v1, 3v3, 4v4, and 11v11 (full game) were investigated. Studies of gaze control in sport tactics have shown that elite players are faster than nonelite players in making decisions and that their decisions are of a higher quality (Helsen & Pauwels, 1992; Williams & Davids, 1998; Williams, Davids, Burwitz, & Williams, 1994), but beyond this it is unclear whether their superior decision-making skills are due to their early detection of cues or their ability to process the fixated information more effectively after it has been fixated.

Helsen and Pauwels (1992) combined elements of the visual-search paradigm with measures of performance in an investigation of soccer offensive tactics. The experimental setup is shown in figure 8.17, including a soccer player with the ball at his feet standing in front of a life-size video projected on a wall. The athlete was fitted with an eye tracker (not shown), and at specific moments during the play, a player in the video directed the ball toward him. When this occurred, the athlete was required to play the ball at his feet and shoot as quickly as possible, make a pass to

a teammate on the screen, or dribble around the defender. Helsen and Pauwels compared the gaze behaviors of expert and novice players and found that highly skilled players not only made better decisions and responded faster, but also had fewer fixations of longer duration to fewer locations.

Williams et al. (1994) and Williams and Davids (1998) found a different result. They used the setup shown in figure 2.3 to determine the gaze of elite and novice soccer players responding to soccer defensive plays (1v1, 3v3, 11v11). The researchers found that skilled soccer defenders were quicker than lower-skilled players in predicting the direction and location of a pass. However, in contrast to Helsen and Pauwels (1992), they found that skilled players directed more fixations of shorter durations to areas that were tactically important, whereas the lower-skilled players were guilty of ball watching and spent longer amounts of time fixating the player in possession of the ball. High- and low-skilled players differed in their ability to anticipate the flow of the plays, but significant differences in fixations were found only in the 1v1 play. The skilled players spent more time fixating the hip region compared with the lesser-skilled defenders, who spent more time fixating the ball.

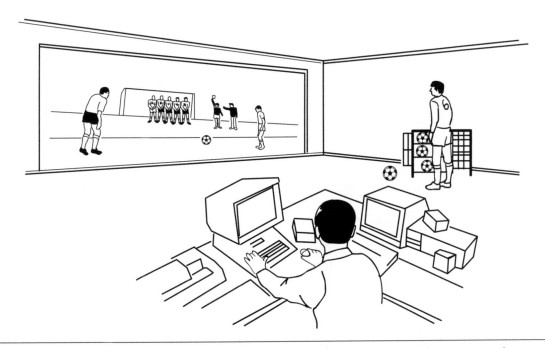

➤ **Figure 8.17** The experimental setup used by Helsen and Pauwels (1992) in examining soccer tactics.

In the following section, it will be shown that one of the reasons for the discrepancy in results may be due to the different task constraints portrayed in the visual-search stimuli used. Helsen and Pauwels (1992) presented soccer plays performed during the final moments when the visual field was restricted and where there was a need to fixate one or two critical cues before acting, while Williams and colleagues used plays of much longer duration encompassing much wider visual fields and gaze locations.

Gaze Control in Ice Hockey Tactics

Studies of gaze control in sport tactics as presented previously in this chapter have shown that elite players are faster than nonelite players in making decisions and that these decisions are of a higher quality (Helsen & Pauwels, 1992; Williams & Davids, 1998; Williams et al., 1994). But, as mentioned, the available research from soccer supports two different views of the temporal regulation of the gaze in sport tactics. According to Helsen and Pauwels (1992), the elite player has fewer fixations of longer duration directed to critical locations viewed late in the action. In contrast, Williams et al. (1994) and Williams and Davids (1998) argue that expertise is dependent on the ability to focus the gaze rapidly on critical locations fixated early in the development of the play. It is therefore unclear how athletes with different skill levels temporally regulate their gaze when performing tactical plays and what the relationship is between their gaze control and their decision making and performance.

In order to explore this problem, Martell and Vickers (2004) recorded the gaze of elite and near-elite ice hockey players as they defended against opponents on the ice. The elite players were members of the Canadian women's team that won the gold medal at the 2002 Olympics, and the near-elite players consisted of five members of the Canadian women's under-22 team that won the Canadian championship in 2001. The analyses focused on the temporal regulation of their gaze, specifically the onset and duration of fixation and tracking during successful and unsuccessful defensive plays.

The players' gaze and skating movements were recorded on ice using the vision-in-action method on ice. A frame of data is shown in figure 8.18. Image A shows the eye of the partici-

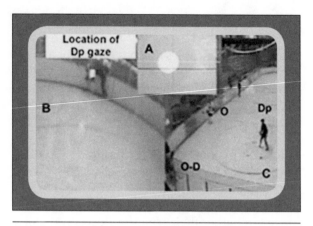

Figure 8.18   A frame of vision-in-action data collected in ice hockey.

Reprinted from Human Movement Science, Vol. 22, S. Martell and J.N. Vickers, Gaze characteristics of elite and near-elite ice hockey players, pp. 689-712, Copyright 2004, with permission from Elsevier.

pant (Dp). Image B shows the gaze of the participant located on a teammate and opponent in the corner. Image C was recorded by an external camera and shows the movements of the participant, teammates, opponents, and puck. The three images were synchronized in time using a time-code generator (not shown) at the rate of 33.33 ms/frame of data.

The participants were required to defend against highly skilled male players in two defensive plays well known in ice hockey. One of these plays is shown in figure 8.19, including the three phases of each trial skated. The three phases (preparation, situation assessment, final execution) were derived from Klein's (1999) RPD model of decision making. The preparation phase was similar to Klein's simple match (variation 1) where perceptual cues are quickly recognized and acted upon using a known course of action. Since both plays were well known to all the players, it was expected that both groups would quickly recognize each play and rapidly initiate skating. The trial therefore began with Dp standing with her eyes closed at center ice in a position to respond to the oncoming rush of O1, O2, D1, and Dt. A whistle from the coach signaled O1, O2, D1, and Dt to begin skating at full speed, while at the same time he shot the puck (P) into the defensive zone. When the first player reached the blue line (BL), a second whistle signaled Dp to open her eyes, read the play, and defend against it in an appropriate manner. The onset of the preparation phase therefore coincided with the first appearance of Dp's gaze, and the offset coincided with

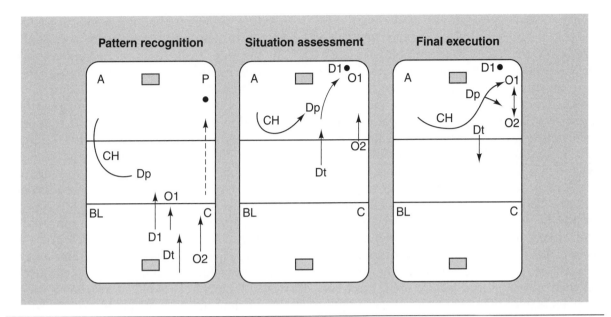

> **Figure 8.19** The three phases of an ice hockey defensive play: pattern recognition, situation assessment, and final execution. Here we see the positioning of the participant (Dp), defensive trailer (Dt), offensive players (O1 and O2), and defensive player (D1), as well as the coach (C), eye-tracker system (A), cable holder (CH), and blue line (BL).

Reprinted from Human Movement Science, Vol. 22, S. Martell and J.N. Vickers, Gaze characteristics of elite and near-elite ice hockey players, pp. 689-712, Copyright 2004, with permission from Elsevier.

the first movement of her skate to defend against the play (see figure 8.19).

The situation phase was based on variation 2 of the RPD model and required "diagnosing the situation" (Klein, 1999, p. 26). During this variation, both familiar and new information must be assessed, but the process ends in a familiar action being taken. In the situation phase, Dp skated rapidly to gain defensive position while at the same time scanning O1, O2, D1, Dt, the puck, and other locations on the ice. During this time both familiar and new information was fixated or tracked; however, given the nature of defensive play in ice hockey, success in each trial required one action to be taken by Dp. She had to engage one of the offensive players in a one-on-one situation and gain control over the puck. The situation phase therefore ended with Dp skating to engage the opposing player (O1 or O2) in the one-on-one situation. The final execution phase followed, and it ended when Dp made first contact with the offensive player or the player eluded her and had an opportunity to score. No shots were taken on goal (backswing only).

Two independent experts in ice hockey rated each trial from the videotaped data, as shown in figure 8.15. Since there were no shots on goal,

the participants were assessed on their ability to prevent a shot on goal or otherwise interrupt the flow of offensive play. The judges' ratings followed preset criteria that defined excellent to poor performance in each play. Only those trials where there was 100% agreement between the two experts were retained.

The results showed that during the pattern-recognition phase, both the elite and near-elite players quickly recognized the type of play and moved to defend in an appropriate manner. In the beginning of the situation phase, the elite group differed from the near-elite group in directing fixations of shorter duration to specific locations as the play developed. The groups did not differ in how quickly they shifted their gaze about the ice, nor did they differ in the number of fixations used or search rates, but they did differ in using a longer final fixation that was located on a single location during the final 30% of the phase. The use of this final long fixation had many of the characteristics found for the quiet eye in the other categories of tasks. It occurred before the final movement that ended each play (contact with an opposing player or the puck or loss of control) and was significantly longer than all other gazes for both groups, averaging 30% of the total trial time.

Overall, the results showed that expertise in ice hockey tactics is defined by the use of two gaze behaviors that occur in temporal sequence. Each trial began with a cascade of fixations of short duration and concluded with a final gaze or quiet eye of long duration to a relatively stable target. A **quick-then-quiet-eye** cascade of fixations occurred where the players quickly fixated critical cues during the early part of the play and concluded with a long duration quiet eye on a final location critical to regaining possession of the puck. These results therefore agreed with the research of Helsen and Pauwels (1992), Williams et al. (1994), and Williams and Davids (1998). Team tactical settings appear to require the use of fixations of short duration early in the play, followed by a single long fixation at the end when the players must take their assignment and gain control of the play.

Klein's RPD model assumes that it is the decision maker's ability to assess the situation, rather than comparative analysis of a number of plausible alternatives, that is critical in understanding typicality and solving the decision problem. This view is supported by the fact that the groups did not differ in the number of fixations or tracking used and their search rates were very similar, but the elite group used significantly shorter fixations during the early part of the situation-assessment phase. The experts' decision-making ability is reflected in a tighter coupling between perception and action than what is found for near-experts. Klein and Hoffman (1993) suggest that the ability to quickly judge what cues are most important in naturalistic environments is an acquired skill that separates many experts from nonexperts.

Klein and Hoffman (1993) summarize as follows: "By quickly seeing which goals are feasible, experts can direct their actions and not waste any effort. By recognizing which cues are relevant, experts can avoid information overload. By anticipating what events to expect, experts can rapidly notice if they have misperceived a situation. And by recognizing a typical course of action, experts can respond rapidly. This type of recognitional decision making enables experts to handle complex cases under time-pressured conditions where analytical methods would not be possible" (p. 211).

Gaze Control in Action

Select a training partner or partners and develop a quiet-eye decision-training program for a tactical task of your choice (select either a locomotion task, an offensive set play, or a defensive set play). Follow these steps:

1. List five quiet-eye characteristics that are needed to perform well in the tactical task. When listing each characteristic, name the cognitive skill that is most important (anticipation, attention, focus and concentration, memory, pattern recognition, problem solving, or decision making).

2. Second, design a drill or progression of drills that will help you and your partner be more successful in the tactical task.

3. Practice the drills for 20 to 30 min per day. Your main goal is to develop the optimal focus as the tactical task is prepared and executed.

Record your results. At the beginning of the first practice, record your pretraining accuracy for the first 10 shots before you do any quiet-eye training. Try to complete five training sessions. At the end of each practice session, record your percent accuracy on the final 10 trials on the blank graph provided on page 157.

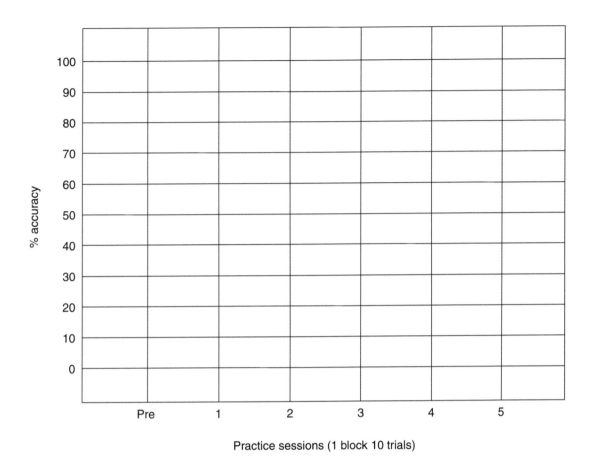

Practice sessions (1 block 10 trials)

From J.N. Vickers, 2007, *Perception, cognition, and decision training: The quiet eye in action* (Champaign, IL: Human Kinetics).

Prepare a short report in which you discuss the following topics:

1. List the five gaze control or quiet-eye characteristics that you selected to work on.

2. Provide a sketch of the drills used to train your quiet eye. Explain how each drill was used to improve your cognitive and quiet-eye focus.

3. What methods of practice did you use? (See chapters 9 through 12 for some ideas about how to vary your methods of training.)

4. Include the figure of results you generated from the blank graph and explain your percentage change over the five practices. Did you improve or get worse?

5. Using information from this chapter, discuss why your results occurred. In your opinion, what were the underlying reasons for your results?

Decision Training in Sport

Part III is concerned with applying many of the cognitive, ecological, dynamic systems, and gaze concepts presented in parts I and II in the everyday practice environment. Chapter 9 presents the three-step decision-training model, which has been used extensively in coaching for 15 y with all ages, abilities, and sport groups. Decision training provides a universal approach for teaching and coaching sport, as well as for physical therapy. Decision training has four major research foundations. These come from the scientific foundations presented in chapters 1 through 8, and also from motor learning studies done that show decision training is effective in improving athlete long-term performance.

Research from motor learning has changed quite dramatically over the past few years in the areas of practice design, feedback, and instruction. In all three areas, current research shows that when athletes experience too much behavioral training, they tend to perform at a high level initially, but these gains are lost both in the long term and when the athlete is placed under pressure. Motor learning research now advocates a change in how athletes are prepared, so that there is more cognitive involvement and shared decision making between the coach and athlete every day in practice. The three-step decision-training model teaches students how this can be done.

Chapters 10, 11, and 12 concentrate on presenting the research foundations for effective practice design, feedback, and instruction. A number of examples are presented in each chapter to highlight the three-step decision-training model, as well as the motor learning tools that exist for practice design, providing feedback, and instruction with a decision-training focus. A number of case studies are presented to provide practical guidance to students. A range of different types of sports are presented in order to illustrate the wide applicability of decision training.

At the conclusion of part III, students should be able to do the following:

➤ Name the four scientific foundations of the decision-training model.

➤ Describe the paradox in motor learning research.

➤ Describe the characteristics of behavioral training and decision training and the strengths and weaknesses of each approach.

➤ Complete the decision-training self-testing questionnaire in order to find out more about your current assumptions about how to best teach or coach.

➤ Name and describe the three steps in the decision-training model, including the seven cognitive skills, seven cognitive triggers, and seven decision-training tools.

➤ Explain how the quiet eye is a key component of decision training.

➤ Explain some of the changes that occur in the training environment when decision training is used. Explain why teachers and coaches must have a sound understanding of the underlying scientific principles from cognition, neuroscience, gaze control, and motor learning research in order to be successful.

➤ Design a decision-training drill in the sport task of the student's choice.

➤ Deliver a decision-training practice in a micro or modified coaching setting and receive feedback from peers and the instructor in a constructive decision-training environment.

Decision-Training Model

◀◀ *Where Have We Been?*

In the introduction and chapters 1 through 3, recent research was presented showing that successful performance in sport requires the optimal acquisition of visual information from complex and dynamically challenging environments. The role that visual information plays in sport performance was explained through scientific developments from cognitive science, ecological psychology, dynamic systems, and the constraints-led perspective. Each of these theoretical perspectives makes a valuable contribution to our understanding of how athletes optimally process information and the effect this has on their performance. Chapters 4 through 8 then concentrated on the new science of gaze control in sport and showed that what was once a hidden world (what athletes see as they perform) is now scientifically revealed, resulting in a new body of gaze control information that not only provides new insights into what underlies elite sport performance, but also provides a new literature that can be used in training.

▶▶ *Where Are We Going?*

In this chapter, a new approach to teaching and coaching sport is introduced: decision training. Decision training incorporates the cognitive and gaze research presented in the first eight chapters, recent developments from applied motor learning, and extensive application in the field. The research foundations are presented, followed by the three-step decision-training model. The chapter ends with a number of studies showing that decision training is effective in improving both performance and the training environment.

Decision training is a new method of teaching and coaching that incorporates into the regular practice environment high levels of decision making within simulated and real sport contexts. Decision training brings the science of how we think, or cognition, to the fore of sport preparation. It is designed to improve the athlete's attention, anticipation, concentration, memory, and problem-solving skills through practices where cognitive training is incorporated with physical and technical training. The overall goal is the development of an athlete who is able to make effective decisions under all the pressures of competition.

Four Scientific Foundations of Decision Training

The first foundation of decision training was presented in the introduction and chapters 1 through 3, where selected concepts from cognitive science, ecological psychology and dynamic systems, and visual attention and gaze were described. Special emphasis was placed on the visual system and visual information, since this has been researched most extensively within various motor and sport contexts. What athletes see when they perform is influenced by the inherent limits of the visuomotor system, specific task constraints, and organismic and environmental constraints. Understanding how these constraints function in real-world sport environments opens a new level of understanding of what underlies decision making and human performance.

The second foundation was presented in chapters 4 through 8, where gaze research in sport was introduced. The gaze and attention of athletes was described in selected targeting tasks, interceptive timing tasks, and tactical tasks. Emerging research from this body of literature shows a strong relationship between shifts of gaze and shifts of attention, thus opening a window that objectively explains how focus and concentration (or lack thereof) contribute to motor performance. In particular, this growing body of research describes how elite athletes control their gaze and how this contributes to their higher levels of decision making and performance.

The third foundation of decision training comes from its extensive use in the field (Vickers, 2000a; Vickers, 2003; Vickers, 1996a, 1996b, 1996c). Decision training has been used for more than 15 y by coaches at all levels in a wide variety of sports, age groups, and ability groups. During this time, the literatures underlying decision training have been put to the test in terms of its applicability to the real world. In some cases (as will be revealed in later chapters), some aspects have been found wanting in terms of transferring from the laboratory to the practice setting, and so adaptations have been made that allow the concepts to successfully work in the field. A number of studies have been completed that have assessed its effectiveness, and these are presented at the end of this chapter (Chambers & Vickers, 2006; Raab, Masters, & Maxwell, 2005; Vickers, Livingston, Umeris, & Holden, 1999; Vickers, Reeves, Chambers, & Martell, 2004).

The fourth foundation will be presented in this chapter, as well in chapters 10 through 12, and comes from motor learning and the emergence of a paradoxical finding from research in practice design, feedback, and instruction. Extensive research in all three areas shows that traditional forms of teaching and coaching, which are collectively called **behavioral training**, are successful in the short term, but athletes trained exclusively under these conditions are unable to perform consistently at a high level in the long term, especially when under pressure. In the following section, these paradoxical developments from motor learning are presented.

Paradox of Modern Motor Learning Research

Until the late 1970s, most researchers in motor learning promoted the use of behavioral training methods where athletes were trained using blocked repetitive practice. During blocked training, complex skills and tactics are broken down through a process called *task analysis* into countless subskills that are then trained using simple to complex progressions of drills (Gagne & Briggs, 1979; Solso, 1995; Vickers, 1990). These procedures are designed to lead learners gradually through a process where the mastery of basic skills occurs before the introduction of complex tactics and decision-making skills. Often the drills are performed under restricted conditions where a specific component of a movement is isolated and repetitively practiced until a state of perfection is achieved. During this process, high levels of technical feedback and specific guidance are provided.

This approach can be traced to a major school of psychology called **behaviorism.** Although behaviorism reached its zenith in the 1950s, it still plays a major role in sport teaching and coaching, as well as in many other areas of education and training. The laws of behaviorism state that a response will become a habit as a consequence of the number of times it is paired or associated with a given stimulus (Skinner, 1953; Thorndike, 1911; Watson, 1924). In order to become proficient in a motor skill, a close association must be fostered between a specific stimulus and response through extensive repetition of the same pairings. Success is measured by visible and immediate changes in physical behavior; there is no concern for the internal thoughts or cognitive processes of the performer. The overarching goal of behaviorism was captured by Watson (1924, p. 11), who stated that "it is the business of behavioristic psychology to be able to predict and control human activity." When a behavioristic approach is used, the mind of the performer is largely discounted as a factor in performance.

Beginning in the late 1970s, however, research began to emerge showing that people trained using behavioral methods were unable to retain the new skills and concepts over an extended length of time. Although the gains in performance were impressive in the short term, they were not sustained over time, especially when new and unusual conditions were encountered (Battig, 1956; Battig, 1966; Battig, 1979; Doane, Alderton, Sohn, & Pelligrino, 1996; Goode & Magill, 1986; Hall, Domingues, & Cavazos, 1994; Shea & Morgan, 1979; Sidaway & Hand, 1993; Swinnen, Schmidt, Nicholson, & Shapiro, 1990; Winstein & Schmidt, 1990).

Figure 9.1 presents an overview of this research and the curious **paradox in motor learning research** that has emerged from the three major areas of practice design, feedback, and instruction (for reviews see Christina & Bjork, 1991; Farr, 1987; Lee, Swinnen, & Serrien, 1994; Schmidt, 1991; Vickers, 1994a). The *y*-axis shows the amount of improvement achieved in a skill or tactic, and the *x*-axis shows the amount of progress made over both the short and long term. The dotted line shows the progress of performers who have been trained using traditional behavioral methods, and the solid line shows the progress of those trained using the newer decision-training methods. Notice that during behavioral training, positive gains occur immediately; therefore this type of training is appealing to many coaches and athletes alike. Coaches feel they are training their athletes correctly and athletes feel they are mastering the sport, but notice what happens in the long term. Performance declines, especially when difficult and stressful conditions are encountered. In contrast, the solid line shows the progress of

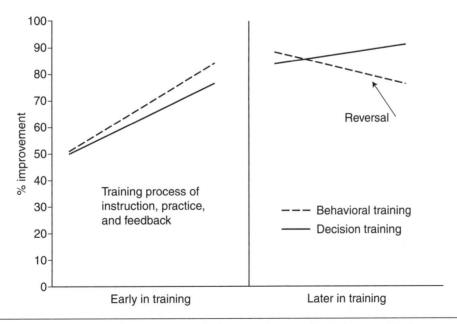

➤ **Figure 9.1** Overview of motor learning research showing the paradoxical reversal in long-term performance that occurs when behavioral training and decision training are used.

those who have experienced decision training. Here we see that although their performance may be depressed initially, in the long term they continue to improve and ultimately perform at a higher level.

Importance of Retention and Transfer Tests

Why have the results shown in figure 9.1 emerged only in the last few years? After all, motor learning is an old field, one that dates back to the 19th century. Before the 1980s, the majority of learning studies, whether in cognition, motor learning, education, or educational psychology, did not test progress after the initial acquisition period. Only short-term learning was assessed and so the reversal that occurs when retention or transfer tests are given was not discovered until recently. **Retention tests** assess the extent that the same skill can be reproduced later on, while **transfer tests** determine if the skill can be used in new situations. Transfer tests are normally more complex than retention tests because they require higher levels of **problem solving** and decision making. Research studies now normally include retention and transfer trials so that both short- and long-term changes in learning and performance can be assessed.

Characteristics of Behavioral Training

The characteristics of behavioral training compared to those of decision training are shown on page 165. The characteristics of decision training and behavioral training are subdivided into the three research areas of instruction, practice, and feedback. During behavioral training, the main emphasis is on the acquisition of technical and physiological skill, and there is little regard for the development of cognitive skills during practices. Behavioral coaching promotes high levels of physical effort but ignores the development of the athlete's perceptual and cognitive processes within regular practices. Instruction follows a path of part-to-whole learning using simple to complex drills. Basic skills are taught before more advanced ones using high levels of repetitive **blocked practice.** The intent is to build the sport gradually so that more complex skills and tactics are introduced

only after the basic skills have been achieved. Practice drills are normally blocked, with the same drills often performed over and over. Technical and physical perfection is the goal.

Coaches who use a behavioral approach immediately provide abundant feedback whenever possible. Athletes are rarely questioned about their performance or expected to detect or correct their own errors or provide solutions. Instead, this is viewed as the primary function of the coach or teacher. There is limited use of video models, where the athletes view other athletes in order to gain insight into how to perform better, or video feedback, where the athletes view themselves in order to detect and correct their own errors.

Behavioral training promotes an internal focus of attention, since coaches continually draw the athletes' attention into their own bodies. Often there is an active attempt to switch the athlete's mind off in favor of the attainment of rapid automaticity. But this approach may be hit and miss, meaning performance is exceptionally good one day and terrible the next. Both the athlete and coach are usually at a loss to know why. Athletes trained in this way do not develop the higher-order cognitive skills needed to understand what underlies their own higher (or lower) levels of performance. This is one reason why they are unable to retain the skill or tactics over long periods of time. This was a point made earlier in chapter 8 by Ericsson (2003), who commented that experts in any field rarely let their actions become fully automatic but constantly find ways to improve using high levels of **cognitive effort** and decision making. In order for the long-term retention and transfer of skills to occur, the athlete has to lay down new neural networks that underlie gains in motor performance.

Characteristics of Decision Training

When a decision-training approach is used, the same emphasis is placed on technical and physiological training, but the cognitive skills underlying higher levels of performance are trained at the same time. Instead of using simple to complex drills, tactical whole training is used where skills are trained within tactically oriented drills that simulate parts of the game. A technique-within-tactics approach is used, where the same technical perfection is sought, but within tactical contexts. Hard-first instruction is used where higher-level tactical concepts are taught in advance of specific skills training. Instead of emphasizing an internal focus of instruction that continually draws the athletes' attention into their bodies and their emotional processes, an external focus is trained where the athletes are encouraged to direct their attention outward to the critical objects, locations, and tactical events in their sport. Communication between the coach and athlete changes from one where the coach tells the athletes what to do to one where the athletes are required to analyze their own performance and provide corrective solutions. This is achieved by deliberately withdrawing and reducing feedback using a bandwidth approach. In order to maintain communication and increase cognitive effort, the athletes are asked questions that probe their understanding and knowledge of the specific skills, tactics, and activities they are engaged in.

When a decision-training approach is used, learning is inferred when there is evidence of two things: the correct decision is being made, and the decision contributes to higher levels of physical performance. As a result, a decision trainer conducts practices where athletes learn to make decisions under the many conditions encountered in the sport or activity. Practices with a decision-training focus help athletes anticipate events, attend to critical cues, retrieve the best response from memory, focus on the appropriate events at the right time, and make effective decisions in both low- and high-pressure settings. Decision training therefore incorporates higher levels of cognitive effort into the practice environment while preserving or increasing the amount of physiological, technical, and tactical training that occurs. Cognitive effort is defined as the mental work that "leads to high levels of decision making . . . anticipation, planning, regulation and interpretation of motor performance" (Lee et al., 1994, p. 328-329). Permanent gains are only achieved when cognitive and physical training occur in concert.

In the next section, the three-step decision-training model is presented in detail. The purpose

Comparison of Behavioral Training and Decision Training

Behavioral Training (Physical, Technical, Noncognitive)

Instruction

➤ Part-to-whole training
➤ Simple to complex drills
➤ Easy-first instruction
➤ Technical emphasis
➤ Internal focus of instruction
➤ Low use of video models

Practice

➤ Blocked practice
➤ Low variability

Feedback

➤ Abundant coach feedback
➤ Low use of questioning
➤ Low use of video feedback
➤ Low athlete detection and correction of errors

Overall: Low levels of athlete cognitive effort

Decision Training (Physical, Technical, Cognitive)

Instruction

➤ Tactical whole training
➤ Competition-like drills
➤ Hard-first instruction
➤ Technique within tactics
➤ External focus of instruction
➤ High use of video models

Practice

➤ Variable practice
➤ Random practice

Feedback

➤ Bandwidth feedback
➤ High use of questioning
➤ High use of video feedback
➤ High athlete detection and correction of errors

Overall: High levels of athlete cognitive effort

of the model is to provide professionals in sport, physical activity, and therapy with research-based strategies shown to improve decision making in sport. The decision-training model can be applied to any sport, age group, or ability group, thus offering a universal approach to coaching science that has been lacking thus far.

Three-Step Decision-Training Model

We saw in the previous section that one of the main reasons that the decision-training approach has been successful is because of a curious paradox that has occurred in the research on motor learning in the past few years. This paradox shows that the traditional approaches to sport training, with their high levels of repetition, feedback, and direct instruction, lead to impressive gains in the short term, but athletes trained exclusively under these conditions often falter in the long term. Research on motor learning now advocates the use of new methods, such as variable practice, random practice, and bandwidth feedback. However, these methods, which are decision-training tools, are not enough to ensure successful performance. Instead, the overall purpose of the practice must be defined first and stated clearly. In the past, instructional designers, curriculum leaders, coaches, and teachers were taught to identify the behavioral goals they wanted their athletes to achieve. Decision training does not follow this approach, but instead requires that the critical athlete decisions underlying successful performance be defined and overtly trained within the practice training environment. The goal is to help the athlete make better decisions, which in turn will lead to greater long term gains in performance.

Instead of leaving to chance the tough job of learning how to make effective decisions, the three steps of the decision-training model bring the training of critical decisions found in each sport to the fore. Figure 9.2 presents the three steps of the decision-training model.

Step 1: Identify a Decision to Be Trained

In step 1, it is necessary to identify the decisions that athletes have to make in competition. Each decision should include one of the seven cogni-tive skills emphasized in this book and shown in the following list. Each decision must also couple one of the cognitive skills with one skill or tactic from the sport. Note that decision training is always applied to specific sports and tactics. It is therefore necessary that teachers and coaches have a good working knowledge of the skills and tactics of their sport. As discussed earlier, the cognitive skills are as follows:

➤ Anticipation is the ability to predict what will occur when preparing to perform a skill or tactic. Before performing, what information must be seen, felt, heard, or otherwise perceived or attended to before acting?

➤ Attention is the ability to select the correct cue from the many that are available before and as an action is performed. What information must be attended to during the performance of a specific skill or tactic?

➤ Focus and concentration refer to the ability to consistently detect the correct cues and not be distracted by irrelevant events over an extended period of time. Specific visual cues that aid anticipation, focus, and concentration in targeting and interceptive timing tasks were identified in chapters 5 to 7.

➤ Pattern recognition is the ability to discern meaning while moving through complex environments. Pattern recognition is required to detect objects and locations during locomotion and in tactical plays that contain expectancies, relevant cues, plausible goals, and actions.

➤ Memory retrieval requires the ability to find the best solutions in memory given the ever-changing conditions found in sport settings. What information must be retrieved? How long does it take the athlete to remember what to do in a specific sport setting? Klein's recognition-primed decision model was presented in chapter 8 as central to this process.

➤ Problem solving is the ability to transform "a given situation into a goal situation when no obvious method of solution is available to the problem solver" (Eysenck, 1994, p. 284). Problem solving occurs constantly in sport and can range from the routine (getting open for a pass) to the novel and complex (executing a

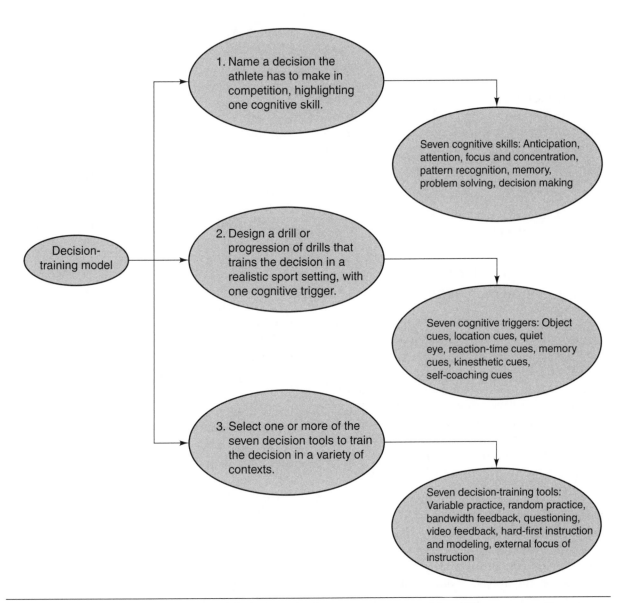

➤ **Figure 9.2** The decision-training model, showing the three steps, seven cognitive skills, seven cognitive triggers, and seven decision-training tools.

completely new play in the final seconds of a game).

➤ Decision making is "the ability to make the best choice between a set of alternatives" (Eysenck, 1994). The ability to make effective decisions is critical in sport and draws on all the other perceptual and cognitive skills discussed earlier.

Many of the foundations for writing the decisions in step 1 were presented in chapters 1 through 8. For example, chapter 5 presented research showing that elite shooters achieve high levels of accuracy in basketball by fixating one location on the hoop within 1° of visual angle for about 1 s before the final extension of the shooting hand. They use this same quiet-eye information in the jump shot and the free throw from different locations on the court and under all types of conditions. Therefore a key decision that athletes have to make when learning to shoot in basketball is to control their gaze and attention so they have the same quiet-eye target information even under the most challenging of conditions. We also saw that specific types of gaze control, attention, and decision making were described in the other categories of targeting, interceptive timing, and tactical tasks.

Practices with a decision-training focus help athletes anticipate events, attend to critical cues, retrieve the best response from memory, focus on the appropriate events at the right time, and overall make effective decisions in both low- and high-pressure settings. As discussed, decision training therefore incorporates higher levels of cognitive effort into the practice environment while preserving or increasing the amount of physiological, technical, and tactical training that occurs. It is only through combined cognitive–motor training that the athletes learn to meet the challenges they will face.

Step 2: Design a Drill With a Cognitive Trigger

Step 2 requires a drill or progression of drills to be designed that best trains the decision identified in step 1. Drills selected in step 2 may be familiar, or they may be new drills developed to train specific decision-making skills. The key is that each drill contains a **cognitive trigger**. A cognitive trigger tells the athlete (and the coach) if the correct decision has been made as the skill or tactic is performed. Seven cognitive triggers that have come from the previous chapters are listed here.

➤ Object cues were defined in chapter 2 (Treisman, 1986a). Athletes are asked to anticipate or focus their attention on a specific object and identify it in some way before performing. These cues function as cognitive triggers the coach can use to see if the athlete is able to detect the cue and use it before performing. For example, in the volleyball training study (Adolphe, Vickers, & LaPlante, 1997) presented in chapter 7, the players had to call out the numbers and letters on the ball before receiving the serve and passing to the setter. This verbal cue not only provided a stimulating challenge for the athlete, but also told the coach whether the athlete was able to track the ball effectively.

➤ Location cues were also defined in chapter 2 (Treisman, 1986a). The athletes are asked to anticipate or focus their attention on a location such as a target area and name it in some way before performing. Gaze locations function as cognitive triggers when athletes have to verbalize or otherwise indicate if they have perceived the cue before executing the skill. For example, in a targeting task, such as basketball shooting, the

athlete may be required to name the final fixation location on the hoop before shooting.

➤ Quiet-eye cues were identified in chapters 5 through 8 in targeting, interceptive timing, and tactical sport tasks. Quiet-eye cues are based on research and contribute to higher levels of skill and performance.

➤ Memory cues are stored in long-term memory and are built up as a consequence of extensive training in sport. Quite often athletes cannot retrieve from memory a solution that is actually well learned, so they need to be trained to get at the right solutions at the right time. Memory-retrieval cues can be trained by asking the athlete to place one skill (which is named) in memory and to hold in memory another skill or skills that may or may not be retrieved by a cue from the coach to switch skills. This type of drill trains the athlete to quickly and accurately retrieve what is needed from memory.

➤ Reaction-time cues require the athlete to switch between skills held in memory within different time constraints. These cues are triggered by a coach's command, external stimuli such as the opponent's movement, or another signal. Information from chapter 3 on the time course of human perception is valuable here because it distinguishes between reaction time and movement time and the thresholds that exist for the sensory systems.

➤ Kinesthetic cues require the athletes to attain a particular feeling for a position, technique, or temporal event.

➤ Self-coaching cues require the athletes to make decisions about how they will train. For example, before practice the athletes may be asked to identify a problem they are having, such as hitting a target (as in shooting in basketball). A day or two before practice, the athletes must submit to the coach one reason why they have this particular problem, as well as identify a training strategy that might help them improve. This is a problem-solving and decision-making exercise that helps the athletes think through their performance difficulties and provide constructive suggestions.

Step 3: Use DT Tools to Train the Decision

In step 3, one or more of the seven tools for decision training are used to train the decision identified in step 1 within the context of step 2. The tools were described earlier and have been derived from extensive research in practice design, feedback, and instruction. The seven decision-training (DT) tools are grouped as follows:

Practice design
- ➤ DT tool 1: Variable practice (smart variations)
- ➤ DT tool 2: Random practice (smart combinations)

Feedback and questioning
- ➤ DT tool 3: Bandwidth feedback
- ➤ DT tool 4: Questioning
- ➤ DT tool 5: Video feedback

Instruction
- ➤ DT tool 6: Hard-first instruction and modeling
- ➤ DT tool 7: External focus of instruction

Modern research on motor learning provides a rich array of tools that allow a decision trainer to design practices where athletes learn to make decisions under the many conditions encountered in sport. For example, in order for athletes to learn to shoot well in basketball using a quiet eye, they need to be trained using variable and random practice conditions (instead of blocked practices), they need to have deliberately delayed and reduced feedback as their skill level improves (instead of abundant feedback), and they need hard-first instruction that helps them direct their attention externally (instead of internally). Each of the training tools is presented in depth in the following chapters, with examples from targeting, interceptive timing, and tactical tasks as found in a variety of sports selected as exemplars. An overview of the decision-training model with its three steps, seven cognitive skills, seven cognitive triggers, and seven DT tools is given on page 170.

Evidence Showing the Effectiveness of Decision Training

Three studies are presented that show the effectiveness of decision training in a number of sport contexts. In the first, a table tennis study by Raab et al. (2005) is presented that compares decision training with behavioral training in table tennis.

In the second, the effectiveness of decision training over behavioral training is shown in baseball hitting (Vickers et al., 1999). Third, 13 coaches in nine sports were analyzed over a full season to see the extent to which they continued to use decision-training methods after first being introduced to the method (Vickers et al., 2004). A fourth study will also be presented in chapter 11 showing the effectiveness of bandwidth feedback with a group of young elite swimmers (Chambers & Vickers, 2006).

Decision Training in Table Tennis

Raab et al. (2005) compared the effectiveness of decision-training and behavioral methods using young, elite table tennis players. At the outset they described decision training as having "integrated the existing motor learning literature and emphasized the training of cognitive aspects involved in decisions rather than only movement execution. In short, this approach proposes that skills should be acquired as a gestalt whole that does not separate declarative from procedural, or technical from tactical, because performance requires efficient integration of all sources of information/knowledge. . . . However, the effectiveness of combining both behavioral and decision strategies into a single training regime has not been assessed. It is possible that behavioral training exerts its influence primarily on 'how' to perform an action, whereas decision training benefits 'what' movement should be performed" (p. 328).

The purpose of the study was therefore to determine which training method (behavioral or decision) would produce the best shot selection in table tennis both in training and also later in game play. Twenty table tennis players (mean age 11.4 y) were recruited from the German Olympic Training Centre and assigned quasirandomly to two groups (behavioral and decision training) so that their performance levels were equivalent. Both groups received the same number of hours of training over 9 wk. The behavioral group received technical (how) training at regular intervals emphasizing targeting accuracy in the forehand and backhand strokes. The decision group received the same training for the first 4 wk but in the remaining 5 wk they were also provided with decision (what) training in the form of video feedback and video modeling oriented toward improving their transitions from the backhand to forehand (or vice

Overview of the Decision-Training Model

Step 1: Decisions

Identify one decision that is to be trained using one of the following cognitive skills.

1. Anticipate what is going to happen
2. Attend to critical cues
3. Concentrate and focus
4. Recognize patterns of objects
5. Retrieve solutions from memory
6. Solve problems in known and new settings
7. Make the best decision in competition and about own and others' training

Step 2: Drills

Design or select a drill or activity that trains the decision in a realistic setting using one of the following cognitive triggers.

1. Object cues
2. Location cues
3. Quiet-eye cues
4. Reaction-time cues
5. Memory-retrieval cues
6. Kinesthetic cues
7. Self-coaching cues

Step 3: Tools

Use one of the training tools to train the decisions using a variety of methods that enhance decision making.

1. DT tool 1: Variable practice
2. DT tool 2: Random practice
3. DT tool 3: Bandwidth feedback
4. DT tool 4: Questioning
5. DT tool 5: Video feedback
6. DT tool 6: Hard-first instruction and modeling
7. DT tool 7: External focus of instruction

versa). Table tennis is a sport where about 550 ms is needed to select a shot and make a hit (Rodrigues, Vickers, & Williams, 2002; Roth, 1989). The training was therefore designed to improve not only the ability to hit the ball but also to select the best shot as quickly as possible. Training this type of movement requires anticipation and decision-making skills mediated by time.

Videotapes were taken of the athletes during competitive matches and rated by two national-level table tennis coaches before, midway, and twice after the training period. The two groups were assessed both on how well they technically performed the strokes and their ability to make the best tactical decisions in terms of shot selection. The results are shown in figure 9.3, which reveals the progress of the two groups in terms of their improvements in both technique (how) and tactical decision making (what). During the delayed posttest the behavior group ranked last in terms of their ability to make tactical decisions (what) and ranked second in terms of their technique (how), while the decision-trained group ranked first in their tactical decision making (what) and

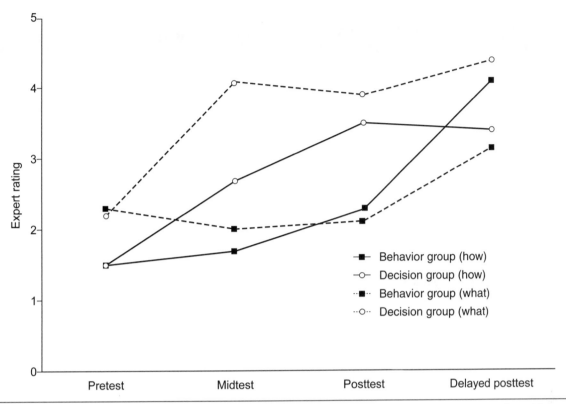

➤ **Figure 9.3** Expert ratings of performance of 'how' decisions (full lines) and 'what' decisions (dotted lines) for the behavior group (black filled squares) and the decision group (white unfilled circles) on a scale of 1 (poor) to 5 (excellent) for pretest, midtest, postest, and delayed posttest.

Reprinted from Human Movement Science, Vol. 24, M. Raab, R.S.W. Masters and J.P. Maxwell, Improving the 'how' and 'what' decisions of elite table tennis players, pp. 326-344, Copyright 2005, with permission from Elsevier.

third in terms of their technique (how). These results show that the combination of technical training and tactical decision training was more successful than technical training alone.

Decision Training in Baseball

Vickers et al. (1999) tested the effectiveness of a decision-training program versus a behavioral training program in baseball hitting. The program lasted 7 wk, and a week-by-week schedule is shown in table 9.1. The participants were undergraduates (137 men and 112 women) aged 18 to 38 y, randomly placed in a behavioral training (BT) or decision-training (DT) group by the registrar's office. Each participant hit a total of 200 pitches during a pretest, 5 wk of training, and a transfer test in week 7. All hits were taken in a professional batting cage maintained by professional staff. The speed of the ball during the pretest and training period was set at a perceived speed of 94 mph (151 kph), or 67 mph (108 kph) real speed.

In week 1, a pretest was given to the BT and DT groups to determine entry-level hitting abil-ity. Three skill levels (novice, intermediate, and advanced) were determined based on the hitting percentages in the pretest. The BT group received abundant feedback from the instructors and peers, whereas the DT group received bandwidth feedback, where feedback was deliberately reduced as their skill level improved. Each participant's swing was videotaped during the pretest.

In week 2, the BT group received easy-first technical instruction from an expert baseball coach who demonstrated the basic components of the baseball grip, stance, and swing. Each participant performed the swing in a simple to complex progression of drills accompanied by feedback from the coach, laboratory instructors, and peers. The practice ended with hitting soft pitches into a net. At the same time, the DT group received hitting instruction using hard-first modeling. They viewed a 30 min video of an expert hitting baseballs in slow motion, in real time, with kinematic overlay, from the left and right perspectives, and with auditory augmentation as the bat contacted the ball. The video also showed the hitting action from behind the hitter as well

Table 9.1   Behavioral and Decision-Training Program for Baseball Hitting

Week	Behavioral training	Decision training
Week 1	Pretest Blocked practice High levels of feedback	Pretest Blocked practice Bandwidth feedback
Week 2	Easy-first instruction Technical model Blocked practice High levels of feedback	Hard-first instruction Holistic model No practice
Week 3	Variable practice High levels of feedback	Variable practice Bandwidth feedback
Week 4	Instructor video feedback Abundant feedback	Self-video feedback Bandwidth feedback
Week 5	Video feedback Variable practice High levels of feedback	Video feedback Variable practice Bandwidth feedback
Week 6	No practice	No practice
Week 7	Competition	Competition

as from the side. From this perspective they were able to attend to the delivery of the pitch, the flight of the ball, the hitter's stance, and the swing through contact with the ball. This group did not swing the bat during the instructional week, a factor that may have harmed the later performance of the DT novices.

In week 3, all groups practiced hitting in the batting cages using variable practice. Variable practice was created by the pitching machines, which delivered the ball throughout the strike zone.

In week 4, both the BT and DT groups analyzed their swings on videotape. The BT group also received feedback from the instructors, who pointed out critical errors and gave directions for improvement. The DT group was required to work independently and compared their hitting frame by frame with that of a hitting model shown on an adjacent monitor.

In week 5, both groups returned to the batting cages and practiced hitting. The BT group received extensive feedback, whereas the DT group reviewed their performance on a monitor compared to that of an expert model.

In week 6, no hits were taken to permit for a transfer delay.

In week 7, the BT and DT groups competed against each other to see who could achieve the highest percentage of hits. The pitching machine was set at a new speed of 104 mph (167 kph), and prizes were made available for each skill group and gender.

Novice Hitting Percentages

Figure 9.4 shows the hitting percentages of the novices over the 7 wk and 200 hits (blocks of 10 hits). As predicted, the BT group hit at a higher level during the training period, but during the final test (t18-t20), the expected better performance of the DT group did not emerge. Instead, the BT group performed at a higher level throughout. The lower performance of the DT group was traced, in part, to the lack of practice opportunities in week 2 when they were given instruction in hitting using an elite video model. If a hitting session similar to what the BT group received had been scheduled following this instruction, then the DT group may have kept pace with the BT group, a result also supported by the Raab et al. (2005) study presented previously. Overall, the results show that when first learning a motor skill, physical practice must occur.

Intermediate Hitting Percentages

Hitting percentages of the intermediate hitters are shown in figure 9.5. As predicted, the BT group hit at a higher level during the training period

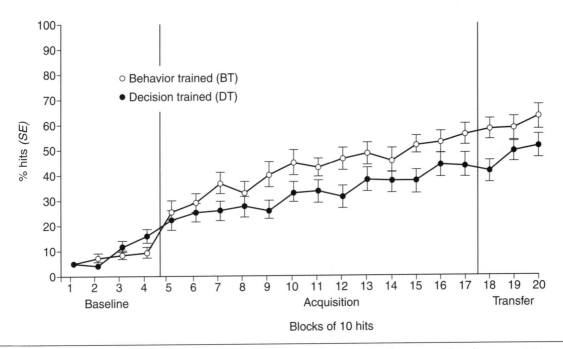

➤ **Figure 9.4** Novice baseball hitting: Percentage of balls hit by BT and DT players over baseline, acquisition, and transfer (20 blocks of 10 trials).

Reprinted, by permission, from J.N. Vickers et al., 1999, "Decision training: The effects of complex instruction, variable practice and reduced delayed feedback on the acquisition and transfer of a motor skill," *J. Sports Sci.* 17(5): 357-367.
http://www.tandf.co.uk/journals

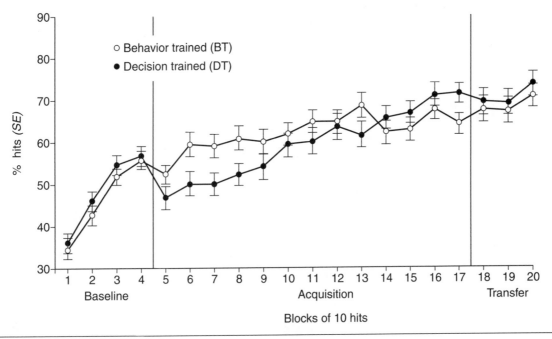

➤ **Figure 9.5** Intermediate baseball hitting: Percentage of balls hit by BT and DT groups over baseline, acquisition, and transfer (20 blocks of 10 trials).

Reprinted, by permission, from J.N. Vickers et al., 1999, "Decision training: The effects of complex instruction, variable practice and reduced delayed feedback on the acquisition and transfer of a motor skill," *J. Sports Sci.* 17(5): 357-367.
http://www.tandf.co.uk/journals

(t5-t13) but were eclipsed by the DT group after hit t14, after which point the DT group maintained a higher percentage. During the final competition, both groups improved equally from t18 to t20. The better performance of the DT emerged as predicted. Note that at t20, the DT group hit at a level higher than at any other time during the study.

Advanced Hitting Percentages

The advanced hitters did not improve to the same degree as the novices and intermediates, but this is to be expected given their high skill level (80%-90%), which led to a ceiling effect. During the acquisition period, the BT group hit at a higher level as predicted, whereas the DT group's performance declined by more than 20% following the hard-first video modeling session (prior to t5). The depression in performance by the elite hitters early on is predicted when decision training is used (see figure 9.6). During the final competition (t18-t20), the DT group hit at a higher level, and the BT group's performance declined to a level lower than what they had achieved during the previous weeks.

Decision-training methods were beneficial for the higher-skilled groups but were not as effective for the novices. Although all the novices improved over the 7 wk, those who experienced BT performed at a higher level than those using DT.

Equal levels of physical practice were not made available to the DT novices during the beginning few weeks, and this worked to the detriment of the group. In addition to showing that novices need the opportunity to physically practice, this study also revealed that the benefits of DT are often delayed. A sustained depression in performance occurred for both the intermediate and elite groups, but this is predicted by the method. Similar delays in improvement were reported by Rothstein and Arnold (1976) in a meta-analysis of the effectiveness of video feedback and in a later study by Selder and Del Rolan (1979), who found improvements were delayed for 5 wk. Reasons for this are elaborated on in chapter 10.

Coaches' Use of Decision Training

Vickers et al. (2004) followed 13 experienced coaches over a full season in order to determine the extent to which they would use the seven DT tools in their regularly scheduled practices. All were full-time coaches (four females and nine males) enrolled in a coaching certification program. The sports they coached included badminton, cross-country skiing, short- and long-track speed skating, squash, men's and women's ice hockey, track and field, and wrestling. The athletes they coached

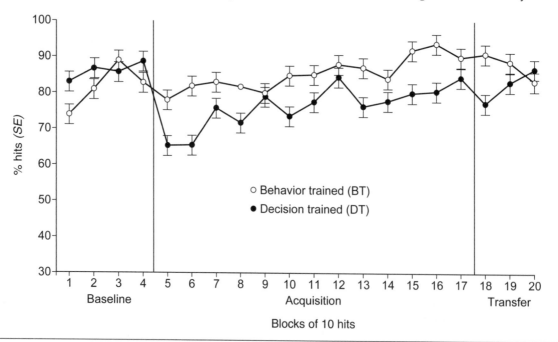

➤ **Figure 9.6**   Advanced baseball hitting: Percentage of balls hit by BT and DT groups over baseline, acquisition, and transfer (20 blocks of 10 trials).

Reprinted, by permission, from J.N. Vickers et al., 1999, "Decision training: The effects of complex instruction, variable practice and reduced delayed feedback on the acquisition and transfer of a motor skill," *J. Sports Sci.* 17(5): 357-367.
http://www.tandf.co.uk/journals

ranged in age from 11 to 30 y, and their skill levels ranged from developmental to seasoned international and Olympic competitors.

The coaches were videotaped during three regularly scheduled practices (P1, P2, P3) spaced across the season. Practice 1 (P1) occurred in the first month and was videotaped before the coaches received any formal education in decision training. In month 2, the coaches took a 1 wk course where the three-step decision-training model was presented. The first 2 days were spent covering the underlying theory and research in a workshop setting, followed by 3 days of microcoaching where each coach assumed three roles: coach, athlete, and peer evaluator. By experiencing these three roles, the coaches were able to learn how to implement decision training as a coach, experience decision training as an athlete, and develop skills in observing peer coaches and providing constructive feedback. Practice 2 (P2) occurred 1 mo after the course during the coaches' regularly scheduled practice with the athletes. Practice 3 (P3) then occurred in month 5 or 6, after all course requirements were completed and no evaluation pressures were present. It was expected that the coaches would improve from P1 to P2 as a result of taking the decision-training course. The critical comparison was therefore from P1 to P3, where no evaluation pressures or observers were present and the coaches were free to conduct their practices as they deemed appropriate.

Two coders familiar with decision training coded the videotapes using the decision-training instrument (Vickers, 2000a; Vickers, 2005). This instrument was developed over many years of working with the coaches and included the three-step decision-training process and the seven DT tools. A 5-point Likert scale was used in which a score of 5 was deemed excellent, 4 good, 3 above average, 2 below average, and 1 unacceptable.

No significant differences were found in any of the practice-management skills. All percentages obtained were within the ranges expected (Seidentop, 1976; Vickers, 1990; Vickers, 2000a), allaying fears that increasing cognitive effort during practices would take away from the time devoted to physical training (Cross & Lyle, 1999; Douge & Hastie, 1993; Seidentop, 1976).

Significant improvements were found from P1 to P3 in using variable and random practice. Improvements were also found in bandwidth feedback and questioning. The coaches reduced the frequency of **corrective feedback** while at the

same time increasing questions asked. Of all the tools, the coaches consistently commented that questioning was the most valuable. One of the coaches put it best when he stated, "If an athlete comes up to me and asks a simple question, I know he or she is looking for a simple answer and the athlete does not understand how decision making operates in our sport. I know now that this also translates into a bad or inconsistent performance in competition. On the other hand, if an athlete asks for verification of their own discovery, then I know that athlete is engaged in developing the decision-making skills needed. Decision training encourages the process of self-discovery and starts the athletes on coming up with well-thought-out questions and solutions and not just looking for answers." From P1 to P2 there was an increase in the use of hard-first instruction and modeling, but there were no increases from P2 to P3. This is appropriate; by definition, hard-first instruction should be provided early in the season and not later in order to maximize the amount of time the athletes have to cognitively incorporate the material into their motor performance. The use of modeling also increased from P1 to P2 but not from P2 to P3. This again was expected since modeling should occur more in the early part of a season as a method of developing analytical and cognitive skills that are sport specific and most effective after long-term use.

The observers also provided a DT index where they measured the extent to which the coaches delivered practices that were perceived to increase the athlete's cognitive effort and decision-making skills. The DT index increased significantly from P1 to P2 and from P2 to P3. The increased use of decision-training methods was observed to help the athletes develop the anticipation, attention, memory, and problem-solving skills needed to perform under all competitive conditions. In the opinion of the observers, the coaching environment improved significantly in that high-level decision-making abilities were being developed.

The coaches were followed for 3 y after the study in terms of their employment and success as coaches. Of the 13 who took part, 4 coached athletes at the 2002 Salt Lake Olympics and two of their athletes won medals, even though they were relatively junior coaches at the time of learning about decision training. In addition, 8 went on to successfully coach at the national or provincial level, 3 at the university or college level, and 2 at the professional or club level.

Decision Training in Action

The following questionnaire (Vickers, 2000a) is designed to tell teachers and coaches if their assumptions about teaching and coaching in sport are rooted in behavioral or decision-training methods. The questions have been designed to help you decide if you are already using decision training or if you are still using the older behavioral methods. It is important to get in touch with your own assumptions about what underlies good teaching or coaching. Before responding true (T) or false (F) to each question, select one of the following roles that best fits your current professional area or area of interest.

> ➤ If you are a coach or teacher, think about how a person holding this position should carry out the role.
>
> ➤ If you are an athlete, think about how you would like to be trained. What do you think the ideal coach should be doing?
>
> ➤ If you are a sport leader, think about the kind of program you want. What do you expect from your coaches and your athletes?
>
> ➤ If you are a parent, how do you want your children coached?
>
> ➤ If you are a therapist, think about how your patients should be treated in terms of their treatment procedures.

Self-Testing Questionnaire: Are You Already a Decision Trainer?

For each question, circle T for true or F for false.

1. It is important to master the fundamental or basic skills of a sport or activity before more complex skills or tactics are introduced. (T or F)

2. A lot of feedback to every athlete or client is required in every practice. More feedback is always better. (T or F)

3. Athletes do not need to be experts at analyzing their own performance—that is the coach's or therapist's job. (T or F)

4. Technical and physical skills should be mastered before decision-making skills are introduced. (T or F)

5. Using video models (athletes view another athlete) or video feedback (athletes view self) as coaching aids is too distracting and time consuming. (T or F)

6. It is critical that the same skills be practiced over and over until perfection is reached; being able to perform without thought is the ideal. (T or F)

7. Using a questioning style where you ask your athletes to think about their movements and suggest improvements is too time consuming and detracts from training. (T or F)

Key to scoring: Add the number of false (F) statements.

1. If you answered false to 7 or more questions, you are using a lot of decision-training methods.

2. If you answered false to 5 or more questions, you are using some decision-training methods.

3. If you answered false to 3 or fewer questions, you are using few decision-training methods.

From J.N. Vickers, 2007, *Perception, cognition, and decision training: The quiet eye in action* (Champaign, IL: Human Kinetics).

CHAPTER 10

Designing Practices With a Decision-Training Focus

◄◄ *Where Have We Been?*

In the last chapter, the three-step decision-training model was presented and the foundations explained. Paradoxical findings that have emerged in research on motor learning over the past 2 decades were highlighted. A number of studies were also presented showing the effectiveness of decision training. Such training can be applied to a wide range of sport activities at any age or skill level. It is a universal approach that can be used by many practitioners of sport and motor behavior—athletes, teachers, coaches, therapists, sport leaders, and parents.

►► *Where Are We Going?*

In this chapter, the decision-training model is developed further within the context of two of the tools for decision training: DT tool 1 (variable practice) and DT tool 2 (random practice). The research behind variable and random practice is explained using both laboratory-based studies and those carried out in applied sport settings. Three examples of the three-step model are presented as exemplars, followed by a number of case studies.

DT Tool 1: Variable Practice (Smart Variations)

During **variable practice,** the athlete practices variations of a single class of skills in a setting that simulates the conditions found in play or competition. Variable practice drills are called *smart variations* when the drills simulate conditions similar to those found in competition. Variable practice is easy to remember if you think of coaching one class or pattern of skills. For example, in badminton, the forehand action is one class of actions used to hit many shots. A variable practice drill would combine a forehand drop, forehand clear, and forehand smash because these all originate from the same basic motor pattern. In golf, instead of taking 100 hits with the same club from a flat surface, practice would occur on a variety of slopes with a number of different clubs, as well as from sand, divots, and bad lies. In receiving the serve in volleyball, variable practice would occur when the same type of serve is received on different parts of the court; and in basketball, it would occur when jump shots are taken from many locations on the floor. In each of these tasks, the basic biomechanical requirements are the same, but the athlete learns to perform the many variations found in the field of play.

DT Tool 2: Random Practice (Smart Combinations)

During **random practice,** the performer learns to combine different classes of movements within settings that simulate the conditions found in play and competition. More than one class or pattern of skills is combined in a tactically relevant way. Random practice drills are called *smart combinations* when the drills simulate conditions that are similar to those found in a play or competitive setting. For example, in golf, a practice session would combine a 9-iron approach shot with the putt; in volleyball, the service reception, set, and attack would be executed; in basketball, a jump shot would occur from a pass, with and without opposition; and in badminton, a forehand shot would be combined with a net shot in a continuity drill with appropriate footwork. Each of these drills combines different biomechanical patterns in ways that occur often in competition.

During blocked practice, the same skill or tactic is practiced over and over with little change in the context. Blocked practice is necessary in situations where a skill is first being learned, as well as later on when the primary goal is to make the skill automatic. When decision training is used, it does not mean that blocked practice is removed completely; it simply means that blocked practice isn't the only type of practice used. Blocked practice is still needed with beginners and very young children until the basic foundations of the skill are understood. However, it is crucial to move on from blocked practice as soon as possible and not keep athletes stuck in one place just because they do not seem to have the basic skills. Instead, variable practice and random practice drills should be introduced as soon as possible. Some athletes prefer blocked practice over variable and random practice because it is easier and more rewarding in terms of short-term success. But remember, research shows that what they are learning will not be retained later on. The following studies illustrate this point.

Research Support for Variable and Random Practice

In this section we now cover some of the studies that have led to the use of variable and random practice. The first study in the motor area was by Shea and Morgan (1979), but the same phenomenon had been shown earlier in studies on reading and mathematics. Battig (1956, 1972, 1979) found that when learning exercises were made more challenging using random techniques, retention and transfer increased. His term for the practice of introducing real-world challenges into the learning environment is **contextual interference.** In Shea and Morgan's (1979) experiment, one group learned a number of arm movements using blocked practice, while a second group learned the same tasks using random practice. The blocked subjects practiced the first arm movement to a high level, and then moved on to the next, and so on. As can be seen in figure 10.1, this worked well and led to high levels of performance during early practice. In contrast, the random group had to learn to perform the skills in any order that was requested. As is evident, they did not achieve the same levels of success as the blocked group during the acquisition phase. Retention tests were then given 10 min and 10 days later. Figure 10.1 shows that although the blocked group did better during the acquisition phase, during the retention tests their performance was lower than that of the random group.

But more interesting are the results shown in figure 10.2, when both groups were required to transfer the initial arm movements to perform a novel action. Notice that the blocked group's performance became much worse, while the random group maintained a high level of performance. This result is critical because it not only shows that the random practice group did better than the blocked in terms of later performance,

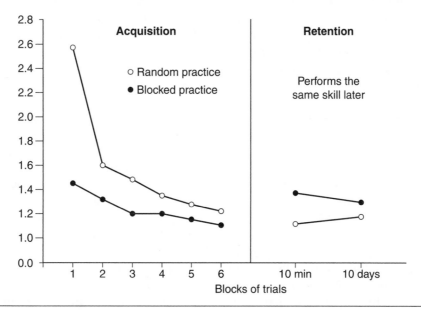

➤ **Figure 10.1**   Time (s) required to perform the barrier knockdown task for the blocked and random groups during initial acquisition and later retention tests.

Reprinted from J. Shea and R. Morgan, 1979, "Contextual interference effects on the acquisition, retention, and transfer of a motor skill," *Journal of Experimental Psychology: Human Learning and Memory* 5(2): 179-187.

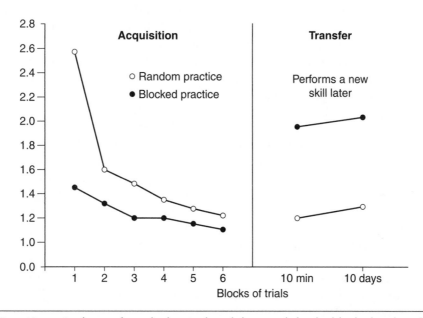

➤ **Figure 10.2**   Time (s) required to perform the barrier knockdown task for the blocked and random groups during initial acquisition and later transfer tests.

Reprinted from J. Shea and R. Morgan, 1979, "Contextual interference effects on the acquisition, retention, and transfer of a motor skill," *Journal of Experimental Psychology: Human Learning and Memory* 5(2): 179-187.

it also shows that the blocked practice appeared to actually be harmful in terms of being able to perform later on. It would appear that too much blocked training creates a mental barrier that prevents the type of decision making needed to handle unusual situations. Since then, numerous studies have been carried out supporting the efficacy of some form of contextual interference under the labels of variable and random practice. A weight of evidence now shows that random and variable practice should be used as soon as is practical (Goode & Magill, 1986; Hall, Domingues, & Cavazos, 1994; Lee & Magill, 1983; Schmidt & Bjork, 1992; Schmidt & Lee, 2005; Ota & Vickers, 1999; Wrisberg & Liu, 1991).

Variable and Random Practice in the Sport Setting

Hall et al. (1994) determined the effects of variable and blocked practice on hitting in baseball. The study was conducted with college-level baseball players during the regular season. The team was first given a hitting test and, based on the number of solid hits made, the players were placed in three batting groups of equal hitting ability (blocked, variable, and control). The control group attended all the regular practices and took the pretest and posttest, but they did not attend any of the extra batting practices, which were held along with the regular practices. The blocked group attended the pretest and posttest and all the regular practices and took 11 extra hitting sessions. During the extra batting sessions, they hit 15 curveballs followed by 15 fastballs and 15 changeups in a set order. The variable group also attended the pretest, posttest, and all regular practices and took 11 extra hitting sessions. But during the extra batting sessions, they hit 45 pitches that were delivered in no set order so that they could not anticipate which type of pitch was being delivered.

In order to understand the cognitive and decision-making differences between blocked and variable practice, imagine being in the blocked group, standing in the batter's box and waiting for the first pitch, which you know will be a curveball. How many of the 15 pitches do you think you will need to focus on? When asked this question, most experienced baseball coaches and athletes say 1 to 3, maximum. They additionally state that during the remaining pitches they like to "switch off their heads" and just "swing away." Many also comment that this is what they have been taught, that an automatic, mindless state is needed in order to become a great hitter. When the next set of pitches (fastballs) is delivered, a similar process is followed. A high level of cognitive effort is needed only during the first few pitches since the flight of the ball is known.

Now place yourself in the random group. You have no idea which of the three pitches will be delivered. Think of the uncertainty and heightened attention needed to perform in this setting. You have to learn to deal with all three pitches at the same time, just like in games. When I ask coaches and athletes how many of these pitches they will have to focus on, they say they have to devote a high level of cognitive effort to most of the pitches because they have no idea what type of ball is going to be delivered.

Think also of the gaze control that is needed to perform in baseball as was described in chapter 7 (interceptive timing tasks). When variable practice is used, athletes are given the chance to develop the anticipation, attention, concentration, and problem-solving skills needed to handle a variety of pitches. They also learn how to adapt their stance, body position, trigger step, swing, and other technical requirements, regardless of the type of pitch being thrown. During each and every pitch, they have the opportunity to develop the important decision-making, biomechanical, and physiological components of hitting into an integrated package. Most important, this is what is required in the game. Athletes cannot simply switch off their mind and assume that any two pitches will be delivered in the same way.

The athletes were assessed on how many solid hits they could make during the pretest, at practice 5, at practice 8, and during the posttest (with both variable and blocked delivery of pitches) in practice 12 (figure 10.3). Three results are important. First, both the blocked and variable groups improved more than the control group over the 12 extra practices. The control group did improve as a result of going to the regular practices, but not as much as the groups that attended the extra batting practices. Second, up to the 8th extra batting practice, the

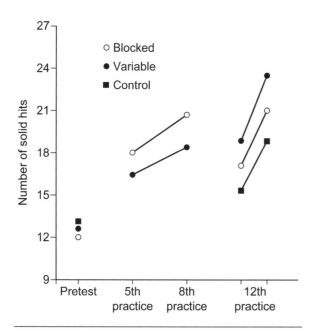

➤ **Figure 10.3** Number of solid hits in extra batting practice as performed by the blocked, variable, and control groups. Subjects were college baseball players (Hall et al., 1994).

Reproduced with permission of authors and publisher from: Hall, K.G., Domingues, D.A., and Cavazos, R. Contextual interference effects with skilled baseball players. *Perceptual and Motor Skills*, 1994, 78: 835-841. © Perceptual and Motor Skills 1994.

blocked group hit at a higher level than the variable group. Third, during the 12th session and final test, the results reversed. The variable group hit at the higher level and the blocked group declined or hit a plateau. Note especially the decline in hitting performance of the blocked group when it had to hit pitches delivered in a random order.

Thus, those athletes who were in the random group did better in the long term. If we do some simple arithmetic on the cognitive effort expended by the blocked and random groups, we see a tremendous difference. As mentioned, it was estimated that the athletes in the blocked group had to concentrate on 3 of the pitches out of every 15 delivered; therefore for this group a high level of cognitive effort was required on only 3 out of 15 pitches per block, or 20%, of all swings. If we do the same math for the variable group, we see that most if not all of the pitches required a higher level of anticipation, attention, memory retrieval, and problem solving. Let's estimate that 80% of all pitches required a high level of cognitive effort. If we compare the two

groups, we see that the variable group expended a high level of cognitive effort on 12 out of 15, or 80%, of their swings; therefore they received 60% more cognitive training than the blocked group, even though both groups hit exactly the same number of pitches.

In the real game of baseball, we know that players can never expect the same pitch twice in a row, and thus they have to know how to handle all the different deliveries. The athlete has to learn to handle a great deal of uncertainty, which should be simulated in practices rather than eliminated or reduced. Variable practice introduces more opportunities for athletes to train the decisions inherent in the sport. When used in the context of daily practice, DT tools like variable and random practice increase the mental workload of players while maintaining or increasing the amount of physical work.

Effects of Variable and Random Practice on the Coach

Using variable and random practice (as well as the other DT tools) changes the training environment, so it is necessary for coaches to be aware of the new conditions that emerge. To illustrate, figure 10.3 shows that the progress of the baseball players who experienced blocked practice was superior to that of the players in the variable group for the first eight practices. Imagine being the coach of the blocked group in this situation. You would probably feel that the extra batting practices were going well, and based on the improvements you could see each day, you would feel pretty good about what was happening. As an athlete, you would also feel that you were being coached in an effective manner. Indeed, anyone observing the sessions would feel that the extra hitting practices were being carried out correctly. And even when performance declined after practice 8, the powerful first impression would remain—blocked practice leads to better results.

Now, imagine being the coach of the variable group. Compared with the blocked group, this group struggled for eight practices, or a full month. As the coach in this situation, you would probably begin to question yourself and what you were doing, and if you were an athlete, you might begin to doubt your coach, especially in light of the better hitting of the blocked group. Unless coaches and athletes have an understanding of the research and theory underlying the use of variable and random practice, there is a strong tendency to abandon the method and go back to blocked training. In truth, blocked training is easier to implement and gives good results immediately, and for these reasons it can be a great seducer of coaches, athletes, and sport administrators.

Variable, Random, and Blocked Practice and Brain Plasticity

In order to understand more about why variable and random training have a better long-term effect on performance than blocked training, this section looks at what may be happening in the brain when a player experiences these forms of practice. We know from the studies on neurogenesis and synaptogenesis presented in chapter 1 that a brain developed within a rich, complex environment differs from one developed within a limited or impoverished environment. Effective neural networks are not developed in restricted environments; instead, the ability to act in an appropriate way is often reduced, behaviors become stereotyped, and the individual does not develop the ability to perceive and act in effective or innovative ways.

Blocked practice environments, with their high levels of automatic repetition, are often achieved at the expense of the inherent complexity within a sport task. When this occurs, athletes are often preparing for events that do not occur or are omitting altogether critical events that will occur. During learning, the brain undergoes neurological changes. To perform well in a sport, the brain has to develop optimal synaptic linkages responsible for the detection and processing of objects, locations, and events both externally within the environment and internally within the athlete. If a practice environment does not provide opportunities for the establishment of the necessary neuronal networks, then the athlete simply does not develop the mental capacity to perform well.

In order to better understand how this occurs in sport, let's revisit the Hall et al. study (1994) in baseball and look at what might have happened from a neural point of view when the players learned to hit under both the blocked and variable practice conditions. During blocked training, the same skill was practiced over and over. The blocked group hit 15 curveballs with little variation in the speed and direction of the

pitch. During blocked training, the brain develops specific but limited associations between neurons that detect the speed, height, direction, velocity, and rate of change of the ball in flight, to name but a few characteristics. Once the flight path of the ball is known, the brain's centers for automaticity, the basal ganglia and the cerebellum, take over and carry out the physical hitting action without much need for thought.

This quick takeover by the lower centers of the brain from the higher was shown in an imaging study by Posner and Raichle (1994), which illustrated how dramatic this effect is. Brain imaging techniques such as PET and fMRI measure changes in blood flow in the brain when attention is heightened, such as when a person is trying to learn a set of words. Figure 10.4 shows the PET scans of a brain learning to associate a particular word (e.g., hammer) with an appropriate action (e.g., hit). Three brain scans are shown: naive, or when the associative word list was first being learned; practiced, or after the list was learned; and novel, or when new word pairs were introduced once again.

Notice that when the associations were first learned, the higher centers had an increased blood flow indicative of increased neural activity (lighter areas) in the frontal areas responsible for making the correct associations. When the associations were learned, the higher centers no longer

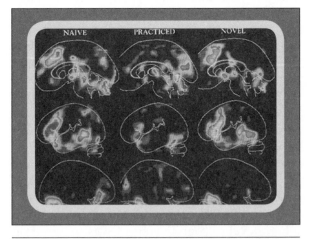

➤ **Figure 10.4**   PET scans of the brain first learning a word-association task (naive, left), when the task is well known (practiced, middle), and when a novel variation is learned (novel, right).

Illustrations from pages 101 and 127 from IMAGES OF MIND by Michael I. Posner and Marcus E. Raichle. © 1994 by Scientific American Library. Reprinted by permission of Henry Holt and Company, LLC.

were engaged; instead, the temporal cortex was involved in terms of making the correct response. When a new list was again presented, the original centers were again activated and the lower centers became inactive. Posner and Raichle (1994) thus show that with practice, the higher centers are no longer needed; the subject can perform well without the direct activation of these areas of the brain. See also a study on juggling that is presented in chapter 1 (Draganski et al., 2004).

Neural Network Development in Baseball

We can use the results found by Posner and Raichle (1994) and speculate that athletes do the same thing when training: They use the higher centers when learning to detect the characteristics of objects in flight (e.g., curve) and the lower centers take over once it is learned. The brain immediately puts itself on autopilot and learning is reduced. The problem with the subconscious centers running the action is that they are unable to detect new cues, which occur all the time in games. For example, if a batter takes 10 curveballs and then is unexpectedly presented with a changeup, the neural centers necessary to see and effect this change may be too slow to respond or may be nonexistent, depending on the training received. Unless the brain is trained to not only see the different variations of pitches but also know how to switch quickly between pitches, it does not have the ability to adapt and respond appropriately. Blocked training does not train the neural ability to rapidly detect changes in ball flight; instead, it prepares the neural system to respond to sameness. To be good in baseball hitting, a brain has to be trained to detect an array of pitches and respond appropriately, and variable and random training conditions are better than blocked training at achieving this.

Example 1: Decision Training in Badminton Tactics

It is now time to present an example of the decision-training model and show how it can be used to design and carry out more effective drills and activities. In this section, the three-step model is applied to badminton tactics. Since a research study has not been carried out that has identified the gaze control, or quiet eye, in badminton, it is necessary to use information from the previous chapters to infer what optimal attention in this sport might be.

Step 1: Define a decision that athletes have to make in competition. The decision should name at least one key perceptual or cognitive skill the athlete needs to master while performing a specific skill or tactic. The seven cognitive skills are anticipation, attention, focus and concentration, memory, pattern recognition, problem solving, and decision making.

In this example, the decision to be trained is the ability to detect (pay attention to) the movement of an opponent across the net before performing a specific stroke or strokes. Quite often badminton players are so involved with executing the strokes of the game that they focus only on the technical aspects of the game. They lose track of the movements of their opponent and develop hitting techniques that make them blind to critical cues provided by their opponent. The ability to perceive the movements of an opponent while performing is important in many sports, and so the following drill has wide applicability to many tactical situations.

Step 2: Design a drill or progression of drills to train the decision in a gamelike situation. As a part of designing the drill, it is also necessary to identify a cognitive trigger that lets both the athlete and coach know if the athlete has made the right decision. Some cognitive triggers include object cues, location cues, memory cues, reaction times, and self-coaching cues.

In badminton, it is common for continuity drills to be used where a feeder places the shuttle to a player so that numerous repetitions of the stroke or series of strokes are performed. In traditional forms of badminton practice, the feeder usually stands in one place and places the shuttle in a predictable manner, as shown in figure 10.5 (left). This traditional drill can be easily modified into a decision-training drill by adding a cognitive trigger. Figure 10.5 (right) shows that the feeder has moved just before the stroke is performed; this movement is the cognitive trigger designed to mimic the movements of an opponent. Two variations of the drill can be used, with the first requiring the athlete to hit to the feeder, and then away from the feeder (as would occur most often in a game). When this type of decision-training

Without cognitive trigger

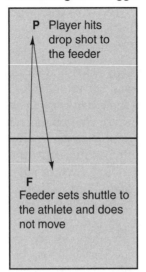

P Player hits
drop shot to
the feeder

F
Feeder sets shuttle to
the athlete and does
not move

With cognitive trigger

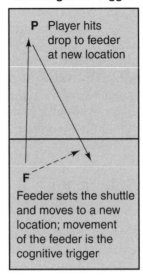

P Player hits
drop to feeder
at new location

F
Feeder sets the shuttle
and moves to a new
location; movement
of the feeder is the
cognitive trigger

➤ **Figure 10.5**   A variable badminton continuity drill (left), and the same drill converted to a decision-training drill with a cognitive trigger (right). The movement of the feeder is the cognitive trigger.

drill is used, many players realize for the first time that they have no awareness of where the opponent is across the net (see case study 10.1). It is also common to find that some athletes are able to see the feeder move, but they have not yet developed the decision-making skills or the strokes needed to perform at the higher level.

Step 3: Select one or more of the seven decision tools to train the decision in a variety of simulated competitive contexts. The seven DT tools are variable practice, random practice, bandwidth feedback, questioning, video feedback, hard-first instruction and modeling, and external focus of instruction.

In this example, DT tool 1 (variable practice) and DT tool 2 (random practice) are used. Variable practice would be present in the drill when a different variation of the forehand action is practiced. For example, the feeder sets the shuttle high and the athlete has to perform variations by returning the shuttle to the new location, or the feeder uses a drop near to or far from the net, a drop left or right, a soft smash left or right, or a clear to back left or right court. All of these strokes are a variation of the same forehand hitting action.

Once the athlete is able to return the shuttle to the feeder when the feeder moves, greater complexity and decision making are added by using random practice. During a random drill, the performer learns to combine different classes

of movements within settings that simulate the conditions found in play. Random practice with a decision-training component occurs when different classes of skills are combined in response to the feeder movement after a number of combinations; for example, the sequence of strokes may combine a forehand drop to the new location of the feeder followed by the feeder setting to the backhand, which requires a completely different motor pattern to be used than the forehand.

CASE STUDY 10.1
Hitting Blind

The decision-training drill outlined previously trains athletes to see the opponent across the net and then make a return in light of this information. I was running this drill in a course where the coaches had been asked to bring along two of their athletes so they could apply some of the concepts learned. One coach brought the current provincial champion (A), who was having serious problems taking his game to the next level, and a second player (B), who had a bad attitude but was a great player. Player B could beat A on most days, even though he was not as fit and did not train as hard.

I asked the coaches to set up the drill as shown in figure 10.5 (left) and then add the decision-training component as shown in figure 10.5 (right). Player B had no problem hitting back to his coach at any location on the court he moved to, but player A could not perform the drill at all. This realization hit player A so hard that when I left the building 2 h later, he was still on court with player B, trying to figure out how he could change his technique so that he could see what was happening across the net. I wished that I had my eye tracker with me, because his problem was probably one of a faulty visuomotor workspace as he hit the shuttle. He had developed the forehand with such a severe shoulder turn that his gaze was oriented so far to the side of the court that he simply could not see across the net with either his focal or ambient system.

Example 2: Decision Training in Freestyle Ski Jumping*

We now look at a second example of the decision-training model applied in a task where the athlete has to be able to retrieve the best movement under temporal, environmental, and competitive pressure. Again, no gaze research has been carried out in freestyle skiing that defines the optimal control of attention prior to a jump, but locomotion information presented in chapter 8 can be used to design an effective decision-training drill. During locomotion, information must be acquired 200 to 300 ms in advance in order to walk over and around obstacles. If this amount of time is needed when simply walking, then even more time is needed to detect critical cues on the course when skiing downhill at high speed. This example from jump training in freestyle skiing was designed to help athletes make decisions when under extreme temporal pressure as well as pressure from coaches and self to complete the run as previously planned.

Step 1: Define a decision that athletes have to make in competition. The decision should name at least one key perceptual or cognitive skill the athlete needs to master while performing a specific skill or tactic. The seven cognitive skills are anticipation, attention, focus and concentration, memory, pattern recognition, problem solving, and decision making.

In freestyle skiing, competitors are required to complete two jumps at strategic locations on the course. In order to be successful, the athlete has to complete the entire run with both precision and speed. Each run is usually choreographed in much the same way as occurs in gymnastics, dance, figure skating, kayak racing, diving, and other judgment sports—by a coach who has high expectations that the jumps be executed as planned. Coaches often expect their athletes to stay as close to the preset choreography as possible, but this creates tremendous stress for many athletes because of the variable conditions that can be present on any day of competition. The course may be rutted from previous skiers, and there may be low light, poor snow, and a host of other factors. The athlete may also experience difficulties due to equipment, anxiety, or other causes. This decision-training drill is designed to help athletes attend to the conditions in the course well in advance and, under reaction-time pressure, select the best jump from a number of preset alternatives stored in memory.

Step 2: Design a drill or progression of drills to train the decision in a gamelike situation. As a part of designing the drill, it is also necessary to identify a cognitive trigger that lets both the athlete and coach know if the athlete has made the right decision. Some cognitive triggers include object cues, location cues, memory cues, reaction times, and self-coaching cues.

Figure 10.6 shows a freestyle skiing drill located on a slope similar to that used in competition. This decision-training drill has been used effectively with children as young as 11 up to Olympic gold medalists. The drill helps athletes make decisions under challenging performance conditions created by the coach in practice. Figure 10.6 shows the location of the athletes and coach and the jump site on the hill. The coach first asks the athlete to name a double jump to be performed. The coach then asks the athlete to select a second single jump that is to be held in memory. As the athlete begins the in-run, if the coach calls "single," then the athlete has to throw the double jump out of memory, prime the single, and perform it under temporal pressure. The call to change to a single under reaction-time pressure is the cognitive trigger. If the coach says nothing, then the original jump

*This decision-training drill was originally designed by Murray Cluff and Julie Stegall, Canadian and Olympic freestyle ski coaches.

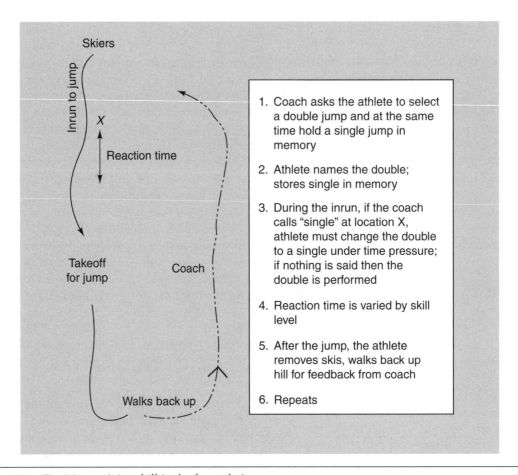

Skiers

Inrun to jump

X

Reaction time

Takeoff for jump

Coach

Walks back up

1. Coach asks the athlete to select a double jump and at the same time hold a single jump in memory

2. Athlete names the double; stores single in memory

3. During the inrun, if the coach calls "single" at location X, athlete must change the double to a single under time pressure; if nothing is said then the double is performed

4. Reaction time is varied by skill level

5. After the jump, the athlete removes skis, walks back up hill for feedback from coach

6. Repeats

➤ **Figure 10.6**　Decision-training drill in the freestyle jump.

(the double) is performed. This drill teaches athletes how to switch quickly to a different move, as well as how to inhibit other moves and carry through with the original plan no matter what the conditions. It also teaches the athletes how to work with their coach in making these kinds of decisions over many practices.

This drill uses auditory reaction time (see chapter 3) to manipulate the amount of reaction time provided. The reaction-time period is the amount of time from when the coach calls "single" until the jump is first initiated. If the skier is a beginner, then the reaction-time period should be longer and occur early in the run. More experienced athletes enjoy a shortened reaction-time period and find this drill both challenging and stimulating. The skier therefore learns to anticipate the conditions in the run, prime the best jump alternatives in memory, and select and execute the best alternative under variable time pressure, and they do all of this with the aid of their coach.

Step 3: Select one or more of the seven decision tools to train the decision in a variety of simulated competitive contexts. The seven DT tools are variable practice, random practice, bandwidth feedback, questioning, video feedback, hard-first instruction and modeling, and external focus of instruction.

The types of jumps that are trained can be increased or reduced in complexity by using variable and random practice. Variable practice is present when the same jump is stored in memory but different degrees of complexity are trained (single to double, double to single, double to triple, and so on). Variable practice is also used when the coach varies the reaction-time period from early to later on. A later cue is more challenging. Random practice occurs when the athlete stores completely different jumps in memory and thus has to learn to quickly shift or transition from one motor program to another.

The drill in figure 10.6 also includes time for bandwidth feedback and questioning (which will be covered in the next chapter). After each jump, the skiers remove their skis and climb up the hill to the location by the coach. It is here that the coach asks questions about the choice of jump and the athlete's ability to handle the time pressure and uncertainty, and then the jumps for the next try are chosen. During this time, the coach and athlete work on their communication skills in terms of the types of jumps to be performed. Together they develop strategies on how to physically and mentally handle challenging conditions. Through decision training, the athlete develops the ability to communicate with the coach and make the decisions required to perform at a high level. Having the athletes climb back up to the location of their next jump adds a physiological training component that is lost if a lift is used. This drill design also increases the number of jumps that an athlete takes in each practice session.

It is through this decision-training process that athletes begin the process of being responsible for their own decisions relative to the choreography of the run. Flexibility rather than rigidity is the goal; exploitation and optimization are the focus rather than artificially imposed restrictions or limitations. To perform well in freestyle skiing under the stress of competition, the athlete has to learn to assess the terrain and retrieve the best jump from memory. Regardless of whether the conditions are poor or excellent, the athlete learns to retrieve the optimal jump and execute it at a high level. Overall, the goal is to exploit the conditions to full advantage on a daily basis. The coach and athlete work together during practices to develop the best decisions together. Over time, this type of decision-training drill improves athlete–coach communication and instills confidence all around.

CASE STUDY 10.2
It's -19 °C and a Perfect Day to Practice

Decision training opens some amazing capacities in young athletes, as illustrated by the following true story about a group of young freestyle skiers who made a decision on their own with far-reaching and positive consequences. The event occurred on a very cold, dark morning at a ski resort high in the Canadian Rockies. Visibility was down, the wind was picking up, and snow was on the way. It was 8 in the morning and the coaches had just finished their morning meeting. Although they had stressed the importance of training under variable conditions, this day was so miserable that they had decided to cancel practice and let their team of freestyle skiers, aged 14 to 17, take the morning off.

There was a knock on the door and there stood the whole team, ready to go. They told their coaches that it was a perfect day to practice; they had checked the instruments. It was -19 °C, the wind speed was 1 km below event cancellation speed, and it was not yet snowing. If it were a competition day, they would have to ski. These teenagers convinced their coaches that this was a day they might not find again—it was a perfect day to practice.

For the past 6 mo, the coaches had been teaching them about decision training—that to be the best in their sport, they would have to learn to make decisions critical to their own success. In order to be the best they could be, they couldn't leave this decision making up to their coaches. Decision training teaches athletes to discern what is important and helps them develop the confidence to make suggestions to their coaches and carry those suggestions out through daily practices. And sometimes, coaches learn from their athletes what is needed most. Decision training helps the coach see that even young athletes can make high-level decisions if given the chance.

Many weeks later came the day of the finals, and you guessed it—the conditions were exactly like those practiced on that bitterly cold morning. The skiers were prepared, elated even, because they had trained for this very day. They were confident that they could handle the bad conditions, while the others teams complained about the wind, the cold, the rules, and their equipment. In the end the team won that championship, and some of those athletes went on to become national, World Cup, and Olympic champions. Decision training changes the relationship between the athlete and coach to one of shared problem solving, responsibility, and decision making. As time goes on, the athletes bring new and exciting challenges to practices and with them, many unexpected rewards.

Told By Murray Cluff, Canadian National & Olympic Freestyle Coach Of Jennifer Heil, Gold Medal Winner, Turin 2006.

Example 3: Decision Training in Golf Putting*

This example is from golf putting and is built upon the quiet-eye results presented in chapter 6, which discussed a study showing the efficacy of quiet-eye training. This decision-training drill builds on the exercise that you completed in chapter 6 using the quiet-eye gaze data in golf. Here we take the information gained in that chapter and implement a decision-training program.

Step 1: Define a decision that athletes have to make in competition. The decision should name at least one key perceptual or cognitive skill the athlete needs to master while performing a specific skill or tactic. The seven cognitive skills are anticipation, attention, focus and concentration, memory, pattern recognition, problem solving, and decision making.

Research presented in chapter 6 showed that golfers often find it difficult to hold their gaze stable on the green during and after the ball has been struck. In particular, many golfers lack the quiet-eye dwell time that has been shown to improve accuracy. The purpose of this decision-training drill is to help golfers maintain their gaze and attention on the green for about 300 ms after the ball has been struck.

Step 2: Design a drill or progression of drills to train the decision in a gamelike situation. As a part of designing the drill, it is also necessary to identify a cognitive trigger that lets both the athlete and coach know if the athlete has made the right decision. Some cognitive triggers include object cues, location cues, memory cues, reaction times, and self-coaching cues.

The drill is performed on the putting green and requires the golfer to perform a number of putts. It is necessary to include a cognitive trigger that will let the golfer and the instructor know whether the gaze remains on the green after contact. An effective cognitive trigger is to place small discs of varying colors, numbers, or letters under a number of balls arrayed on the green. As the golfer

executes each putt he or she must correctly name the color, number, or letter hidden under the ball after the ball is contacted and before looking to the hole.

Step 3: Select one or more of the seven decision tools to train the decision in a variety of simulated competitive contexts. The seven DT tools are variable practice, random practice, bandwidth feedback, questioning, video feedback, hard-first instruction and modeling, and external focus of instruction.

In this example, DT tool 1 (variable) and DT tool 2 (random practice) are used. During a variable practice drill, the performer practices several variations of a single class or patterns of skills in a setting that simulates the conditions found in play. A variable practice drill is one in which a line of golf balls is set up with the distance between the hole and the ball greater on each putt. In this case the golfer has to change the pace and weight on the club head in order to handle the different distances. The golfer begins with the ball closest to the hole and then continues to the ball farthest from the hole. This drill is effective when there is only one hole or there are limited holes to aim at. Variable practice occurs in the drill when a golfer performs putts on different slopes, at different distances, under different environmental conditions, and with and without distractions. In each case, the golfers need to show that they are able to attend to the ball using a quiet-eye dwell time that does not change even though variable conditions are encountered.

During random practice, the performer learns to combine different classes of movements within settings that simulate the conditions found in play or competition. Random practice would occur in the drill when different strokes are practiced. The golf instructor may design a practice where the golfer first performs a chip shot and then a putt. In this case, two classes of action are being trained (chip and putt) in a realistic setting. In this case the colored discs could be placed under the balls that are to be chipped, thus extending the quiet-eye dwell time to another stroke.

---

*This quiet-eye decision-training drill was designed by Dr. Nancy Buzzell, counseling psychologist, University of New Brunswick, and certified decision trainer.

Decision Training in Action

Design, and deliver if possible, a 15-minute decision-training drill using the three-step decision-training model.

> ➤ Step 1. Name a decision the athlete has to make in competition. The decision should name at least one key perceptual or cognitive skill the athlete needs to master while performing a specific skill or tactic. The perceptual and cognitive skills are anticipation, attention, focus and concentration, pattern recognition, memory, decision making, and problem solving.

> ➤ Step 2. Design a drill or progression of drills or activities to train the decision. As part of designing the drill, identify a cognitive trigger that lets both the athlete and coach know if the athlete has made the right decision.

> ➤ Step 3. Select one of the two decision tools discussed in this chapter to train the decision in a variety of simulated competitive contexts.

The following case studies demonstrate several real-life examples of how different athletes and coaches have used blocked, variable, or random practice methods and the effects these have had on their performance.

Case Study 10.3   Blocked and Defeated

Henry had the dubious distinction of making it to the finals only once in his 20 y of basketball coaching. This occurred despite his being at a large university with every advantage in terms of recruiting and budget. He had a reputation as a coach who knew every nuance of the game. He demanded technical perfection and it was not unusual to go to his practices and see his players performing set plays perfectly at any location on the court. He taught a disciplined, tough game and demanded full compliance. So why did his teams constantly knock at the door and never make it to the finals?

There were some clear signs pinpointing his difficulties. He was constantly at loggerheads with many of his players who felt stifled and held back. One year he succeeded in recruiting some of the very best players in the country, but one after another they rebelled against his perfect system. During the last year of his career, he happened to hear about decision training. Suddenly he knew that the perfection he was getting within his practices was achieved at the expense of his players developing the decision-making skills they needed for handling the unexpected events of actual games. He realized that he spent virtually all his time running artificial repetitive drills that had little carryover to what happened in games. The big games were always unpredictable, so instead of training a rigid system that was easily read by his opponents, he changed to practices that featured more and more of the events the athletes had to face. His practice drills became variable and random; thus he introduced into practices the conditions he knew his players would have to face, rather than shielding them from this reality. Henry's team finally went on that year to win their first championship.

Case Study 10.4   Gymnastics Paralysis

An example of how debilitating blocked practice can be occurred during my gymnastics class while an undergraduate in university. Three times each week for 2 h we practiced gymnastics. In the first class, our instructor made it clear that the perfect progression he used had been carefully thought out in order to help us move forward faster from the floor exercise to the more complicated equipment. For example, we were not to attempt a handspring off the box until we could do a handspring (kip) off the floor. He insisted on this, so the whole class practiced the handspring off the floor every practice for 3 mo with ragged success.

The final week, I thought, the heck with this. I tried the handspring over the box and much to my surprise landed it without too much trouble. I remember being mildly annoyed that most of us had spent months on a basic move when we probably could have done a lot more advanced skills instead of being stuck in his so-called perfect progression. How many times have you found yourself in this situation—or unwittingly placed your athletes in this situation? How many times have you found yourself running out of time late in the season still stuck on the basics?

This negative cycle occurs because of the erroneous belief that foundation skills must always be mastered before more advanced ones can be learned. But this is not the case—each person learns in a unique way and the more smart variability and smart combinations you include in your practices, the quicker you will prepare your athletes mentally and physically to perform.

Case Study 10.5   If They Would Just Pass Me the Ball!

Jill was an above-average basketball player who worked hard every day in practices and also on her own for hours with a teammate who fed her the ball from her four or five favorite spots. She would religiously do the same routine every day. And every day when she left practice, she knew that if she ever received the ball in any of those spots she would score for sure. As the season passed, Jill became increasingly frustrated that no one passed her the ball when she was in one of her favorite spots. Instead, she always seemed to be in the wrong place at the wrong time. Even the teammates she practiced with could not get the ball to her even though she ran the same patterns over and over.

What Jill did not realize was that within 10 min of a game beginning, the opposition knew what she was going to do and effectively shut down any passing lanes to her, let alone shooting opportunities. And because she spent all her time practicing just a few things, she was a predictable player who could not respond to what was around her. Jill would have been much better off if she had spent the extra hour of practice each day playing in pickup games with players equal to or better than her. She might have also benefited from realizing that her blocked practice style was wiring her brain to become more rigid rather than flexible and adaptable. She was teaching herself to be inner directed, that is, controlled by her internal focus of attention rather than the external events of the actual game. Jill's brain was not learning to see and exploit the weaknesses of her opponents. Instead, her practice regime made her increasingly oblivious to those events.

Case Study 10.6   My Evolution as a Decision Trainer

This case study tells the story of my evolution from behavioral trainer to decision trainer. It was the late 1980s and I was a professor who specialized in preparing coaches and teachers for public schools, sport teams, and clubs. It was at this time that the new literature on variable and random practice was just coming out. I remember not really believing it at first. Although I taught it to my students in lectures, I was still a behavioral trainer in my badminton classes. I used high levels of blocked training, repetition, and direct feedback. I had developed a number of perfect progressions that seemed to work magic right before my eyes and those of the students. I was very reluctant to give up a system that seemed to be working just fine (see Vickers, 1990).

But one year I had a group of students who not only took my first class, but also took a second class scheduled 4 mo later. The first course was structured so that all the basic skills were taught gradually in 18 classes over 6 wk. I used blocked practice extensively until perfection was achieved on those skills. I had also developed a software program (Vickers, 1990) that allowed the students to check off when they had completed 20, 30, 50, and 70 repetitions. Most students in this particular class achieved an *A* by the end of the course in almost all the skills.

A few months later, I was pleased to see that a good number had signed up for the next level of the course. Since this new class was a mix of those who had achieved a high level of performance and new students with unknown skill level, I decided to rerun the final test from the first course. Much to my amazement, the students who had achieved 100% just 4 months earlier were only marginally better than the new students!

This incident, in combination with the emergence of the new research from motor learning about variable and random training, was a turning point for me. I had just assumed that what I was teaching in drills would be retained over time. Now I knew that to foster long-term retention and transfer, I had to make some fundamental changes in how I taught. With time, I made three changes in the course. First, I changed the drills to be more gamelike—active simulations of what occurred in games. This added great interest to the course, which became more challenging in terms of the thinking skills needed to perform the sport at a high level.

Second, the students were no longer tested in set drills but during gamelike drills. What a difference this made! On one occasion I had a student suggest that I was not spending enough time evaluating him because a number of his skills were not checked off. After talking with my assistant, we both realized that we had watched this student countless times but he could not perform the skills under game conditions—only in drills. Once he came to realize this, he was motivated to make the changes needed to perform better in gamelike conditions.

Third, I no longer used simple to complex progressions as the best way to teach; instead I had the students experience hard-first training that required playing modified games against different opponents from the beginning. The motivation of the students improved, which was an added bonus. Finally, because the games were physically taxing, the fitness benefits of the class also increased.

This story captures my own journey from behavioral trainer to decision trainer. Even though I was reading about the new research in motor learning and indeed teaching it, it took events within my own teaching to see the deficiencies of a purely behavioral approach. I realized that it is relatively easy to design drills that achieve short-term perfection, but it is a completely different thing to teach and coach for long-term success.

CHAPTER 11

Providing Feedback With a Decision-Training Focus

◄◄ *Where Have We Been?*

In the last chapter, the three-step decision model was presented within the context of DT tool 1 (variable practice) and DT tool 2 (random practice). Research studies supporting both tools were presented, along with information about the effects of using variable and random practice on the coach and the effects of variable, random, and blocked practice on neural network development and the practice environment. Various examples of the three-step model were presented, along with case studies.

►► *Where Are We Going?*

In this chapter, the three-step decision model is presented within the context of DT tool 3 (bandwidth feedback), DT tool 4 (questioning), and DT tool 5 (video feedback). The term *feedback* is first defined, along with the various forms it takes in sport coaching. The way a teacher or coach provides corrective feedback has a profound effect on how well athletes learn and perform. Two applications of the three-step model are presented, one a research study with swimmers, and the second a study in biathlon skiing. The chapter concludes with DT tool 5 (video feedback) and a number of case studies.

Feedback Defined

There are two main classes of feedback. The first arises internally from the production of the movement and is referred to as internal, inherent, or **intrinsic feedback.** Schmidt and Lee (2005, p. 464) define this simply as "sensory information that arises from movement." The effect of sensory feedback on motor control was presented in chapter 3, particularly in the sections on open- and closed-loop motor control and the role of the M1, M2, TR, and M3 feedback loops in motor control.

The second source of feedback comes from external sources, such as feedback from a teacher or coach, videotape, or formal analysis of movements, as occurs in biomechanics or motor control. In this chapter we concentrate on the effect of **extrinsic feedback** on the athlete. Sources of extrinsic feedback may be grouped into two categories: knowledge of results and knowledge of performance. Knowledge of results refers to the outcome of a movement (e.g., race time, percent shots made, trial success or failure), while knowledge of performance refers to the characteristics of the movement itself (e.g., technical components, kinematics or kinetic information derived from biomechanical analysis). Often the term **augmented feedback** is used to refer to any combination of knowledge of performance and knowledge of results.

In addition to these terms, many other terms have evolved to explain the various ways extrinsic feedback is provided. The following definitions are used in this book:

> ➤ **Corrective feedback** refers to technical, tactical, and other sport-specific information provided to the athlete with the aim of improving performance.

> ➤ **Summative feedback** is a form of corrective feedback that is given only after a number of attempts are performed. In summative feedback, the coach tries to sum up what occurred in terms of major technical, tactical, or other cues.

> ➤ **Positive feedback** is any form of verbal or nonverbal feedback that contributes to the achievement of the goals of the practice.

> ➤ **Negative feedback** is any verbal or nonverbal statement that detracts from the achievement of the goals of the practice.

> ➤ **Frequency of feedback** refers to how often feedback is provided to an athlete or a group within a specific period of time.

> ➤ **Instantaneous feedback** is a form of corrective feedback that is given immediately, before athletes have time to think about their performance.

> ➤ **Delayed feedback** is a form of corrective feedback provided after a delay so that athletes have time to think about their performance.

> ➤ **Faded feedback** occurs when a high frequency of feedback is given early on and then gradually reduced as skill level develops.

> ➤ **Bandwidth feedback** incorporates a number of the previous characteristics (reduced frequency, delay, fading) into one comprehensive approach to providing feedback as skill level develops.

DT Tool 3: Bandwidth Feedback

In the past, researchers recommended providing feedback "as soon after performance as possible, as often as possible, and in such a way as to reduce performance errors as efficiently as possible" (Lee, Swinnen, & Serrien, 1994, p. 332). It has long been the tradition in sport to provide abundant levels of corrective feedback, regardless of age, skill level, or competition level. But research now advocates reducing and delaying feedback as skill level improves (Lavery, 1962; Lee & Carnahan, 1990; Winstein & Schmidt, 1990; Schmidt, 1991; Sherwood, 1988; Swinnen, Schmidt, Nicholson, & Shapiro, 1990; Janelle, Barba, Frehlich, Tennant, & Cauraugh, 1997). To achieve high levels of performance over the long term, bandwidth feedback should be used where feedback is gradually reduced and delayed as skill level increases (Sherwood, 1988). When bandwidth feedback is used, the athlete has a chance to function more and more in an independent way, free from constant external guidance and correction provided by the teacher, coach, parents, peers, or others involved in the athlete's training.

Research Support for Bandwidth Feedback

One of the first studies to show that a change was needed in the provision of feedback was by Lavery (1962). In his study, three groups practiced a pinball task over 3 mo, as shown in figure 11.1. One group received summary feedback, another received immediate feedback, and a third received both immediate and summary feedback. This meant that they received feedback on every trial as well as a mean score after a number of trials. During days 1 through 6 the groups practiced with feedback, and during days 7 through 10 all feedback was withdrawn and they had to perform on their own. Retention tests were also carried out on days 37 and 97 where no feedback was provided.

Figure 11.1 shows that the two high-feedback groups (immediate and immediate plus summary) increased the number of targets hit correctly to around 80%, but the summary group struggled. The rapid improvement of these two groups shows that high levels of feedback can create large increases in performance. This is one reason why high levels of feedback have been advocated so much in the past—they definitely work in the short term, so positive effects are seen immediately, giving both the athlete and the coach encouraging signals that the training

is appropriate. In contrast, those in the summary group lagged well behind throughout the 6 days of training. After each trial, this group had to determine the next correction on their own, and they improved very slowly over the 6 days. Imagine being the coach of the groups that received lots of feedback, and then of the summary group that received very little. It certainly would be easier to coach the high-feedback groups. Six days of poor performance is a long time for performers to struggle and for coaches to endure their struggle. It is easy to see why many coaches abandon a bandwidth strategy and retreat to giving a lot of feedback when their athletes begin to struggle.

Figure 11.1 shows the three groups' performance on days 7 through 10, when no feedback was provided. The high-feedback groups suffered an immediate and serious decline in accuracy to levels lower than what they were clearly capable of, whereas the summary group continued to improve. Imagine this occurring to you and your athletes in the real world of sport. It would be frustrating to be in one of the high-feedback groups, because you would know that your performance should be better. The tendency in this situation is to return to what seemed to work in the past—high levels of feedback. But we now know this is not the best strategy. To improve

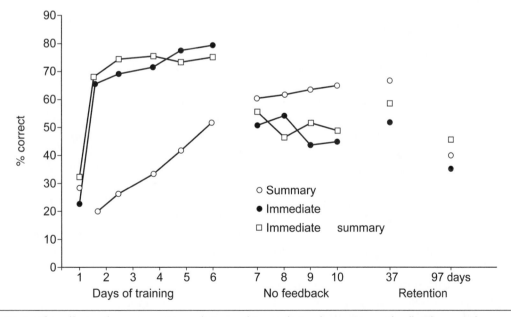

➤ **Figure 11.1**   The effects of summary, immediate, and immediate plus summary feedback on performance.

Reprinted from J.J. Lavery, 1962, "The retention of simple motor skills as a function of type of knowledge of results," *Canadian Journal of Psychology* 16: 300-311.

in the long term, athletes need a period of time where they must solve problems on their own, without relying on external sources.

Note that the summary group continued to improve to the 37th day. For this group, the psychological dynamics of getting better day after day must have been very positive, while the declines in performance that occurred with the high-feedback groups must have had the opposite effect. Finally, the results show that all the groups fell back in their performance after 97 days, suggesting that a complete withdrawal of feedback is not a good idea in some tasks. Overall, these results show that it is important to reduce and delay feedback as skill develops. It is also important to use summary feedback rather than constantly providing correction on every attempt. Athletes quickly become dependent on such feedback and do not go through the internal mediation and processing steps required to learn the task so that they know they can perform it on their own later on.

Importance of Fading Feedback as Skill Improves

We've seen that motor learning is enhanced when a lower frequency of corrective feedback is provided. But the complete withdrawal of all feedback can be upsetting for many athletes, so a better strategy is to fade feedback gradually over time (Swinnen et al., 1990; Winstein & Schmidt, 1990). In the beginning when the task is first being learned or reviewed, giving high levels of feedback is fine, but it is important to fade feedback as performance improves over time. One of the first studies to show this was by Winstein and Schmidt (1990), who provided feedback on 100% of all trials to one group and faded feedback from 100% to 50% of trials to a second group. No differences appeared between the groups during the acquisition period, but in retention tests given later the 50% group outperformed the 100% group. When athletes are given a chance to correct their own errors cognitively, they experience changes in attention, memory retrieval, problem solving, and decision making that are retained over time.

There are also different ways that feedback can be reduced, as is illustrated by a study of golf putting by Goodwin and Meeuwsen (1995) where different feedback strategies were used. Participants were college students with no previous golf experience who completed 100 putts to a distance of 15 ft (4.5 m). A professional player performing putts at a similar distance in competition would be expected to make 10% of these putts. Participants were placed in four feedback groups: (1) a group that received feedback whenever they missed, (2) a group that received feedback only when their putts were more than 18 in. (46 cm) off the target line, (3) a group that received less feedback at the beginning and more at the end of the 100 putts, and (4) a group that received less feedback at the beginning and more at the end.

During a 48 h retention test without any feedback, the participants that did best were those who received feedback only when their putt was more than 18 in. (46 cm) off target and those whose feedback was faded so that they were more on their own at the end of the study. This study shows that receiving too much feedback as occurred with the first group is not a good idea, and neither is receiving too much feedback at the end as skill develops. Instead, feedback should be gradually reduced and delayed over time as performance improves with practice. The goal is to help athletes achieve a point where they can comfortably diagnose their own mistakes and perform with little external guidance.

Importance of Delaying Feedback as Skill Improves

In the past, coaches were told that they needed to provide feedback immediately, as soon as athletes had performed a skill. But now research shows that a delay should be permitted between the time when the athlete finishes performing and the next attempt. This delay allows the athletes to think about what they have done and to formulate a solution for the next attempt. If the coach jumps in too rapidly and provides feedback, athletes have no time to think about their performance and solve problems on their own.

Figure 11.2 shows the results of a study by Swinnen et al. (1990) where participants learned to anticipate when a light reached the end of the runway. A handheld stylus was used to anticipate the arrival of the light and a score was given signifying if their movements were too early, too late, or at the right time. Participants in one group were given their scores instantaneously, whereas the others were given their score after a delay of 3.2 s. During the first acquisition period, the delay in feedback had

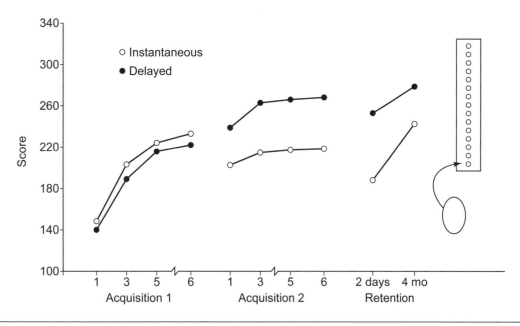

➤ **Figure 11.2**   The effect of a feedback delay on learning a complex timing skill.

Reprinted from S. Swinnen et al., 1990, "Information feedback for skill acquisition: Instantaneous knowledge of results degrades performance," *Journal of Experimental Psychology: Learning, Memory and Cognition* 16: 706-716.

little effect on performance. However, by the end of the retention period, which was 4 mo later, it was clear that allowing a delay in feedback had a positive effect on performance, while the instantaneous group performance declined or reached a plateau after the acquisition period. This study shows that giving performers even a few seconds to think about their performance provides a mediation period that is beneficial in improving performance.

Importance of Reducing the Frequency of Technical Feedback

Most of the studies presented thus far have manipulated the provision of knowledge of results (e.g., accuracy, time, precision), but should knowledge of performance or frequency of technical feedback be reduced as well? Weeks and Kordus (1998) conducted a study in soccer where the participants were boys (mean age 12.3 y) attending a baseball camp. Although the boys were excellent baseball players, none had played soccer. The task they learned was the soccer throw-in, which was taught by expert soccer coaches who used a list of 8 technical cues identified as critical to throw-in success. The boys practiced the skill in two feedback groups. The 100% group received technical feedback on every trial from a list of

eight cues, whereas the reduced-feedback group received the same type of feedback on only 33% of trials. All trials throughout the experiment were videotaped, and independent experts graded the throw-ins to assess improvement on the basis of the eight technical cues stressed in training. Throw-in accuracy was also assessed immediately, as well as 24 and 72 h after the initial training to a new target distance that was smaller than any used in training.

The accuracy scores did not differ between the two groups, but figure 11.3 shows that the 33% group was significantly better in technical skill, as assessed by the experts from the videotapes. The results showed that although both groups were equally accurate, the 33% group developed significantly better technique than the group that received 100% feedback on every trial. Reducing the amount of technical feedback contributed to the 33% group having a better ability to maintain form even under the pressure of hitting new targets, whereas the 100% group appeared to sacrifice form in order to maintain accuracy. This study showed that reducing the frequency of technical feedback leads to greater gains in technical performance, even for young athletes. We now know that too much feedback creates a dependency within the athlete that is detrimental to later performance, and this often occurs when the pressure to perform is greater.

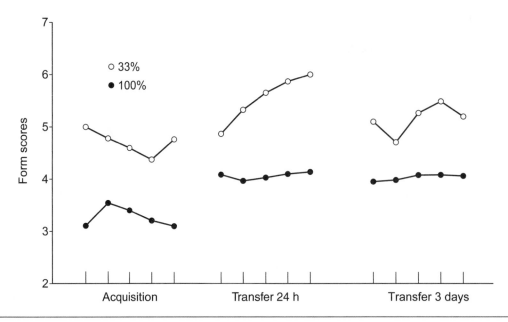

> ➤ **Figure 11.3** The effect of reducing technical feedback on throw-in accuracy.

Reprinted, by permission, from D.L. Weeks and R.N. Kordus, 1998, "Relative frequency of knowledge of performance and motor skill learning," *Research Quarterly for Exercise and Sport* 69(3): 224-230.

Bandwidth Concept: Putting It All Together

The previous sections have presented evidence explaining why feedback should be reduced, faded, and delayed over time as performance increases. Bandwidth feedback puts all these characteristics together into a comprehensive feedback strategy (Sherwood, 1988; Schmidt, 1991). Figure 11.4 shows the bandwidth strategy at work in a hypothetical situation where an athlete or group of athletes is learning to perform a skill or tactic. The line through the middle of the figure shows what the coach ideally wants, given the task, age, and skill level of the athlete. The ideal performance will have subjective and objective qualities that are based on the coach's amount of knowledge, experience in the sport, and expectations for the athlete. The ideal standard is therefore both subjective and objective, and it represents both the art and science of teaching or coaching. The two lines on each side of the middle line represent a hypothetical bandwidth set by the coach.

Notice at the bottom of the figure that five attempts are performed and the athlete's performance is both inside and outside this bandwidth. On trials 1 and 2, the athlete's performance is outside the coach's bandwidth and therefore feedback is given. Feedback should always be given when performance is within this region, even with elite performers. For example, there may be a safety concern or deeper problems related to stance, posture, and specific techniques. On trials 3, 4, and 5, the athlete's performance is inside the bandwidth and closer to the ideal. The coach does not give any feedback on these trials; instead the athlete is asked to diagnose the errors and formulate a solution.

As is evident, bandwidth feedback requires that performers be intentionally left to solve technical and performance problems on their own when their performance falls within a bandwidth of acceptance set by the coach. Feedback is provided only when performance falls outside this level. Again, where the bandwidth is set is based on the coach's knowledge and experience, the objective standards that exist for the skill or tactic, the age and ability level of the athlete, and the intention and motivation of both the coach and athlete. In order to make the bandwidth concept work, all these factors need to be applied.

Bandwidth Feedback and Athlete Dependency

Athlete dependency occurs when there is too much reliance on the coach for feedback. Schmidt and Lee (2005, p. 398) state that "when augmented feedback

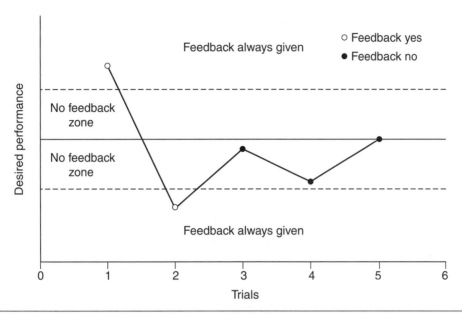

> **Figure 11.4** Hypothetical bandwidth feedback over five trials.

is provided frequently, immediately, or otherwise in such a way that various processing activities are not undertaken, then there will likely be a decrement in learning." The use of a bandwidth strategy allows performers to develop the skills and confidence to solve problems on their own, and it combats the dependency that arises when too much feedback is provided. In other words, gradually delaying and reducing feedback promotes self-reliance and lowers the level of dependency on the coach. A process of empowerment occurs where athletes begin to feel more confident, begin to push forward, and want to do more and more, and coaches find that they have to accelerate the content and sophistication of their programs. Perhaps the most intriguing part of bandwidth feedback is that it takes wisdom on the part of the coach to determine how best to apply a bandwidth for each skill and tactic for each athlete during various parts of the season.

Effects of Using Bandwidth Feedback in the Field

In the introduction to decision training in chapter 9, it was mentioned that some of the new findings on motor learning work well in the laboratory but need to be adapted to work in the field. This is the case with bandwidth feedback, where a number of problems can arise related to communication with athletes, parents, and administrators. Using a bandwidth can cause some athletes to feel

neglected, while others may think the coach has stopped doing the job that is expected. Parents often equate good coaching with high levels of verbal feedback, and they may not understand why feedback is being reduced. Some coaches also find it difficult to reduce the amount of feedback they give. Since coaching has traditionally involved high levels of both direct instruction and feedback, many coaches find it very hard to withdraw, delay, and reduce feedback.

A number of things can be done to alleviate such problems. First, in order to make the bandwidth concept work, it is necessary to tell the athletes at the outset that a reduction in feedback means their performance is nearer to what is expected, whereas the constant provision of feedback means their performance is still quite far from what is needed or desired. Not receiving feedback from the coach is actually a good thing. Second, it is important to stress that feedback is being intentionally delayed and reduced in order to give the athletes time to solve performance problems on their own since during competition they will need to be able to perform without external guidance. The goal is to help the athletes develop self-reliance and confidence that transfer to games. It is only when the coach changes the feedback strategy that the athletes have a chance to solve problems on their own and learn to think and act as they need to during the stresses of competition. Third, although the research advocating bandwidth feedback is correct, the use of a bandwidth does reduce communication in real-world sport environments and creates unnecessary problems that must be alleviated. DT tool 4, questioning, is the solution to this problem, as explained in the next section.

DT Tool 4: Questioning

In the last section we saw that a growing number of studies in motor learning have supported delaying and reducing feedback in order to affect long-term changes in performance (Goodwin & Meeuwsen, 1995; Lavery, 1962; Lee, White, & Carnahan, 1990; Sherwood, 1988; Weeks & Kordus, 1998). Based on the research, bandwidth feedback is a highly effective method of improving long-term performance, particularly when self-regulation is emphasized and participants are encouraged to ask for their own feedback.

However, in our extensive use of bandwidth feedback in the real world of coaching (Vickers et al., 1999; Vickers, 2000a; Vickers et al., 2004; Vickers et al., 1996a, 1996b, 1996c), three problems surfaced that require a solution. First, because bandwidth feedback is a technique that affects long-term retention and transfer performance, successful transfer performance requires increased cognitive effort and engaged mental work over time. Just as early studies neglected to uncover the efficacy of such methods because the techniques did not produce immediate results, coaches have been hesitant to employ techniques that did not produce rapid improvements in athlete performance (Lee et al., 1994; Vickers, 2000a).

Second, bandwidth feedback, by definition, results in the gradual reduction of input from external sources (e.g., the coach) and increases the responsibility of the athletes to monitor and modify their personal performance. Based on this reasoning, one might assume that athletes would grow more autonomous through increased perceptions of self-responsibility and control. Although this does occur with some athletes, others have commented they feel neglected when their coach reduces and delays feedback. Coaches who used bandwidth feedback techniques also experience communication problems with some athletes who reported feeling ignored. In some instances this grew to include parents and administrators who interpreted a reduction in observ-able feedback as a failure on the part of coaches to provide the continual support long associated with traditional methods of coaching.

Finally, when a coach withdraws feedback, and an athlete engages cognitive processes designed to maximize their motor performance, how can a coach determine if athletes are, in fact, making correct decisions and solving relevant problems? Athletes may not involuntarily initiate thought processes related to their performance. The evidence presented earlier suggests that athlete cognitive effort may well focus on the coach's lack of interaction, not on improving sport performance. A method was therefore needed that enabled coaches to ascertain whether their athletes are cognitively engaged in the skills and tactics being trained.

Questioning has not been recognized as a parallel tool in coaching, despite representing a fundamental instructional tool in education, counseling, psychology, outdoor leadership, and medicine (Knight, Guenzel, & Feil, 1997; Metzler, 2000; Otero & Graesser, 2001; Sachdeva, 1996). Questioning techniques have the potential to remedy the problems cited previously. Questioning provides coaches with a method of encouraging active learning through problem solving, discovery, and performance awareness. As feedback is reduced, coaches can elicit intrinsic awareness through questioning while maintaining, even increasing, productive communication with athletes.

Bandwidth Feedback and Questioning

When a bandwidth strategy is used, a feedback delay occurs that should be filled with questions from the coach to the athlete. This strategy increases verbal communication in a way that is consistent with increasing athlete cognitive effort and decision training. Bandwidth feedback and **questioning** form a handshake in the decision-training approach—one goes naturally with the other.

Questioning is one of the most challenging tools to implement because it requires a high level of knowledge in the sport and the development of listening skills that are often new for coaches. Developing the ability to ask sport-specific questions and also to listen for answers and respond in an encouraging but task-effective way takes time and practice. The goal is to develop a repertoire of questions that explore the critical dimensions needed to perform at a high level. Instead of coaches always telling the performers what to do in the form of direct instruction and feedback, they should ask questions that probe what the performers understand about the drills, skills, and tactics being taught, or the decisions being trained.

Research Support for Questioning

Research in nursing, family therapy, psychology, education, and health counseling has shown that questioning is an effective communication and learning tool (Dozier, Hicks, Cornille, & Peterson, 1998; House, Chassie, & Spohn, 1990; Otero & Graesser, 2001; Sachdeva, 1996; Schell, 1998; Wink, 1993). Paramount in these studies is the use of questions in order to promote self-regulation, as well as what Dozier et al. (1998) call a *therapeutic alliance* between the therapist and the family or individual. Dozier et al. developed a questioning approach to help families in crisis. Videos were made of hypothetical family therapy sessions using one of the four questioning strategies. Participants, 40 triads of families, were randomly assigned to watch one of the videos. The results showed that questioning techniques that helped the participants understand the underlying causes of the dysfunction led to higher rankings of perceived alliance with clients than did questions that were perceived to be confrontational or contain strategies imposed by others. The authors suggest that the type of questions asked is a critical factor in determining the level of cooperation that occurs between the therapist and patient.

The need to create an alliance between client and patient is important in providing therapy as well as in establishing an effective coach–athlete relationship. One of the goals of decision training is to promote the ability of coaches and athletes to work together, even in stressful settings such as competition. Few studies have looked at the efficacy of a questioning strategy in the context of sport coaching. The coach's role is similar to that of a therapist in that the coach imparts knowledge to the athlete, often to remedy incorrect technique or tactical errors. This is similar to the role of the therapist in providing interventions that may help clients improve their health. One of the best methods for imparting this informa-

tion is to involve the athletes in analyzing their own performance, with the intent of guiding them toward solutions they discover on their own. In other words, it is helpful to involve the athletes in a guided process that facilitates the self-regulation of behavior.

Self-Regulation of Feedback

The chain of events from a situation where the coach provides direct feedback to one where the coach asks questions and the athlete provides more and more input to the correction of errors is called **self-regulation.** Janelle et al. (1997, p. 270) comment that research on feedback has focused primarily on extrinsic sources of feedback while neglecting the "active role of the learner." They conducted a study where participants attempted to learn a new skill (throwing with the nondominant hand to a target) under four different feedback conditions: (a) a knowledge-of-results (KR) group that received no feedback; (b) a summary group that received feedback after every five trials; (c) a self-controlled group that received feedback only when they requested it; and (d) a yoked group that received feedback only when the self-controlled group requested it. The critical groups were therefore the final two in that the self-controlled group regulated when they received feedback, and the yoked group received feedback only when the self-controlled group did and therefore had no control over the information provided to them.

The results showed that the self-controlled group achieved the highest scores on both technique and accuracy in the transfer condition. Even more interesting was that the self-controlled group chose feedback on only 11% of all the acquisition trials, much less than what was expected. In addition, they created a faded feedback schedule on their own, requesting 72% of all feedback in the first five trial blocks. Since the yoked group did not improve to a similar degree even though they received similar feedback at the same time, it was clear that the lack of personal control was critical in leading to higher levels of performance. It is now recommended that self-regulation feedback strategies be used, since these increase self-control and enhance learning as a result of the extent that "individuals are meta-cognitively, motivationally, and behaviorally active participants in their own learning" (Zimmerman, 1994 in Janelle et al., 1997, p. 270).

Research Support for Bandwidth Feedback and Questioning

Although studies in nursing, medicine, psychology, and education have shown that questioning and self-regulation are effective treatment interventions, the effectiveness of bandwidth feedback and questioning have not been explored in sport coaching. Chambers and Vickers (2006) carried out a study where the goal was to determine the effectiveness of a combined bandwidth feedback and questioning strategy on the development of swim technique and speed of swimmers aged 13 to 17 y. Two teams were randomly selected from the five competitive clubs in the city of Calgary. The objective was to determine if using bandwidth feedback and questioning would significantly improve the swim times and technique of the team receiving bandwidth feedback and questioning (BF-Q) compared with a control (C) team that continued to use their traditional approach.

The training of the BF-Q coach included an instructional seminar, a 1 wk practical application, and a feedback session (video and discussion) related to the use of bandwidth feedback and questioning techniques. The C coach received equivalent time in swim discussion but no training. Both coaches were videotaped at two randomly selected practices each week throughout the intervention period (from pretest to posttest) in order to monitor compliance of the BF-Q coach and consistency of the C coach in adhering to the original coaching style. It was confirmed that both coaches maintained consistent coaching styles throughout.

The study spanned one competitive winter season of 4 mo. A pretest of swim technique and time was carried out at the outset, followed by a 6 wk intervention and a posttest and transfer test after 2 wk. The coach of the BF-Q team gradually withdrew feedback over the training period while at the same time asking the athletes specific questions about the effectiveness of their current technique. All athletes provided suggestions on how they could improve their technique in that and subsequent practices. The coach of the C team continued to coach in his traditional manner but was provided with an equal number of minutes of instruction on the organization of the study

and related topics. Integrity of the interventions was maintained over the training and transfer period using videotape and direct observation to measure feedback and questioning styles of both coaches.

Differences in competitive swim times (*d*-scores) were determined from pretest to posttest and from posttest to transfer test, with the transfer test being the final competition of the year. Technical evaluations were carried out by independent experts from swimming, who watched videotapes taken at similar intervals in order to determine changes in swim technique.

Improvement in Swim Technique

Figure 11.5 shows the *d*-scores for swim technique for the two groups. A score of zero meant no change in technique, while a plus score signalled an improvement and a negative score a decline in form. The BF-Q group improved in technique more than the C team during the early season (from pretest to posttest) and showed a modest improvement later in the season (from posttest to transfer test), whereas the C group showed an opposite profile. Their technique improved less

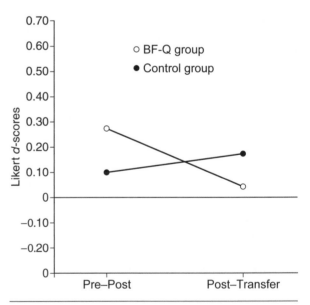

➤ **Figure 11.5** Improvement in swim technique, as indicated by the Likert difference scores from pretest to posttest and from posttest to transfer test. A higher score indicates greater improvement in technique.

Reprinted, by permission, from K.L. Chambers and J.N. Vickers, 2006, "The effect of bandwidth feedback and questioning on competitive swim performance," *The Sport Psychologist* 20(2): 184-197.

during the early season (pretest to posttest) and more during the latter part of the season (posttest to transfer test). These results showed that using bandwidth feedback and questioning led the BF-Q athletes to make changes in their technique that were apparent to the judges of the videotapes. The C group did not undergo any alteration in technique until late in the season, and overall their changes in technique were less than those observed for the BF-Q swimmers.

Improvement in Swim Times

Did a change in the coach's feedback style and subsequent change in swim technique also contribute to improvements in the athletes' swim times? There was no significant improvement in swim times when measured during practice meets, but figure 11.6 shows that during competition, the BF-Q group's swim times improved least from pretest to posttest and most from posttest to transfer test. Note that a decrease in swim time meant an improvement in races. The C group showed an opposite profile, experiencing their

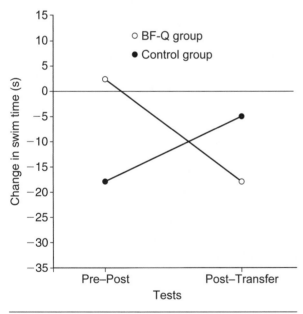

➤ **Figure 11.6** Improvement in swim times as recorded during competition. Difference scores from pretest to posttest and from posttest to transfer test are shown. A negative score means a faster time was achieved.

Reprinted, by permission, from K.L. Chambers and J.N. Vickers, 2006, "The effect of bandwidth feedback and questioning on competitive swim performance," *The Sport Psychologist* 20(2): 184-197.

greatest improvements during the early season and their least improvements in the final competition. In terms of absolute competitive swim times, the times of the two groups did not differ during the early part of the season, but by the end of the season (posttest to transfer test), the BF-Q group recorded faster times than the C group, although not significantly so.

According to these results, the use of bandwidth feedback and questioning contributed to different learning and performance effects compared with the traditional form of coaching where the athletes were coached in a direct way. The use of bandwidth feedback and questioning early in the season contributed to the BF-Q athletes changing their technique, which led to decrements or a plateau in their swim times early in the season. But by the end of the season, their changes in technique resulted in greater improvements in competitive swim times than when the traditional coaching approach was maintained. These results for both technique and time are therefore consistent with those found in many other studies on motor learning in both the applied and laboratory settings, where improvements are often delayed. This study also agrees with Janelle et al. (1997) in showing that athletes involved in self-regulation of their own performance do better than those denied this opportunity in training. A final result in the study was also intriguing—the dropout rate was lower for the BF-Q group than for the C group.

In summary, techniques that affect long-term retention and successful transfer require cognitive effort, and cognitive effort requires arduous mental work and time. Early studies neglected to uncover the efficacy of such methods for good reason: The techniques did not produce immediate results (Lee et al., 1994; Vickers, 2000a). "Learners need to . . . be prepared for the effortful nature of [cognitive work] so they do not abandon the process too soon, believing that thinking should have been easier or accomplished more quickly. The development of expertise in any area requires deliberate, effortful, and intense cognitive work" (Wagner in Halpern, 1998, p. 452). However, as the study by Janelle et al. (1997) shows, infusing instruction with techniques that increase athlete autonomy may temper the negative effects of cognitive effort. Allowing athletes a degree of control over their thought processes and development may positively affect their performance.

Questioning is a technique designed to share control with athletes, or with patients and their families in the case of health research. Self-reflection, self-regulation, and superior problem-solving abilities have been linked to the use of questioning in nursing and health counseling (Dozier et al., 1998). These outcomes are similar to the goals of decision training, where athletes are encouraged to self-regulate and consider their own solutions as opposed to relying on the coach for all answers.

Enhanced communication between the coach and athlete emerges from these diverse research areas. In an effort to circumvent problems associated with bandwidth feedback, coaches should use questioning to fill the feedback delay. These questions not only allow coaches to monitor and assess athlete cognitive effort, they also stimulate athlete self-reflection, self-regulation, and problem solving. As athletes become more actively engaged in their learning through these processes, they adopt more control over their development. Concurrently, questioning can maintain and even improve coach–athlete relationships and improve performance outcomes.

DT Tool 5: Video Feedback and Self-Regulation

During **video feedback,** athletes view their own performance on videotape and analyze their movements with the intent of gaining new insights that will aid their performance. Video feedback occurs when athletes observe their performance, which differs from video modeling, where the athlete views another person demonstrating a skill or tactic. Some controversy exists concerning the efficacy of video feedback. Schmidt and Lee (2005) state that little evidence exists to support the notion that videotape replay by itself is effective. Research shows that simply showing athletes a video of themselves is of little value because videotaped events occur too fast and there is simply too much information available for the untrained eye to interpret. But when video feedback is presented and interpreted by a knowledgeable individual, beneficial effects have been found.

This was shown in a meta-analysis of 50 studies by Rothstein and Arnold (1976), who found that beneficial effects occurred in all sports and at all

skill levels when guidance was provided for a period of time exceeding 5 wk. In agreement with these findings, Selder and Del Rolan (1979) found that gymnasts needed at least 5 wk to incorporate new techniques into existing routines. This was also a result of a study of elite, intermediate, and novice baseball players (Vickers, Livingston, Umeris, & Holden, 1999). All of these studies have shown that video feedback is indeed beneficial, but only when the attention of the performer is directed toward certain cues and when this process is carried out for a period exceeding 5 wk.

Despite research support for video feedback (Hodges, Chua, & Franks, 2003; Raab, Masters, & Maxwell, 2005), it is not used as extensively as one might expect, especially at the lower levels of sport where the number of athletes tends to be higher, thus precluding individual video analysis by a teacher or coach. Many coaches find the process too time consuming and so abandon the use of video feedback or use it too sporadically for it to be useful.

One way to alleviate this problem is to adopt a bandwidth feedback and questioning strategy similar to that described earlier. In the beginning, a video modeling session is led by the coach, who identifies critical cues and makes suggestions for improvement. This is then followed by video feedback sessions where the athletes are required to analyze their own videotapes relative to the video model and answer questions posed by the coach. For example, the athletes might be asked to detect the differences between their technique, timing, or decision making and that of the model. Finally, the athletes learn to analyze the performance of their teammates and opponents. This type of self-regulation of feedback is consistent with that proposed by Janelle et al. (1997) as described earlier in this chapter. This is also the procedure followed in the quiet-eye training studies in volleyball (Adolphe, Vickers, & LaPlante, 1997; Harle & Vickers, 2001).

Example 1: Decision Training in Biathlon Skiing*

This example comes from biathlon ski racing. During a biathlon race, participants cross-country ski and take rifle shots at set intervals to targets

---

*This decision-training drill was designed with Gail Niinimaa, junior provincial biathlon coach, the Nordic Centre, Canmore, Alberta.

located at 50 m. For every target missed, the athlete must ski a penalty distance. Both male and female elite athletes hit more than 90% of the targets, which is necessary to win races. A study in biathlon shooting was presented in chapter 5 (Vickers & Williams, under review), where it was shown that elite ski racers who maintain a quiet eye appear to be resistant to the type of choking witnessed in skiers who lose their focus on the target. In this decision-training drill, the goal was to increase the quiet-eye duration to an optimal duration of near-elite skiers aged 16 to 19 y. Most of the team members were fast racers, but many had problems shooting accurately.

Step 1: Define a decision that athletes have to make in competition. The decision should name at least one key perceptual or cognitive skill the athlete needs to master while performing a specific skill or tactic. The seven cognitive skills are anticipation, attention, focus and concentration, memory, pattern recognition, problem solving, and decision making.

In biathlons, problems with inaccuracy can arise for many reasons. Primary reasons may be failing to maintain a quiet eye on the target long enough to ensure accuracy or failing to regulate breathing and heart rate correctly. Athletes might also not take the wind and other factors into account as they shoot. Given that there may be many reasons why inaccuracy occurs, the athletes were asked 2 days before a major practice to make a decision about why they personally were inaccurate. All athletes were asked to think about the competitions they had been in recently and identify the main reason (in their view) for their shooting errors. Then they were asked to think about one way this one error could be alleviated in the next training session.

Step 2: Design a drill or progression of drills to train the decision in a gamelike situation. As a part of designing the drill, it is also necessary to identify a cognitive trigger that lets both the athlete and coach know if the athlete has made the right decision. Some cognitive triggers include object cues, location cues, memory cues, reaction times, and self-coaching cues.

The following exercise was carried out: 2 days before a major training session, the coach sent an e-mail to the athletes, asking them to identify one reason for the shooting problems they were experiencing. They were also asked to make one deci-

sion about how they would correct that problem in the next practice. They had to respond by e-mail a day before practice. In this decision-training drill, the coaches wanted to give all athletes time to think about their past competitions and arrive at one solution to both the error and correction. The practice drill was a simulated race, with time and penalty minutes added as in competition.

Step 3: Select one or more of the seven decision tools to train the decision in a variety of simulated competitive contexts. The seven DT tools are variable practice, random practice, bandwidth feedback, questioning, video feedback, hard-first instruction and modeling, and external focus of instruction.

The DT tools used in this example were bandwidth feedback and questioning. At the outset of the practice, all the athletes were first asked to identify their error, as shown in figure 11.7. This was then followed by the athletes each presenting their self-coaching cue. The athletes had no difficulty sharing their errors; many seemed relieved to identify these problems to their coaches and the other athletes. They also identified more reasons for their inaccuracy than the coaches had imagined. Three were very concerned about the competitor beside them as they shot, and this anxiety worsened if they started to miss. One skier, who was exceptionally fast on his skis, stated he actually had no idea how to shoot accurately. For him, hitting the target was simply a matter of chance, and he really needed help. A number of athletes mentioned that they needed to regulate their breathing and heart rate better. Two mentioned that although they knew

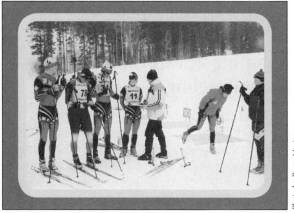

Photo by Barry Morton

➤ **Figure 11.7** Feedback and questioning session before a simulated biathlon race.

it was critical to check the windsock located near the targets, they often forgot to do so. One athlete stated that if she checked the windsock and concentrated on what that was telling her, she rarely missed, and indeed she shot over 95%. A great number of the athletes approached her after the practice for advice.

This example contains many of the self-regulation strategies advocated by Janelle et al. (1997) and included bandwidth feedback and questioning. What differed here was the reflective nature of the question-and-answer sessions. The athletes were asked 2 days before the practice to identify what they thought was their main problem; therefore they had a lot of time to think about their shooting difficulties and how to correct them. They were also asked to share this information with their teammates, as well as the solution they had developed for their problem. After practice, they were then given a chance to debrief and discuss how their self-coaching strategy worked. As is evident, decision-training drills often seek to empower athletes to be more responsible for their training and performance and that of others on their team.

But did this approach work beyond the one training session? Several results suggest that it did. First, the athletes reported a renewed interest in training for a big race, which was in 2 mo. Second, the coaches had more insight into what each athlete needed to improve and were better able to provide individual help. Third, the athletes enjoyed training in areas they personally identified. Fourth, the athletes continued to help one another. And finally, for the first time one of the skiers qualified for an international race, and the reason was her superb shooting. She therefore provided a model that the others could follow.

Example 2: Decision Training in Counseling*

Many of the skills required in giving bandwidth feedback and questioning are similar to those found in counseling psychology. In this example, a decision-training exercise was used to prepare masters and PhD students enrolled in graduate training in psychology.

Step 1: Define a decision that athletes have to make in competition. The decision should name at least one key perceptual or cognitive skill the athlete needs to master while performing a specific skill or tactic. The seven cognitive skills are anticipation, attention, focus and concentration, memory, pattern recognition, problem solving, and decision making.

In this decision-training exercise, the goal is to help counselors select and execute the most appropriate counseling skill within a simulated counseling interview. The cognitive skill selected for this activity is memory retrieval. Student counselors are asked to select one or more basic counseling skills from memory and effectively apply the skills in a simulated counseling interview. Basic counseling skills included the following: attending to cues from the client, using open and closed questions, encouraging, paraphrasing, summarizing, and reflecting on feelings.

Step 2: Design a drill or progression of drills to train the decision in a gamelike situation. As a part of designing the drill, it is also necessary to identify a cognitive trigger that lets both the athlete and coach know if the athlete has made the right decision. Some cognitive triggers include object cues, location cues, memory cues, reaction times, and self-coaching cues.

The activity selected to help the students develop their cognitive skills was 10 min of role-play, followed by a 10 min debriefing that included video feedback targeting the student performing in the role of counselor. The class was first organized in dyads. One student assumed the role of the counselor and the other that of the client. The dyads then switched roles and repeated the activity. Triads can also be used with the third student in the observer role. The instructor provided each dyad with two scenarios so that each student counselor had a different scenario from which to respond. Following are two examples:

➤ *Scenario A.* Mark is a 21-y-old university student who lives in residence. He is a proctor and one of the leaders in his house. Lately, there have been rumors in the house regarding several of the other students who seem to have eating issues. According to Mark, these residents are

---

*This decision-training drill was developed by Dr. Nancy Buzzell, counseling psychologist, University of New Brunswick and certified decision trainer.

always talking about calories and purging after meals, and it's upsetting him as well as the other students in the house. The difficulty for Mark is that he knows something should be done about this situation, but he feels in a bind because he's best friends with a couple of the students who are central figures in the situation.

➤ *Scenario B.* Denise is a 32-y-old woman who recently married a man she met through an Internet dating service. She has always wanted to be married and is excited about the prospect of creating a life and family with her new husband. Denise reports coming home from work one night to a message on the answering machine from her husband. The message said he is leaving her and is leaving the country by the next day. Denise alternates between being in shock and feeling completely devastated by this news. She says her husband refuses to come home or make any attempts to work it out.

The cognitive trigger selected was a self-coaching cue. Before each role-play session began, the students were told they would need to coach themselves in terms of the following questions: Did their intervention facilitate the client's exploration of the concern? How would they be sure that they helped the client identify the problem, why the problem was occurring, and how to solve the problem? Was the counselor also able to help the client identify an area of strength, why the client has this strength, and how the client can continue to use this strength?

If the instructor wishes to use a second cognitive trigger, a memory cue could be used to enhance the cognitive skills training. The student counselor is asked to hold in memory one counseling skill as well as a second skill that may be switched when cued by the instructor. The class instructor can remind students that the goal of the role-play activity is to facilitate the client's exploration of the concern more fully and that they have seven basic counseling skills from which to choose. In addition, the students are informed that the instructor will be interrupting their dyad from time to time in order to provide the client or counselor with additional instructions designed to challenge the counselor's ability to adapt quickly within the counseling interview.

Step 3: Select one or more of the seven decision tools to train the decision in a variety of simulated competitive contexts. The seven DT tools

are variable practice, random practice, bandwidth feedback, questioning, video feedback, hard-first instruction and modeling, and external focus of instruction.

The DT tools used in this example were bandwidth feedback, questioning, and video feedback. Each 10 min counseling interview was videotaped. At the end of the 10 min role-play, students used video feedback to identify the counselor's strengths and areas for improvement. Video cameras with external microphones and playback monitors were set up in each room. Students were instructed on how to use the equipment and how to focus the camera so that both client and counselor were captured in the scene.

Students were also instructed to identify an individual counseling skill they performed, as well as to note what happened immediately following their individual intervention. Whether the counseling skill was effective or not was decided based on the client's response following the intervention. Did the counselor's intervention encourage the client to continue exploring the concern or did it shut the client down? Did the intervention increase the client's self-awareness of cognitive, emotional, and spiritual reactions to the concern? Did the intervention facilitate the client–counselor relationship? Students were asked to identify several counseling interventions and to identify areas of strength as well as areas for improvement in their execution of basic counseling skills.

Some beginner counselors are too active in their interviews. They ask too many questions, pile one or more questions on top of a question (multiple questions), and even answer their own questions, which results in decreased involvement by the client. Generally, the correction is for counselors to slow down the interview process so that clients have time to think and become more aware of their beliefs, values, and emotional reactions. Counselors can facilitate the client's exploration process by selecting skills such as open-ended questions, paraphrases, and reflections of feelings.

Beginner counselors also tend to stay at the cognitive level in their interviews. They attend predominately to what their clients think and believe, which allows clients to intellectualize their concern rather than go deeper into their emotional reactions, conflicting values, and spiritual dilemmas. As in the previous case, the correction to this problem is for the beginner counselor to slow down the process and encourage clients to explore all sides of their concern, including the emotional, spiritual, intellectual, and behavioral aspects.

Using decision-training techniques helps the counselors in training identify their strengths and weaknesses in the safety of simulated counseling sessions. These sessions allow the course leader to identify the main areas each student has to work on. They also set up a system where the counselors learn to help one another not only during the course, but throughout their professional career.

Decision Training in Action

Design, and deliver if possible, a 15-minute decision-training drill using the three-step decision-training model.

➤ Step 1. Name a decision the athlete has to make in competition. The decision should name at least one key perceptual or cognitive skill the athlete needs to master while performing a specific skill or tactic. The perceptual and cognitive skills are anticipation, attention, focus and concentration, pattern recognition, memory, decision making and problem solving.

➤ Step 2. Design a drill or progression of drills or activities to train the decision. As a part of designing the drill, identify a cognitive trigger that lets both the athlete and coach know if the athlete has made the right decision.

➤ Step 3. Select one of the three decision-training tools discussed in this chapter to train the decision in a variety of simulated competitive contexts.

A number of case studies are now presented about athletes and coaches who used or experienced bandwidth feedback, video feedback, or questioning.

Case Study 11.1   Video Feedback and the Power of Training Multiple Minds

The scene is the dying minutes of a tied American football game that is the national final. I am watching the game on television and how the two teams are behaving on the sidelines. There are about 2 min left in the game and Peter's team is clustered in calm, small groups—the offensive line, defensive line, special teams, and so on. Many of these groups have no coaches in sight; indeed, Peter is topside calling down plays. The atmosphere around Peter's team is one of a businesslike calm that contrasts starkly with that of the opponent. On that sideline, there are no groups of athletes; each athlete is alone looking out on the field or sideways at the coaching staff that is gathered around one another.

Peter's groups were exactly the same as the ones I had seen countless times throughout the season in our media center, huddled around video machines without a coach in sight. It was his practice to expect the different specialist groups to analyze the game from the last week and present to their teammates what they had learned. During the dying minutes of the game, the groups were working in the same manner as they had all season, using the same skills they had developed together—how to solve problems under pressure. They went on to win the championship and many more, and one of the reasons this occurred was the team problem-solving abilities they had learned using videotape analysis.

Case Study 11.2 Questioning and the New Coach

Several years after learning about decision training, Neal Marshall recounts this story about his evolution as a coach. He had just retired as an elite athlete and, based on his success at the international and Olympic levels, he had enrolled in the National Coaching Institute–Calgary and had taken the decision-training courses. He had also been given his first speed-skating team to coach. But much to his dismay, he found he did not know what to say to his athletes. Although he was an expert skater himself, he had not yet translated his extensive athlete knowledge into the specific coaching knowledge he needed to do the job.

He found that the combination of bandwidth feedback and questioning saved the day for him during the first few weeks. Instead of telling his skaters how to perform every aspect of the stride (which he had not yet sorted out), he asked them what they thought was most important when they entered a corner, when they skated the apex, when they exited, and so on. Gradually he built his own repertoire of verbal knowledge, all the richer for the insights that his athletes provided. Today he is a top international coach. Indeed, one of his athletes (Cindy Klassen) went on to win five gold medals at the 2006 Turin Olympics.

Story told by Neal Marshall, National Olympic Coach, Team Canada Speedskating

Case Study 11.3 Questioning as a Language Bridge

Xiuli (Julie) Wang won a gold medal for China in long-track speed skating at the Nagano Olympics in 1998. She had skated at the highest level for more than 10 y and was now training to be a coach. Julie took part in a research study (Vickers, Reeves, Chambers, & Martell, 2004) where each coach was videotaped during four practices: once prior to taking the course, twice during the course, and once afterward. Julie's frequency of questioning on these four occasions increased from virtually no questions in practice 1 to a very high number in practices 3 and 4.

More important was her own description of why she changed and the effect this had on her coaching. She mentioned that in her training in China, a very traditional approach was used where the coach directed every aspect of the athlete's performance. In her first few months of coaching in North America, she found that the athletes resisted her traditional style, which was the one she had experienced as an athlete. Therefore, adopting a bandwidth feedback and questioning approach was a major change from anything she had experienced before. Using bandwidth feedback and questioning allowed Julie to direct probing questions to her athletes, and this caused them to be more fully engaged in the training process. It also allowed her to share her vast knowledge and insights within a context that the athletes appreciated. And using a questioning style also eased some of the pressure of learning to speak English. Xiuli is a head coach with Team Canada Speedskating. She coached Cindy Klassen from 2002 to 2004 and contributed to her winning five medals at the 2006 Turin Olympics. At Turin she coached Clara Hughes to a gold medal and Kristina Groves to a silver medal, as well as contributed to the men and women winning silver medals in team pursuit.

Story told by Xiuli (Julie) Wang, National Olympic Coach, Team Canada Speedskating.

CHAPTER 12

Providing Instruction With a Decision-Training Focus

◄◄ Where Have We Been?

In the last chapter, DT tool 3 (bandwidth feedback), DT tool 4 (questioning), and DT tool 5 (video feedback) were presented within the context of the three-step decision-training model. Research supporting the tools was discussed, along with examples and case studies on how to implement each tool in the field.

►► Where Are We Going?

In this chapter, we cover the last two tools: DT tool 6 (hard-first instruction and modeling), and DT tool 7 (external focus of instruction). Several converging lines of research support a change in how instruction is provided to athletes, including the use of hard-first rather than easy-first instruction, the extensive use of modeling, and instruction where an external rather than internal focus of instruction is emphasized. A number of decision-training applications and case studies are presented at the conclusion of the chapter.

DT Tool 6: Hard-First Instruction and Modeling

There is an old adage in education that you only get to teach something once. Regardless of age and ability level, there comes a time when each major element of your program has to be taught well, and if this does not occur, it is surprisingly difficult to go back and do it again. For this reason, experienced coaches develop sophisticated progressions of skills and tactics and they teach in focused and engaging ways. In most cases they begin with simple components and progress to more difficult ones. These so-called perfect progressions often use artificial drills that bear little semblance to how the sport is actually performed in real life. In many cases, these progressions take the learners' mind into their body and technique. Some coaches may also become obsessed with their athletes achieving the fundamental skills of their sport first and often never get to the higher-level skills and tactics that their athletes need to perform. This type of instructional strategy results in an easier learning experience initially, but we now know that it actually hinders long-term performance and prevents athletes from progressing as quickly as they might.

In this chapter, we learn that although emphasizing the fundamental skills of a sport is still important, coaches should not believe that a basics-only approach will guarantee success. Instead, they should seek to develop a balanced instructional approach where both the basics and higher-level concepts are taught together from the outset. The reason this strategy should be followed is the convergence of three lines of evidence. The first is the efficacy of hard-first instruction versus easy-first instruction (Doane, Alderton, Sohn, & Pelligrino, 1996). The second was introduced in chapter 1 and is the discovery of mirror neurons that fire when we observe another person move (Rizzollati, Fadiga, Gallese, & Fogassi, 1996). The existence of mirror neurons provides a foundation for using modeling as an instructional aid. The third is research encouraging an external focus of instruction rather than an internal one provided by Wulf and colleagues (Wulf, McConnel, Gartner, & Schwarz, 2002; Wulf, McNevin, Fuchs, Ritte, & Toole, 2000; Wulf, McNevin, & Shea, 2001; Wulf, Mercer, McNevin, & Gaudagnoli, 2004; Wulf, Prinz, & Hob, 1998). Related to this is training a quiet eye, which is an objective indicator of external focus known to improve performance.

Easy-First Versus Hard-First Instruction

In Doane et al.'s (1996) experiments, participants were placed into two groups. One group received **easy-first instruction** and the other received **hard-first instruction,** and their progress was assessed over a number of training sessions. The experiment required the discrimination of complex visual shapes (polygons) shown in figure 12.1. The hard-first polygons were similar in shape and therefore hard to discriminate, whereas the easy-first polygons were easy to discern. Reaction time and errors were assessed across the training sessions.

Figure 12.1 shows a typical experiment in which an easy-first group and a hard-first group experienced three training sessions. In the first block of trials (1-3), the easy-first group was presented with polygons that were easy to tell apart. Consequently, they responded quickly and achieved high scores (percent accuracy of 92%-96%). Meanwhile, the hard-first group was presented with polygons that were difficult to discriminate, and they were both slower and their accuracy was lower (81%-93%). The two groups were then switched (training blocks 4-6), and the easy-first group now had to distinguish the hard stimuli and the hard-first group the easy ones. The group that started the experiment with complex visual stimuli now scored 100%, but the easy-first group's accuracy was much lower (69%-81%). This is an intriguing result in light of the other group's performance in the easy-first condition. The final session (blocks 7-9) required both groups to identify complex stimuli. When this occurred, the group that began with easy-first instruction never performed at a level as high as that achieved by the group that began with hard-first training.

This study is important in sport coaching for a number of reasons. In order to perform in a sport, the skills and tactics that comprise the sport must be perceived and translated into motor codes for action. This is a critical first step in all motor skill acquisition and has been termed the *perceptual* or *cognitive phase* (Fitts & Posner, 1967). In sport, simple components have usually been taught first, with the notion that this not only makes

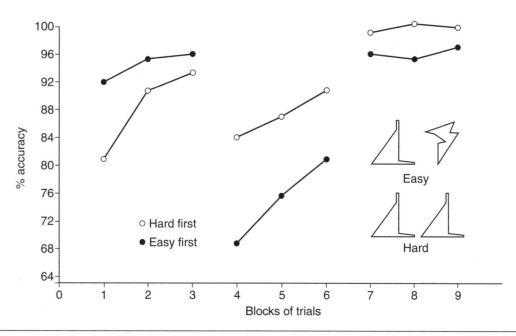

> **Figure 12.1** Three stages of easy-first and hard-first training, as used by Doane et al. (1996).

Adapted from S.M. Doane et al., 1996, "Acquisition and transfer of skilled performance: Are visual discrimination skills stimulus specific?," *Journal of Experimental Psychology: Human Perception and Performance* 22(5): 1218-1248.

learning easier, it is also safer and developmentally more appropriate. There is a measure of truth in this, but Doane et al.'s (1996) research shows that if learners are initially introduced to easy material, then they develop a learning strategy that is hard to change later on and also leads to lower levels of long-term performance. Doane et al. (p. 1241) state that once a group has been exposed to easy-first training, their performance can be improved, but

> this modification takes many sessions and is still inferior to that of participants who start with initial difficult training, even when they have less experience with the transfer stimuli. This is very important: We are showing that training in one environment can actually be a hindrance to transfer performance for an extended period.

In a later study, Doane, Sohn, and Schreiber (1999) showed that when easy-first instruction is used in situations where the essence of what has to be learned is complex, learners develop a functional fixedness that is difficult to change later on. Not only does this instructional strategy deny learners the knowledge and insight needed to move ahead as fast as they might, but it also creates a mindset that makes it more difficult to learn complex skills and tactics later on. In contrast, if complex cognitive information is presented from the outset, it appears that performers select a more appropriate level of cognitive effort that ensures a higher level of long-term learning and success in the long term.

Implementing Hard-First Instruction

When hard-first instruction is given, it is critical that the teaching environment always be safe and that developmentally appropriate drills and exercises be used at all times. Two rules apply:

> ➤ Hard-first instruction for the complete beginner should be primarily cognitive and conceptual. The teaching of physical skills should remain safe and appropriate at all times while at the same time beginners are exposed to complex models and simulations of high-end performance. This is achieved through the use of video models, take-home projects where skills and tactics are analyzed, assignments over the Internet, and question-and-answer sessions where the learners are asked to analyze a situation and provide solutions. An example of a hard-first application in sport is the football playbook. Beginners are often given the whole playbook and told that they have to know it within a week, even though it will take many years for them to master the skills within.

➤ As the skill level of the performer improves, hard-first instruction should include performing the skills within tactical settings. Basic skills should always be taught within microsimulations of actual games, which are achieved through the use of tactical simulations, small-sided games, and lead-up games. If a drill does not capture the essence of what happens tactically in a game, it should be used sparingly, if at all. For example, instead of having children in soccer learn to pass and receive in lines of players, grids should be set up where two players first learn to pass and receive and score by placing the ball into a goal, which may be a hoop, cone, or other target. They then progress to a 2v1 setting and then 2v2, always ending with a scoring attempt. In other words, the skills of passing and receiving are learned within a context where offensive and defensive plays are oriented toward a target. Above all, coaches should not use lines that do not lead to scoring attempts, passes where players stand still, or other drills that teach skills that actually detract from playing the game.

Does Modeling Improve Performance?

Modeling is a form of hard-first instruction that occurs when the athlete views another performer in order to learn about the different technical and tactical skills required. Models come in the form of live demonstrations by a coach, teacher, or other athlete, or in videotapes, computer simulations, pictures, photographs, and other portrayals. When an athlete models the performance of others, the mirror neuron system is used, which is located in the frontal and parietal lobes (see chapter 1). The ability to mimic or copy another person's movements is present from the time we are born.

Rizzolatti, Fogassi, & Vittorio (2006) explain that "much as circuits of neurons are believed to store specific memories within the brain, sets of mirror neurons appear to encode templates for specific actions" (p. 54). This leads to the possibility that the mirror neuron system is one of the most critical in terms of undergoing change as a result of motor skill acquisition.

Calvo-Merino, Glaser, Grezes, Passingham, and Haggard (2004) used fMRI to determine differences in the mirror neurons of members of the Royal London Ballet compared with elite capoeira dancers. Capoeira is a Brazilian martial art developed over four centuries by ex-slaves who had to fight for their freedom without the benefit of weapons. They learned to defend themselves with their hands and feet and created a style of self-defense that today has achieved national and international recognition as a dance, sport, game, and artistic expression of freedom.

Expert ballet dancers and expert capoeira practitioners were shown video clips of ballet and capoeira dancers while their brains were scanned. Activation was higher for the ballet dancers when watching ballet sequences and lower when watching capoeira, whereas the opposite effect was found for the capoeira dancers. Normal controls, participants who had no training in either movement form, had little activation while viewing either sequence. When a person is engaged in modeling, the mirror system in the premotor and parietal cortices is activated and integrates the observed actions with the person's motor representations.

But how effective is viewing a model in learning a motor skill? One view is presented in a humorous way by a television advertisement where Tiger Woods goes to the driving range. As soon as he begins to hit the ball, the whole line of golfers behind him begins to hit perfectly as a result of watching and modeling his perfect swing. Then when Tiger leaves the range, their hits disintegrate into chaos. Research shows that video modeling can indeed have a beneficial effect on performance, but unlike this advertisement, the effect is not immediate. It takes time, sometimes 4 to 7 wk or more (Schmidt & Lee, 2005; Sidaway & Hand, 1993; Vickers, Livingston, Umeris, & Holden, 1999).

Sidaway and Hand (1993) trained novice golfers in the chip shot by having them view a model presented on a video monitor, as shown in figure 12.2. One group was shown the expert model before every shot (1 to 1), while the other groups had less exposure to the model (1 in 5 strokes, 1 in 10 strokes, and no model). After the initial training sessions, there was no difference in the performance of the groups, and it appeared that those who viewed the expert model on every stroke were no more accurate than those who had limited or no access to the model. But in a later transfer test, those who had viewed the model on every trial (1 to 1) were significantly more accurate than those who had limited or no access.

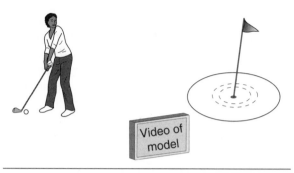

> **Figure 12.2** Video modeling as a form of instruction in golf.

This result shows that video models can have a positive effect, but it takes time for the beneficial effects to emerge.

These results can be related to the hard-first training experiments of Doane et al. (1996). When the 1v1 group viewed the model before every shot, they had to discriminate what was important in the stroke before performing; the other groups viewed the model less often and therefore were not given a similar opportunity to perceive and physically adopt the movement characteristics of the expert model. It would appear that continual exposure to complex motor information early in training leads to the development of strategies that transfer to later use. DT tool 6, hard-first instruction, therefore requires the presentation of complex instructional information right from the beginning and the use of extensive modeling that lets athletes get a more accurate mental picture of what they need to do.

Does Modeling Create Athlete Dependency?

One of the downsides to using modeling, or guided practice as it is also called, is that it can create athlete dependency on the modeled information. This was shown by Weeks, Hall, and Anderson (1996) in a study on sign language. Three novice groups were instructed in sign language using different types of modeling. One group learned to sign by watching an expert and performing the movements at the same time. A second group watched the expert and then repeated the signs after a 10 s delay. The third group performed the signs using both procedures. After similar amounts of instruction and practice time, the second group did better recalling the signs than the first and third groups. Delayed

modeling throughout acquisition generally facilitated retention later on than learning with the aid of a model. The authors explain that the presence of the model does not require the same amount of cognitive effort to be expended than when the various hand shapes have to be recalled from memory without the use of an external aid. A similar type of dependency occurs in aerobics classes where everyone follows the steps of an instructor. So although modeling is very useful in helping people understand what needs to be done in order to perform well, it is important to also use learning exercises that require independent performance.

DT Tool 7: External Focus of Instruction

In traditional forms of coaching, instruction is often phrased so that attention is drawn to the internal requirements of the skill—the technical aspects, the physiological demands, and the emotional requirements. Most statements made in coaching, whether for the purposes of feedback or for instruction, are about how to control movements of the body. This process creates an internal focus where the athlete's attention is drawn into the body and its processes. Recent research by Wulf and colleagues shows that when an **internal focus of instruction** is used, gains in long-term performance are lower than when an **external focus of instruction** is used (Wulf, McConnel, Gartner, & Schwarz, 2002; Wulf, McNevin, Fuchs, Ritter, & Toole, 2000; Wulf, McNevin, & Shea, 2001; Wulf, Mercer, McNevin, & Gaudagnoli, 2004; Wulf, Shea, & Park, 2001). When a coach uses an internal focus, the emphasis is on the body and on the techniques to be performed. When a coach uses an external focus, the emphasis is on the goals of the task and specific objects and locations in the environment.

Research Support for an External Focus

In Wulf et al.'s experiments, the effectiveness of promoting an internal and external focus during instruction was assessed in slalom-type movements on a ski simulator (Wulf et al., 1998), on a stabilometer (Wulf, Shea, & Park, 2001), and in tennis and golf (Wulf et al., 2000). In a typical experiment, participants were instructed to focus either on some aspect of their body movements (internal focus) or on an external goal or target (external focus). Across these studies, consistent support has been found for using an external focus of instruction in terms of improving retention and transfer. This effect was also found in a rehabilitation study where the incorporation of attentional focus, self-control, and practice in pairs resulted in greater improvements than those found with traditional forms of therapy. McNevin, Wulf, and Carlson (2003) state that "directing learner's attention to the effects of their movements can be more beneficial for learning than directing their attention to the details of their own actions," and that "furthermore, giving learners some control over the training regime has been found to enhance learning" (p. 373).

Not only is an external focus needed to perform well, but it is also the **preferred focus** when moving from a novice to more proficient state. Figure 12.3 shows the results of a study by Wulf, Shea, and Park (2001) where they determined the preferences and advantages of an internal or external focus over a training period of 3 days in a stabilometer balance task. On day 1, the participants were instructed to alternate their focus so that during one trial they attended to their feet (internal focus) and during the second they focused on markers placed in front (external focus). On days 2 and 3, they were asked to select the focus they preferred on day 1 and practice using this focus. Finally, at the end of day 3 they were asked to indicate what ultimately was their preferred focus.

On day 1, when focus alternated from internal to external, we see that the ability improved quickly. On day 2, the external- and internal-preferred focus groups continued to improve, and it appeared that there was no difference in terms of one group being better than another. But when asked what attentional focus they preferred at the conclusion of day 3, we see that those who adopted an external focus performed at a higher level.

Wulf, Shea, and Park (2001, p. 342) explain their results using the **constrained action hypothesis,**

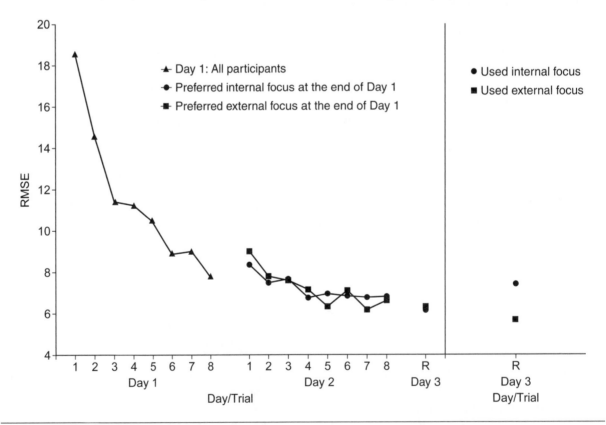

> **Figure 12.3** Performance on a stabilometer and preferences for using an internal or external focus of attention.

Reprinted, by permission, from G. Wulf et al., 2001, "Attention and motor Performance: Preferences for and advantages of an external focus," *Research Quarterly for Exercise & Health* 72(4): 335-344.

which states that "conscious attempts to control movements interferes with automatic motor control, while focusing on the remote effects of the movement allows the motor system to self-organize more naturally unconstrained by conscious control." This implies that an external focus frees the internal systems to function at a more optimal level. The constrained action hypothesis may also explain why the quiet eye is so effective. The quiet eye is not only directed toward the information critical to performing well in targeting, interceptive, and targeting tasks, but is also turned to accomplish the goals of the task.

Training an External Focus Versus Sport Vision Training

Training an external focus, or quiet eye, departs from the type of sport vision training that is carried out in optometrists' offices or other clinical settings. Sport vision training is designed to improve the hardware of the visual system, such as visual acuity, depth perception, and contrast sensitivity (Abernethy, 1986; Abernethy, 1996). Sport vision training is controversial, with serious challenges to its effectiveness (Abernethy, 1986; Abernethy & Woods, 2000; Vinger, 1996). Part of this controversy comes from the use of artificial training tasks that are performed in the office or clinical setting. Sport vision training has been shown to be largely ineffective beyond the office where the training occurs (Abernethy, 1986; Abernethy & Woods, 2000; Vinger, 1996). Abernethy (1986) and others (Druckman & Bjork, 1991; Helsen & Pauwels, 1993) have argued that training the ocular system to respond in environments that differ from those encountered in the real world of environmental stimuli are of limited value. Vinger (1996) states that "the key question remains: will equivalent time spent with a good coach or instructor result in better final performance?" (p. 77).

When an external focus is trained, as in quiet-eye training, the testing and training occur on the court, on the ice, or wherever the athlete performs. The perceptual and cognitive systems are trained, as well as how they interact with the motor system within the visuomotor workspaces found in the sport or activity. In combination with decision training, an external focus helps athletes answer many questions central to improving their performance: What are the critical objects, people, or events that I must see to perform well? To what extent must I perceive objects or locations before a movement occurs? To what extent must the input of new visual information be prevented or controlled due to its distracting or interfering nature? What exactly am I looking at during each phase of the movement? How can I improve?

Example 1: Decision Training in Cycle Racing*

This example was developed to prepare young riders for riding in the pack as found in cycle riding. In this decision-training exercise, 14- to 17-y-old junior elite cyclists were taught what to attend to externally when racing in a line or in a pack formation where considerable jostling occurs.

Step 1: Define a decision that athletes have to make in competition. The decision should name at least one key perceptual or cognitive skill the athlete needs to master while performing a specific skill or tactic. The seven cognitive skills are anticipation, attention, focus and concentration, memory, pattern recognition, problem solving, and decision making.

Cycle racing requires riding in lines and packs where it is common for the rider to be bumped and obstructed by others. The successful rider is able to detect the movements of other racers well in advance and to handle being hit or bumped while riding. The decisions made are therefore to anticipate the movements of the other racers and attend to specific cues known to improve balance and concentration while being obstructed.

Step 2: Design a drill or progression of drills to train the decision in a gamelike situation. As a part of designing the drill, it is also necessary to identify a cognitive trigger that lets both the athlete and coach know if the athlete has made the right decision. Some cognitive triggers include object cues, location cues, memory cues, reaction times, and self-coaching cues.

---

*This decision-training drill was designed by Dan Proulx, junior national cycling coach.

The training session occurs on free rollers that are moved into various line and pack configurations. Figure 12.4 shows a pack configuration. The racers use their own bikes, which are not locked into or stabilized in any way on the rollers. The cognitive cues are the specific locations that require focus and attention, as well as the kinesthetic cues that signal safe riding under control. The cognitive triggers are object and location cues known to improve anticipation and attention.

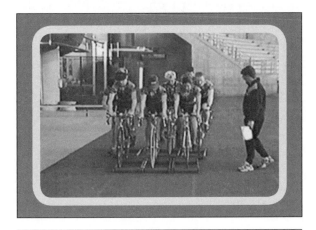

► **Figure 12.4**   A pack-riding drill in cycling with riders aged 14 to 17 y in which hard-first instruction, an external focus, bandwidth feedback, and questioning are used.

Step 3: Select one or more of the seven decision tools to train the decision in a variety of simulated competitive contexts. The seven DT tools are variable practice, random practice, bandwidth feedback, questioning, video feedback, hard-first instruction and modeling, and external focus of instruction.

The DT tools used in this drill are hard-first instruction, external focus of instruction, bandwidth feedback, and questioning. The drill involves hard-first instruction because the riders begin with the rollers, rather than leaning against wall or using systems that lock their bikes down. This drill is therefore appropriate only for skilled riders and not novices. While cycling, the coach asks questions such as "Where should you focus when following the bike in front? What is the best way to counter being hit, obstructed, and so on?" The performers answer these questions while biking and experiencing the various con-

figurations (loose pack, close pack, line) over an extended period of time. This drill helps the riders to anticipate being hit and teaches them how to direct and redirect their focus when obstructed, how to control their center of gravity in numerous simulated conditions, how to use a teammate for support, and how to solve other typical problems in road racing. This drill can only be carried out using rollers and should only be used in a safe setting. It is also the only way this type of bumping and jostling can be simulated in training. Coaches comment that the athletes find the drill challenging and also confidence building as they learn that they can handle quite a bit of jostling without losing their balance or getting upset.

Example 2: Decision Training in Speed Skating

In this section, four decision-training drills are presented that together provide a comprehensive overview of certain decision-making skills required in long-track speed skating. These drills were selected to cover the main events that occur in a speed-skating race where errors in decision making often occur. They also were selected because they cover the four major phases that occur in all speed-skating races. The first drill concentrates on the start, the second on entering the turn, the third on exiting the turn, and the final on pacing. These drills can be applied to sports that have similar events, such as those found in track events, short-track speed skating, cycling, and so on.

Drill 1: The Start*

Speed-skating races are won in milliseconds; therefore any time that can be saved is critical. In chapter 3, reaction time and movement time were presented. Success in speed skating and in many other races is dependent on who has the best reaction time and movement time. Most coaches concentrate on the movements of the start, but an equally good place for an athlete to gain time is the reaction-time phase. This is the 150 to 200 ms that occur from the time the gun sounds until the skater's first observable movement. This drill

---

*These four decision-training drills were developed with Debra Fisher, Director of Developmental Speed Skating, Olympic Oval, Calgary. Debra is a certified decision trainer.

presents the type of decision making required to minimize reaction time.

Step 1: Define a decision that athletes have to make in competition. The decision should name at least one key perceptual or cognitive skill the athlete needs to master while performing a specific skill or tactic. The seven cognitive skills are anticipation, attention, focus and concentration, memory, pattern recognition, problem solving, and decision making.

A study by Buckolz and Vigars (1987) determined whether a sensory set or a motor set provided faster reaction times. An athlete who starts using a motor set is focusing internally on the muscles and limbs responsible for an explosive start. Motor sets tend to be slower than sensory sets because they encourage the performer to focus internally on the details of response execution, which slows reaction time. In chapter 3, the different thresholds for reaction time were presented, and it was shown that auditory reaction time was fastest. The decision to be trained therefore is attention to the auditory cue, even as the gaze is focused externally on the entrance to the turn. This gives racers total visual control over the entry to the turn, even as they devote their attention to the starter's gun.

Step 2: Design a drill or progression of drills to train the decision in a gamelike situation. As a part of designing the drill, it is also necessary to identify a cognitive trigger that lets both the athlete and coach know if the athlete has made the right decision. Some cognitive triggers include object cues, location cues, memory cues, reaction times, and self-coaching cues.

The drill is similar to the start in races, complete with a starter who calls the correct commands. Three commands are normally given: go to the start, ready, and go. The goal is to have the athletes experiment with the different attentional sets, which serve as different cognitive triggers.

➤ Auditory cue—Attend to the "go" signal (voice, gun, other sound).

➤ Visual cue—Attend to the movements of the skaters beside you.

➤ Motor set—Think about pushing off the back skate or other internal motor behavior.

The coach begins the starting drill by asking the skaters to completely clear their minds of all thoughts and focus on each cue as the starting commands occur. The skaters go through a number of starts with the coach presenting various cues on the command of "go."

Step 3: Select one or more of the seven decision tools to train the decision in a variety of simulated competitive contexts. The seven decision-training tools are variable practice, random practice, bandwidth feedback, questioning, video feedback, hard-first instruction and modeling, and an external focus of instruction.

The DT tools used in this drill are hard-first instruction, external focus of instruction, bandwidth feedback, and questioning. Bandwidth feedback, questioning, and video feedback were used as follows. Each start is videotaped so that both reaction time and movement time could be determined. Reaction time was from the sound of the gun to the racer's first observable movement. Movement time was from the first observable movement until the completion of one full stride or when the forward skate reached a near point on the track. The skaters were shown their starts and were asked questions about what they thought was the cue that allowed them to have a faster start. They also were required to determine their own reaction time and movement time from their videotapes following the same procedures as used in the analysis of Mark McGwire in chapter 3. Over a series of starts, the athletes were trained to attend to the auditory cue, even as they held their gaze on the entry block to the turn.

Drill 2: Entering the Turn

Speed skaters have to enter each turn and begin the crossover steps that allow them to build speed as they skate the apex and exit the turn. In chapter 8, the gaze of elite speed skaters was described as they entered and exited the turn. Here that research is applied in a decision-training drill. This drill may be used in both long- and short-track speed skating. Short-track speed skating differs from long track in that the racers can move out of their lanes and obstruct one another within certain limits.

Step 1: Define a decision that athletes have to make in competition. The decision should name at least one key perceptual or cognitive skill the athlete needs to master while performing a specific skill or tactic. The seven cognitive skills are anticipation, attention, focus and concentration, memory, pattern recognition, problem solving, and decision making.

The decision to be trained is concentration and visual focus on the correct entry point of the turn (see chapter 8). In short-track racing, since athletes are also required to start at different locations along the start line, it is critical that they focus on the correct point of entry to the turn.

Step 2: Design a drill or progression of drills to train the decision in a gamelike situation. As a part of designing the drill, it is also necessary to identify a cognitive trigger that lets both the athlete and coach know if the athlete has made the right decision. Some cognitive triggers include object cues, location cues, memory cues, reaction times, and self-coaching cues.

The skaters do two sets of three starts from different positions on the starting line looking toward the entry of the turn. The cognitive trigger is different blocks placed at different locations on the entry, each with a number. The blocks are cues for the athletes' external focus and attention, but they also serve as a cue for when the crossover steps begin.

Step 3: Select one or more of the seven decision tools to train the decision in a variety of simulated competitive contexts. The seven DT tools are variable practice, random practice, bandwidth feedback, questioning, video feedback, hard-first instruction and modeling, and external focus of instruction.

The DT tools in this example are variable practice, bandwidth feedback, questioning, and video feedback. After each entry, the coach probes the athletes' understanding of the best entrance cue and optimal focus and concentration points after the start. The skaters perform a number of entries, focusing on a different block and entry point each time. The athletes are also required to do an assignment where they analyze their best and worst entrances on videotape.

Drill 3: Performing the Crossover in Long Track

Speed skaters in long track always race another skater. In order to make sure each skater skates the same distance, they have to accommodate one another in a tricky crossover maneuver that occurs on the backstretch. Often they get into trouble and inadvertently drag race one another

down the backstretch. The inside skater has to give way to the outside skater at some point, and both end up losing time. The following decision-training drill helps both skaters anticipate when the crossover occurs and attend to the correct cues under time pressure.

Step 1: Define a decision that athletes have to make in competition. The decision should name at least one key perceptual or cognitive skill the athlete needs to master while performing a specific skill or tactic. The seven cognitive skills are anticipation, attention, focus and concentration, memory, pattern recognition, problem solving, and decision making.

The decision to be trained occurs when exiting the turn in Olympic-style speed skating. The athletes not only have to build speed out of the turn, but they also have to learn to execute crossovers to the correct lane on the backstretch. This maneuver has to be coordinated with another skater who has the right of way. The decision the athletes have to make is to attend to the cue for each crossover and execute it in the variable times given.

Step 2: Design a drill or progression of drills to train the decision in a gamelike situation. As a part of designing the drill, it is also necessary to identify a cognitive trigger that lets both the athlete and coach know if the athlete has made the right decision. Some cognitive triggers include object cues, location cues, memory cues, reaction times, and self-coaching cues.

The drill occurs on ice and requires two athletes to enter the turn and exit into a crossover as in a race. The cognitive trigger is different timing cues given by the coach from different points on the track.

Step 3: Select one or more of the seven decision tools to train the decision in a variety of simulated competitive contexts. The seven DT tools are variable practice, random practice, bandwidth feedback, questioning, video feedback, hard-first instruction and modeling, and external focus of instruction.

Variable practice is used as follows:

➤ The first cue is given as the athletes enter the turn, thereby giving the athletes a long reaction time. A cue card is flashed that signals which skater should take the inner or the outer lane depending on designated lane change following the exit of the turn.

> ➤ The second position is from the top of the turn and the skaters are given a verbal cue from the coach to go either inner or outer. In this case the reaction-time phase is shortened.

> ➤ The third position is from the coach's box on the backstretch, where the coach points to go either inner or outer (shortest reaction time). The athletes have little time to make the crossover efficiently.

Drill 4: Pacing in Long-Track Speed Skating

Each race in long-track speed skating requires a different pace. Athletes also skate a number of races in a meet and have to get the pace correctly each time. If athletes make a mistake and get the pace wrong, then they cannot maintain their optimal speed to the end of the race. This decision-training drill is designed to help the athletes learn the pacing of the many different events.

Step 1: Define a decision that athletes have to make in competition. The decision should name at least one key perceptual or cognitive skill the athlete needs to master while performing a specific skill or tactic. The seven cognitive skills are anticipation, attention, focus and concentration, memory, pattern recognition, problem solving, and decision making.

All speed skaters must develop the ability to pace themselves during a race. Elite skaters are able to estimate their lap times within a few milliseconds. Since skaters often skate different events that require different pacing, in this drill the athletes must retrieve from memory the correct pacing information and skate laps at these times.

Step 2: Design a drill or progression of drills to train the decision in a gamelike situation. As a part of designing the drill, it is also necessary to identify a cognitive trigger that lets both the athlete and coach know if the athlete has made the right decision. Some cognitive triggers include object cues, location cues, memory cues, reaction times, and self-coaching cues.

This drill occurs on ice where the skaters skate 3 sets of 5 laps (15 total). The cognitive trigger is a different pace (500 m; 1,500 m; 3,000 m, etc.) that is cued (cognitive trigger) by the coach from the side of the ice. Times are recorded for each lap per event.

Step 3: Select one or more of the seven decision tools to train the decision in a variety of simulated competitive contexts. The seven DT tools are variable practice, random practice, bandwidth feedback, questioning, video feedback, hard-first instruction and modeling, and external focus of instruction.

In this example, variable practice, bandwidth feedback, and questioning are used. On the first set, the coach shows the skaters the lap times relating to a specific distance they should skate on particular laps. On the second set, the pace for sprinting or endurance laps is shown. On the third interval, the skaters must hit the time without any cues being given. The skaters must retrieve from memory what it feels like to skate at the requested pace. At the conclusion of the practice, the skaters are asked if they felt they skated close to the prescribed time. They see their actual lap times and compare these with their own perceptions of pace. With training, the skaters learn to retrieve the correct pace for each event.

Decision Training in Action

Design, and deliver if possible, a 15-minute decision-training drill using the three-step decision-training model.

> ➤ Step 1. Name a decision the athlete has to make in competition. The decision should name at least one key perceptual or cognitive skill the athlete needs to master while performing a specific skill or tactic. The perceptual and cognitive skills are: anticipation, attention, focus and concentration, pattern recognition, memory, decision making, and problem solving.

> ➤ Step 2. Design a drill or progression of drills or activities to train the decision. As part of designing the drill, identify a cognitive trigger that lets both the athlete and coach know if the athlete has made the right decision.

> ➤ Step 3. Select one of the two decision tools discussed in this chapter to train the decision in a variety of simulated competitive contexts.

The case studies provided here show how hard-first instruction, or an external quiet-eye focus, has proven to be beneficial for those who have used it. In the first, an elite speed skater is introduced to quiet-eye training just prior to the national trials and the Turin Olympics. In the second, Cirque d'Soleil decides to apply hard-first instruction in their training studios in Montreal.

Case Study 12.1   Improving an External Quiet-Eye Focus Leads to Increases in Speed and an Olympic Medal

For many years I watched Dr. Vickers and her research team conduct studies with the basketball players and hockey players. Every time I told myself if one day we could somehow do the same with our speed skaters it would definitely help me understand and possibly answer some questions that I've been trying to find answers to for many years. Finally, my prayers were answered back in February of 2005 when Dr. Vickers announced to me that it was now possible to test my speed skaters on ice. With the Turin Olympic Games 12 months away, I knew that improving their focus as they skated had some real potential to help my skaters perform better at the Games.

One skater in particular was, in my opinion, a primary subject for quiet-eye testing and training: a young 20-year-old female skater who had been skating on long-track speed skating for only 2 seasons and was progressing really fast despite her lack of experience in the sport. Her progression was mainly due to the fact that she was getting fitter and technically skating better. But at the same time, she was having a hard time executing the perfect lap. In speed skating it is very important for a skater to be able to select the best line both into and out of the turn in order to skate the fastest lap possible. That particular skater wasn't able to execute the right pattern on a regular basis. Mainly, her corner entrance and corner exit were all over the place, making it hard to carry any speed in the straightaway and making her sometimes skate 450 m on a track of 400 m. Was the problem a lack of focus, or was it a biomechanics or some other problem? After using many different approaches to correct her problem it was still very much present in her way of skating and especially when she was racing.

Then came the quiet-eye testing and training. After only one test on ice I got the answer I was looking for. I knew at that point that her problem was an easy fix after all. But, before jumping to any conclusions, we did a multitude of tests and they all showed us the same result. What that skater was failing to do was focus in a way that allowed her to enter each turn with the most optimal line leading to the exit. When she first reviewed her quiet-eye results with Dr. Vickers, she had no idea that her gaze control was leading her to skate the way she was. For her it was quite a shock and very revealing for me in terms of finally being able to help her correct it. After being made aware of the problem and learning what to do to correct it she was able to execute a better lap and carry that speed going into the corners and coming out of those corners with more speed.

An optimal quiet-eye focus became part of her mental preparation before each training session and before each race leading up to the Turin Olympic Games. I can honestly say that the quiet eye helped me and my athletes understand the reason why she was not skating to her potential.

Story told by Marcel LaCroix, head coach, Team Canada Speedskating, and coach of many medal winners at the 2006 Turin Olympics. The athlete he speaks of, Christine Nesbitt, won a bronze medal in Turin, even though she was a B skater when she first started using quiet-eye training. She has since gone on to win a number of World Cup races.

Case Study 12.2   Hard-First Instruction for Cirque d'Soleil

I was brought in to help the coaches of Cirque d'Soleil with decision training. "Your mission is a simple one," said Bernard Petoit, the director of the performance studios of the Cirque d'Soleil in Montreal. "We need to accelerate how quickly we can get the performers from the training studios here in Montreal out to the shows. Right now it is taking us 6 to 8 mo and we need to reduce this 4 to 6. Cirque d'Soleil is expanding from seven shows worldwide to double this, so we need to be that much better at what we do. We need to have everyone working together sooner and better." This included choreographers, voice coaches, dance coaches, dramatists, and comics in all disciplines from gymnastics, tumbling, diving, dance, drama, and art.

The facility in Montreal is ultra modern, huge, bright, and dynamic—everything you would expect. On my first visit I presented an overview of decision training. Although I was working with some of the best coaches in the world, I quickly saw that they were feeling the same pressures as everyone who works in high performance sport. There is often too much to do and not enough time.

At the Cirque, champion athletes come from around the world and are given 4- to 8-mo contracts to find their place in one of the shows. The most difficult step for them, and the Cirque, is to identify those who not only perform superbly in a physical way, but also have the aesthetic qualities that radiate from the stage through movement, emotion, feeling, humor, beauty, adventure, and creativity. This is a tough job because most of the athletes have learned not to express their own creativity, and the coaches have very little time to help them find their aesthetic physical selves while producing a show.

I met with Bernard and his other performance directors after my session, and they decided to implement hard-first training as soon as the athletes arrived! I couldn't imagine how what the Cirque did could be harder! Their solution is so typical of what I see so often in elite sport. Once the ideas of decision training are grasped, then the coaches find a way to implement an aspect into their world. The coaches decided the best way to implement this new training was to create a new structure within the program. Instead of the athletes spending the first two months with the different sport coaches reviewing and learning the acrobatic components of the different routines, the athletes began to work with a coach and a choreographer immediately who had to learn to work together to quickly bring out the best in the athletes. The hard-first training aspect the Cirque introduced was aesthetic athleticism because that is so critical to their shows. The benefits of this new training were obvious to Bernard and his colleagues, but they all knew it presented its own challenges. When I returned later on, most of the coaches and choreographers had found a new way to work together, and the benefits were what they had expected. The Cirque was able to identify the hidden qualities in their performers faster and bring forth those qualities in their shows.

GLOSSARY

abstract targeting tasks—A subcategory of targeting tasks, where the best target for the gaze and objects is not easily perceived but requires higher order cognitive processes to discern (e.g., golf putting on a sloped line, playing billiards).

affordances—A term coined by Gibson (1979), "the affordances of an environment are what it offers the animal" (p. 127).

alternative models of visual awareness—Visual awareness is flexible and situation-dependent rather than hard-wired (Tononi & Edelman, 1998).

ambient system—Includes the areas on the retina that are not within the fovea. The ambient system is specialized for motion and the rapid detection of information and for perception during low light conditions.

amygdala—Located at the tip of the hippocampus and plays a major role in emotional control and memory formation. The closeness of the amygdala to the center of memory formation partly explains why even one devastating experience seems to stay with us forever; memories are formed along with their emotional consequences.

anosognosia—A rare disorder where a stroke in the right hemisphere of the brain leads to a complete paralysis of the left side of the body.

anterior executive network—Responsible for bringing into consciousness critical aspects of what is being fixated. This network interprets what is being viewed and imposes a higher-order understanding on the task based on past experience and knowledge. Skilled players bring a richer knowledge base and more refined rules than less skilled performers, who are often unsure of what they need to see as they perform.

anticipation—Directing attention to a stimulus prior to its presentation, thus better preparing the body and mind to act.

athlete dependency—Occurs when too much external feedback is provided to an athlete by a coach, thus preventing the athlete from developing the problem solving, decision making, and coping strategies needed for high-level performance.

attention—Explains how we select information for more extensive processing in thresholds that minimally range from 120-200 ms depending on the sensory modality (i.e., vision, hearing, touch, smell, or taste). "Everyone knows what attention is. It is the taking possession by the mind, in a clear and vivid form, of one out of what seem several simultaneously possible objects or trains of thought. Focalization and concentration of consciousness are of its essence. It applies withdrawal from some things in order to deal effectively with others, and is a condition which has a real opposite in the confused, dazed, scatter brained state which in French is called distraction, and Zerstreutheit in German" (James, 1890/1981, p. 381-382).

auditory reaction time—The time it takes from the presentation of a sound until the first observable movement for a naive participant to respond to the stimulus (average 140-160 ms).

augmented feedback—Used to refer to any combination of knowledge of performance and knowledge of results.

autism—A cognitive disorder characterized by greatly impaired social interaction; a narrow range of interests; deficits in language and communication; and fixed, repetitive movements.

axon—The part of a neuron that conducts nerve impulses or messages over distances between neurons.

bandwidth feedback—Refers to deliberately reducing and delaying feedback as skill level improves.

basal ganglia—A group of nuclei located deep in the forebrain that coordinates voluntary movement of the limbs and body.

behavioral training—Method of training where the coach or teacher is concerned only with observable changes in the physical movements of the athlete and not the athlete's thinking and decision-making skill.

behaviorism—A response will become a habit as a consequence of the number of times it is paired or associated with a given stimulus (Skinner, 1953; Thorndike, 1911; Watson, 1924).

binding problem—"Concerns our capacity to integrate information across time, space, attributes and ideas . . . . [it is] required when we select an action to perform in a particular context. We must, for example, reach in the right direction, lift the glass with the correct muscle tension, and drink the water it contains rather than eat or inhale it" (Treisman, 1999, p. 105).

binocular fusion—Occurs when slightly different images from the two eyes fuse into a single stereoscopic perception, simply called fusion or binocular interaction. The slight difference in the images, which arises from binocular disparity, is important because it provides the cue we use for depth, yet we still see a single, stable image. Gregory (1997, p. 60) states, "A remarkable thing about the visual system is its ability to combine the two somewhat different images into a single perception of solid objects lying in three-dimensional space (stereoscopic perception)."

binocular vision—Occurs when an object is viewed with both eyes.

blinks—Occur when the eyelid covers the eye. Blinking is essential for refreshing the cornea and lens and for maintaining vision. During blinks, information is also suppressed (Volkmann, Riggs, & Moore, 1981).

blocked practice—The same skill or tactic is practiced over and over with little change in the context. Blocked practice is necessary in situations where a skill is first being learned, as well as later on when the primary goal is to make the skill automatic.

bottom-up processing—A form of attention that proceeds in a "single direction from sensory input, through perceptual analysis, towards motor output, without involving feedback information flowing backwards from 'higher' centers to 'lower' centers" (Corbetta & Shulman, 2002, p. 201).

breakpoint—A location of the gaze found in golf putting on a sloped line that identifies where the ball will begin its roll to the hole.

cerebellum—Also known as the hindbrain, the cerebellum is located at the back of the head and is involved in motor coordination and the timing of movement.

change blindness—A phenomenon that occurs when humans often fail to notice critical changes in their environment. It is "the failure of observers to detect large, sudden changes in a display. Although such changes are readily seen under normal conditions, change blindness is easily induced if the changes are made simultaneously with an eye movement, film cut, image flash, or other transient that masks the motion signals normally accompanying the change" (Rensink, 2002, p. 1469).

choking—The "failure to perform up to whatever level of skill and ability the person has at the time" (Baumeister, 1984, p. 610), it occurs in high pressure performance settings when the athlete allows internal thoughts (or self-focus) or external distractions to disrupt well-learned automatic routines developed through extensive practice.

chunking—Through learning and experience, seemingly diverse pieces of information are grouped together into fewer but more meaningful ideas or concepts that enhance the control of action.

closed-loop control—A mode of motor control where the movement can be influenced by feedback arising from the muscles and external stimuli. Skills are often classified as under closed-loop control when the movement time phase is more than 200 ms.

cognitive anxiety—An athlete who is cognitively anxious has "negative expectations and cognitive concerns about oneself, the situation at hand, and potential consequences" (Martens et al., 1990a, p. 541). Performers who experience high levels of cognitive anxiety are worried about their ability to perform and are fearful of the consequences of not performing well.

cognitive effort—The mental work that "leads to high levels of decision making . . . anticipation, planning, regulation and interpretation of motor performance" (Lee et al., 1994, p. 328-329).

cognitive neuroscience—Describes the structure and function of the brain. Recent brain imaging techniques, such as fMRI (functional magnetic resonance imaging) and PET (positron emission tomography), permit scanning of the brain when different types of information are processed under different conditions. These methods permit identification of the areas of the brain involved in processing different types of information and the effect this has on behavior movements.

cognitive psychology—The formal study of how the brain functions in terms of information processing. Sternberg (2003, p. 527) defines cognitive psychology as "the study of how people perceive, learn, remember, and think about information." Solso (1995, p. 2) explains that "cognitive psychology is the scientific study of the thinking mind and is concerned with how we attend to and gain information about the world, how that information is stored in memory by the brain and how that knowledge is used to solve problems, to think and to formulate language."

cognitive trigger—A visual, verbal, or kinesthetic cue strategically placed by a coach within a drill to help the athlete (and coach) know if the correct decision has been made as the skill or tactic is performed.

consciousness—Explains why we are aware of some things but not others and the effect this has on learning and performance. This "is both the most obvious and the most mysterious feature of our mind" (Dennet, 1987, p. 160).

constrained action hypothesis—States that "conscious attempts to control movements interferes with automatic motor control, while focusing on the remote effects of the movement allows the motor system to self-organize more naturally unconstrained by conscious control" (Wulf, Shea, & Park , 2001, p. 342).

constraints-led perspective—As proposed by Newell (1986) and Newell and McDonald (1994), holds that motor coordination can only be understood when three categories of constraints (organism, task, and environment) are taken into consideration that "interact to determine for a given organism, the optimal pattern of coordination and control for any activity" (Newell, 1986, p. 348). The model also includes a perception–action cycle that actively seeks information from the perceptual-motor workspace, resulting in motor coordination.

contextual interference—The practice of introducing real-world challenges into the learning environment.

cornea—The transparent surface of the eye.

corrective feedback—Refers to technical, tactical, and other sport-specific information provided to the athlete with the aim of improving performance.

covert orienting of attention—The gaze is located on one object or location and the attention on another. Think of a basketball player looking in one direction while attention (and a pass) is made to another direction.

creativity—Explains how the human mind generates original thought.

decision training—A new method of coaching that incorporates into the regular practice environment high levels of decision making within simulated and real sport contexts. Decision training brings the science of how we think, or cognition, to the fore of sport preparation. It is designed to improve the athlete's attention, anticipation, concentration, memory, and problem-solving skills through practices where cognitive training is incorporated into physical and technical training. The overall goal is the development of an athlete who is able to make effective decisions under all the pressures of competition.

degrees of freedom—Of a movement is the number of separate independent elements that must be controlled in the body to produce a coordinated action.

delayed feedback—A form of corrective feedback provided after a delay so that athletes have time to think about their performance.

dendrite—A branch of neurons that greatly increases its area.

direct perception—As proposed by Gibson (1979), actors perceive the environments in which they perform unaided by inference, memories, or other neural representations as suggested by cognitive psychology.

distraction models of choking—A model of choking due to cognitive deficits that arise when the athlete's attention is diverted away from the primary task, causing a cognitive deficit that impairs performance

(Bleilock & Carr, 2001; Eysenck, 1992; Eysenck & Carvello, 1992; Wine, 1971).

dorsal stream—The pathway that conducts signals from the occipital cortex to the parietal lobe and is responsible for orienting the gaze and sustaining attention at one location (Posner & Raichle, 1994). It is also responsible for the rapid processing and updating of information that is important for orientation in space and movement. The dorsal stream is also known as the "where pathway" because it directs attention to locations in space.

dynamic systems—This perspective grew out of the work of Bernstein (1967), and later that of Turvey (1977a, 1977b), Kelso (1982), and others. In a dynamic systems approach, "movement patterns arise from the synergistic organization of the neuromuscular system based on morphological factors (i.e., biological constructs), biomechanical factors (i.e., Newtonian Laws), environmental factors (i.e., spatial and temporal configuration of events), and task constraints (e.g., walking at slow or fast speeds)" (Kurz & Stergiou, 2004, p. 93).

easy-first instruction—Refers to an instructional method in which easy conceptual material is presented early in training.

ecological psychology—Founded by James Gibson (1966, 1979), and is also called direct perception. It is identified as direct because it is believed that people perceive the environments in which they perform unaided by inference, memories, or other neural representations as suggested by cognitive psychology (Michaels & Carello, 1981). Movement through the world is dependent on the establishment of direct optical relationships that develop without any apparent need for the many processing stages described in cognitive psychology.

ecological validity—The methods, materials, and setting of an experiment approximate the real-life situation that underlies the study. Findings in the experiment are shown to apply to real world settings.

electroencephalography (EEG)—Noninvasively records electrical brain activity through electrodes placed on the scalp. These electrodes summate postsynaptic potentials in the cerebral cortex and other areas of the brain.

electromyography (EMG)—Recording of the electrical activity from the muscles.

elite athlete—An athlete who consistently achieves the highest statistics in a specific task in his or her sport, as documented by external authorities such as statisticians, league officials, as well as by testing in the experimental environments.

environmental constraints—External to the body and include "gravity, natural ambient temperature, natural light and other environmental features that are not usually simply adaptations of the task" (Newell & McDonald, 1994, p. 350).

error correction phase—A final period of time in a movement when feedback is used to hone or refine the movement.

external focus of instruction—The coach directs the athlete's attention toward the outcome of the task or the goal being pursued.

extrinsic feedback—Feedback from external sources such as a coach, teacher, videotape, or computer.

eye-in-head system—Tracking of the object occurs using both head and eye movements and the image is maintained on the fovea longer.

eye–head stabilization—During interceptive timing tasks, the period of time when the gaze and head are stable as the moving object is controlled.

faded feedback—Occurs when a high frequency of feedback is given early on and then gradually reduced as skill level develops.

feature integration theory—When an object is fixated, the stimulus properties are encoded into separate neural pathways, each of which generates a feature map for color, orientation, size, distance and stereo distance, and other factors. Selected features from these maps are then integrated onto a master map where one object or location among many becomes the spotlight for the attention and pops out more than anything else.

feedback—Sensory information that arises from movement.

feed-forward—Information is sent ahead from the higher neural centers and is incorporated into incoming sensory information for use in motor planning.

fixations—Occur when the gaze is held on an object or location within 3° of visual angle for 100 ms or longer (Carl & Gellman, 1987; Carpenter, 1988; Fischer, 1987; Optican, 1985).

fixed targets—A fixed object or location in space toward which an object is normally aimed, such as a basketball hoop, a bullseye, or a rifle target.

focal vision—Used when fixated or tracked information falls on the fovea and aspects of an object or location are viewed with full acuity or detail.

fovea—A small area at the back of the eye in the retina that is responsible for visual acuity, or the ability to resolve small details and thus see objects or locations clearly.

fractionated reaction-time paradigm—A method of dividing a motor response into temporal components, such as (1) a warning signal to get ready; (2) a signal to start the movement, or "go" signal; (3) the first moment of observable movement; and (4) the time when the movement ends.

freezing, freeing and exploiting the degrees of freedom—A theory of motor skill acquisition proposed by Bernstein (1967) and Vereijken, van Emmerik, Whiting, and Newell (1992), who further explained that when we first learn a skill, we tend to freeze the degrees of freedom in a way that limits coordination and control. Then as a skill is acquired, we free some of the degrees of freedom, thus allowing the movement to be performed more efficiently and accurately. Finally, we learn to exploit the degrees of freedom, an evolution in skill development that is needed to perform at a high level in any context. Freezing, freeing, and exploiting the degrees of freedom therefore can be viewed as stages the performer goes through in the attainment of higher levels of skill.

frequency of feedback—Refers to how often feedback is provided to an athlete or a group within a specific period of time.

frequency of fixation—The average number of fixations per unit of time.

frontal cortex—Also known as the executive of the brain and coordinates advanced thinking, planning, and language. It is where goals and intentions are formulated for the specific event that is occurring.

gaze control—The process of directing the gaze to objects or events within a scene in real time and in the service of the ongoing perceptual, cognitive, and behavioral activity (Henderson, 2003).

gaze control framework—Describes control of the gaze in three major categories of motor tasks (targeting tasks, interceptive timing tasks, and tactical tasks). Within each category, the available gaze research shows that the function of the gaze differs, as does the number and type of visuomotor workspaces and the spotlight of attention underlying optimal performance.

glial (or glia) cells—These cells lack the membrane properties required to fire action potentials as in neurons, but they communicate with one another and with neurons chemically rather than through electrical signals. Glial cells play a major role in information processing in the nervous system, and they may one day provide a greater understanding of how information is processed. During development "glia have a powerful role in setting up the basic scaffolding of the brain" (Fields & Stevens-Graham, 2002, p. 561) in that they extend the influence of axons and dendrites in forming synaptic connections.

handicap—A handicap of 0 in golf means that a player is able to play a complete round of golf in the number of strokes determined by the course designer. Normally a round of golf has 18 holes, each of which requires 3 to 5 strokes. The optimal number of strokes is usually around 72 on most 18-hole courses. A related system is called the index, which takes into account the type of course that the handicap is earned on. In this case, the handicap is adjusted to reflect the difficulty of the course.

hard-first instruction—Refers to an instructional method in which difficult conceptual material is presented early in training.

Hick's law—States that the amount of time it takes to prepare a response is dependent upon the number of stimulus–response (SR) alternatives that are present.

hierarchical models of visual awareness—Visual awareness occurs only when visual information reaches the higher cortical level areas (Crick & Koch, 1995).

hippocampus—A large forebrain structure that is responsible for cell genesis, learning, and memory formation. Damage to the hippocampus prevents the retention and transfer of short-term memories to long-term memory centers that are located throughout the brain.

image–retina system—The eyes and head remain motionless as an object washes over the retina.

impulse phase—Similar to the initiation phase, or the first observable movement in a motor task.

inattention blindness—"Denotes the failure to see highly visible objects we may be looking at when our attention is elsewhere" (Mack, 2003, p. 180).

indirect perception—The cognitive process of perceiving the world in which we move without the intervention of memories and knowledge representations stored in the brain.

information processing—The study of the flow of information through the neural and motor systems and the effect this has on cognitive processing, the acquisition of knowledge, and behavior.

inhibition of return—The process whereby a currently attended location is prevented from being attended to later on. If an object or location is viewed on one occasion, then there is a lower probability that an attempt will be made to fixate that location again.

in situ—A Latin term that means in its original place.

instantaneous feedback—A form of corrective feedback that is given immediately, before athletes have time to think about their performance.

interactive models of visual awareness—Visual awareness occurs in V1, or very early in the visual pathway (Buller, 2001; Pollen, 1999).

interceptive timing tasks—An object travels toward the performer and the gaze and attention systems are used to read the object as it is delivered, track it as it approaches, and then control it as it is received or controlled in some way.

internal focus—The performer's available attentional resources dwell on an aspect of technique, physiology, or emotional control rather than task and environmental factors.

internal focus of instruction—The coach directs the athletes' attention to their technique, physiology, or emotions related to the activity.

in the zone—A feeling experienced by performers when their thought and body processes are in perfect synchronization, resulting in excellent performance.

intrinsic feedback—Feedback that arises internally from the production of a movement.

invariants—Any aspect of the environment (or people or events) that does not change but retains the same qualities in all situations. Michaels and Carello (1981) define an invariant as a constant pattern, usually amid change in other variables of stimulation" (p. 31). Invariances are "those high-order patterns of stimulation that underlie perceptual constancies, or more generally, the persistent properties of the environment that an animal is said to know. Invariant structures in light and sound not only specify objects, places and events in the environment, but also the activities of the organism… Thus invariants are, by virtue of the laws that support them, information about the environment and the animal's relation to it usually amid change in other variables of stimulation" (p. 40).

kinesthetic reaction time—The time it takes from the presentation of a perturbation (e.g., vibrating key) until the first observable movement for a naive participant to respond to the stimulus (average 120-140 ms).

knowledge of performance—A form of external feedback that is usually concerned with technique and form. This information is normally provided by a coach, video, or other aid.

knowledge of results—A form of external feedback that arises from the outcome of the movement (e.g., hit or miss, a fast time or a slow one, a good judges' score).

language—Explains the nature of speech, audition, comprehension, writing, and other forms of literary expressions.

line of gaze—Originates from each eye, passes through the appropriate field, and intersects in front. The line of gaze is defined as "the absolute position of the eyes in space and depends on both eye position in orbit and head position in space" (Schmid & Zambarbieri, 1991, p. 229).

locations—Distinct from objects in that they are topographically defined and therefore rarely move, but they are similar to objects in that they are psychological representatives affecting the sensory receptors of the performing player. The perception of locations allows the performer to determine the relative position of the body and other objects in space. The spaces within which locations occur can span 360° around the performer and are three-dimensional in nature, possessing height, width, and depth. Spatial locations in sport therefore include all the surfaces that athletes perform on, whether horizontal, vertical, or possessing depth (e.g., ice, snow, grass, greens, floors, walls). Locations also include lines or other marks on playing surfaces, goals, hoops, nets, and similar equipment.

location–suppression hypothesis—A hypothesis of gaze control that states that during the location phase, the athlete focuses on the most critical location on the target for about 1 s before the execution of the skill. Fixation is held at that location until an object (such as a ball) enters the athlete's visuomotor workspace, during which vision is suppressed in order for the task to be performed accurately.

locomotion—In biology, the self-powered movement of the limbs found in movements such as walking and running. Locmotion is "the movement of one's body around an environment, coordinated specifically to the local or proximal surrounds—the environment that is directly accessible to our sensory and motor systems at a given movement (or, at most, within a few moments). When we locomote, we solve behavioral problems such as identifying surfaces to stand on, avoiding obstacles and barriers, directing our movements toward perceptible landmarks, and going through openings without bumping into various things" (Montello, 2005, p. 258-259).

M1 (monosynaptic) loops—Are brief (30-50 ms) and relay sensory information from the muscles to the spinal cord and then back to the same muscle. They automatically maintain balance and stability without conscious awareness.

M2 loop—Longer (50-80 ms) than M1 loops, and goes from the muscles up the spinal cord to the brain to stored plans and programs for the actions we are performing. We are also not aware of this feedback; the time period is too fast to permit conscious awareness.

M3 loop—The longest loop, it requires conscious perception and attention to what we feel, see, hear, or otherwise sense. The latency of the M3 loop varies by the sensory system being used. The fastest is that of kinesthetic reaction time, which, as we saw in table 3.1, has a latency of about 120 ms. Next is the auditory reaction time, which requires 140-160 ms. The slowest of all the reaction times is vision, which requires 180-220 ms to see a stimulus and produce an action.

memory—Describes how information is stored in the brain, how we access it and represent it as knowledge, and how we use it to guide our actions.

mirror neurons—Located in the frontal cortex and the parietal cortex and responds when an action performed by another person or animal is observed. Rizzolatti (2006, p. 54) states that, "sets of mirror neurons appear to encode templates for specific actions."

modeling—A form of hard-first instruction that occurs when the athlete views another performer in order to learn about the different technical and tactical skills required.

monocular vision—Occurs when an object is viewed with one eye.

motor control—The ability to plan and produce a movement that successfully achieves a particular goal.

motor control neural areas—Located at the top of the head (i.e., the primary motor cortex, the supplementary motor area, and the premotor area) and are responsible for the control of movements.

motor learning—The process of going through a set of internal processes, phases, stages, steps, or transitions on the way to becoming proficient in a motor skill. Motor learning requires physical practice and is affected by age, maturation, amount of time devoted to practice, plus a host of other factors.

motor performance—A final stage of motor learning when most of the learning of the skill has been done and the challenge is now one of motor control, or producing the same optimal outcome each time.

motor phases—"Describe the temporal structure of a sequence, usually measured by the ratios of element durations and the overall movement duration" (Schmidt & Lee, 2005, p. 466).

motor program—"An abstraction representation, that when initiated, results in the production of a co-ordinated movement" (Schmidt & Lee, 2005, p. 466).

motor time—Within the fractionated reaction paradigm, the period of time from the onset of a motor response as detected by internal methods such as EMG until the first observable movement.

movement kinematics—"As applied to movement behavior, describes the movement of the limb, the entire body, or both. The locations of the various parts of the body during movement, the angles of the various joints, and the time relations between the movement of one joint and the movement in another are examples of the many ways movement kinematics can be recorded (Schmidt & Lee, 2005, p. 36)."

movement time—The time from the first observable movement of the effector until the end of the response.

moving targets—A location of the gaze found in the subcategory of targeting tasks where the target is in motion (e.g., passing to a receiver).

near-elite athlete—An athlete who has all the attributes of an elite athlete (same age and physiological characteristics, technically similar, same coach, training time, and regime), but is unable to achieve top statistics in a task in the sport (e.g., shooting free throws, putting, shooting on goal).

negative feedback—Any verbal or nonverbal statement that detracts from the achievement of the goals of the practice.

neural plasticity—The capacity for neurons to change in response to experience. Neurophysical and neurochemical changes enhance the ability of the brain to compensate and adapt to environmental change and injury. Two major processes are involved called synaptogenesis and neurogenesis.

neurogenesis—The birth of new neurons. It is important to note that there is still some controversy surrounding whether neurogenesis occurs in humans, although it is widely accepted in animals and birds (Kalat, 2004).

neurons—Composed of a cell body, dendrites, a main axon covered with a myelin sheath, and terminal buttons that connect with other neurons. Neurons are responsible for carrying nerve impulses throughout the nervous system and for communicating with other neurons through synaptic junctions. Neurons acquire information from the sensory receptors (sight, hearing, touch, smell, taste) and pass this information to other neurons that send the information to the muscles to produce movements. Neurons communicate with one another through neurotransmitters and the transmission of electrical signals or action potentials.

object-control phase—During interceptive timing tasks, fixation and tracking gaze are used to stabilize the eyes and head as the object is caught, kicked to a teammate, hit as in baseball or cricket, passed to a teammate as in volleyball, and so on.

object fixations—The gaze is directed toward objects in space, thus allowing the detection of new information. During object fixations the gaze is stationary on objects or locations, even as the feet continue walking or running.

object-recognition phase—During interceptive timing tasks, fixations and pursuit tracking are used to study the movements of the object and the individual propelling the object as it is pitched, bowled, kicked, shot, or otherwise propelled toward the athlete.

objects—"An object in the real world is a physical entity that has, at any given time, a defined location, mass, volume, shape, and other physical properties. It may reflect or generate light, sound waves, or chemical stimuli; it may move or be moved; and it has some degree of temporal continuity. A perceptual object is a psychological representative of a physical object that is currently affecting the sensory receptors of the perceiving organism" (Treisman, 1986a, p. 1). Objects within the performance environment include balls, pucks, shuttles (or similar), rackets, and all other equipment; as well as opponents, teammates, officials, coaches, judges, spectators, and all other persons. Objects may also have subcomponents, such as a player's head, torso, or feet, or a specific part of a piece of equipment (e.g., stick handle, stick blade).

object-tracking phase—During interceptive timing tasks, smooth pursuit-tracking gazes are used to maintain the image of the object on the fovea in order to detect if it spins, accelerates, or decreases in speed; changes direction; or is affected by wind, sun, or a host of other factors that can occur.

occipital lobe—The visual cortex comprised of areas V1 to V5. Each of these areas is specialized for processing different visual inputs. Tong (2003, p. 219-220) states that V1 is "uniquely positioned as the primary distributor of almost all visual information that reaches other cortical areas. About 90% of projections from the eye are channeled through lateral geniculate nucleus (LGN) to V1."

occlusion period—In vision-in-action studies, occlusion occurs when the athlete's limbs, an object, or implement blocks information in the visuomotor workspace. Occlusion techniques are also used to mask or remove aspects of the visuomotor workspace or video display.

open-loop control—A mode of motor control in which motor commands are prepared in advance and executed without any influence from muscle feedback. Skills are classified as under open-loop control when the movement time phase is under about 200 ms.

optic array—In Gibson's (1979) theory, these are projections of the surrounding visible environment.

optic flow—In Gibson's (1979) theory, these are changes in the optic array created by observer movement and include how visual information is perceived as it moves toward or by us as a consequence of our own movements.

optic tract—The part of the brain comprised of the optic nerves that extend from each eye through the lateral geniculate nuclei to the primary visual regions or occipital cortex, which are located at the back of the head.

organismic constraints—Include various biological and functional aspects of a person, such as body weight, height, and shape, as well as synaptic connections that control cognitive and body functions.

Organismic constraints are inherent in the person and are affected by genetics, nutrition, development, and training experiences.

overt orienting of attention—Both the location of the gaze and the locus of attention are directed to the same location or object in space. For example, a basketball player using overt attention will look directly at the player and also think about passing the ball to that player.

paradox in motor learning research—Recent developments in motor learning research in practice design, feedback, and instruction. Extensive research in all three areas shows that traditional methods of teaching and coaching, which are collectively called behavioral training, are successful in the short term, but athletes trained exclusively under these conditions are unable to perform at a high level in the long term, especially when under pressure.

parietal lobe—Located at the back of the head and responsible for the orienting of the gaze and attention in space.

pattern recognition—The ability to discern meaning from configurations of stationary or moving objects (such as players in a team game), as well as when navigating a cluttered environment.

perception–action cycles—Link information perceived in the environment to specific physical behaviors in time-dependent ways.

perceptual-motor workspaces—"Nonstationary, that is, the nature of the workspace changes over time because of a variety of influences, including ongoing interactions of the performer with the environment" (Newell & McDonald, 1994, p. 527). It is within perceptual-motor workspaces that visual information is acquired and critical decisions are made that affect sport performance.

plasticity—Refers to the brain's ability to change over time as a result of neurogenesis and synaptogenesis.

positive feedback—Any form of verbal or nonverbal feedback that contributes to the achievement of the goals of the practice.

posterior orienting network—Responsible for controlling the gaze and attention in space. This network, which is located in the parietal region, directs the gaze to specific locations of importance in a task. It is also responsible for preventing the disengagement of the gaze to other locations.

predictable object motion—When the flight of the object is relatively constant.

preferred focus—The focus of attention when executing a motor skill. The preferred focus may or may not be an optimal one for the individual.

preparation phase—The period of time in a movement when the movement is organized; therefore it is akin to the reaction-time phase.

premotor time—The period of time from the presentation of a stimulus to the onset of a motor response as detected by EMG or other internal methods.

pressure—Often leads to choking and is composed of "any factor or combination of factors that increases the importance of performing well on a particular occasion" (Baumeister, 1984, p. 610). High-pressure environments are those where the performer perceives the stakes to be high and where poor performance may lead to a loss of position or stature. In contrast, low-pressure environments are those that contain few risks and the pressure to perform well is low, as is the tendency to choke.

problem solving—Explains how we use perception, attention, and other cognitive abilities to arrive at solutions in both old and new situations.

pupil—The opening in the iris of the eye that adjusts the amount of light and becomes smaller in bright light and larger in low light.

pursuit tracking—Occurs when the gaze follows a moving object, such as a ball or a person. The 100 ms threshold is used for pursuit tracking for the same reason it is used for fixations; it is only when the gaze is stabilized on the moving object or person that the individual is able to process the information provided by that object or person.

questioning—One of the seven decision-training tools that is used by the coach to determine the level of understanding the athlete has of a technique or tactic. Sentences are worded to seek information in a nonthreatening but probing way. Proper use of the language in the sport and in sport science is encouraged.

quick-then-quiet-eye—In tactical settings, where the gaze dwells for a short time (quick) on aspects of the evolving play in order to read the pattern, and then hones in on one critical assignment as the play nears the scoring zone (quiet eye).

quiet eye—A fixation or tracking gaze that is located on a specific location or object in the visuomotor workspace within 3° of visual angle for a minimum of 100 ms. The onset of the quiet eye occurs prior to the final movement in the task; the quiet-eye offset occurs when the gaze moves off the location by more than 3° of visual angle for a minimum of 100 ms. The quiet eye is therefore a perception–action variable, in that its onset is dictated by the onset of a specific movement in the task.

quiet-eye dwell time—Occurs in golf putting when the fixation on the ball is maintained on the green after the ball has been struck.

quiet-eye training—Involves using both video modeling and video feedback to help athletes develop the same quiet-eye focus and motor control as found in elite performers.

random practice—The performer learns to combine different classes of movements within settings that simulate the conditions found in play and competition. More than one class or pattern of skills is combined in a tactically relevant way. Random practice drills are called smart combinations when the drills simulate conditions that are similar to those found in a play or competitive setting.

rate of perceived exertion (RPE)—As developed by Borg (1971), is our understanding of the subjective sensation of the amount of physical work being performed. The Borg scale quantifies the extent an exercising person perceives there is little or no work being done.

reaction time—The period of time from the presentation of a stimulus until the first obsevable movement to complete the response.

recognition-primed model of decision-making—As proposed by Klein (1999), experts are better at making decisions in high-pressure environments than non-experts due to their ability to detect the most important environmental cues without hesitation and in a way that leads to decisive and appropriate actions.

relative time—Defined as the "fundamental temporal structure, organization, or rhythm of a movement . . . this structure remains the same even when people decide to make changes in the flexible features of the pattern" (Schmidt & Wrisberg, 2004, p. 157). Relative time is often expressed as a set of ratios or percentages that defines the durations of several phases of a movement, or time intervals.

retention tests—Assess the extent that the same skill learned earlier can be reproduced later on.

retina—The surface of the back of the eye that converts light into energy that results in neural activation. The retina is lined with two types of visual receptors called rods and cones. Cones are located within the fovea and are responsible for the detection of color and light and for resolving detail. The proportion of rods increases in the periphery of the retina, which is specialized for detecting low light and motion.

saccades—Occur when the eyes move quickly from one fixated or tracked location to another. Saccades are rapid eye movements that bring the point of maximal visual acuity onto the fovea so that it can be seen with clarity. During saccades, information is suppressed.

salient features—Those features that are intrinsically conspicuous in a given context and that preattentively affect the orientation of attention. A salient feature also tends to be "independent of the nature of a particular task, operates very rapidly, and is driven in a bottom-up manner, although it can be influenced by contextual, figure-ground effects. If a stimulus is sufficiently salient it will pop out of a visual scene. This suggests that saliency is computed in a preattentive manner across the entire visual field . . . the speed of this saliency is on the order of 25-50 ms per item" (Itti & Koch, 2001, p. 194).

scan path—A series map of eye movements that shows how a performer fixates or tracks the objects and locations in a perceptual-motor workspace.

self-focus models of choking—One of the two models of choking; performance decrements occur when attention is directed inward to technical, physiological, or emotional aspects that are normally automated (Baumeister, 1984; Lewis & Linder, 1997; Masters, 1992; Masters & Maxwell, 2004).

self-organization—Kelso (1995, p. 1-2) describes this as existing in all forms of life "without any agent-like entity ordering the elements, telling them what to do and where to go." Self-organization is often used to describe the process of development, where humans grow from infants to crawlers to toddlers to children to adolescents to adults and finally to elderly adults without any external agent appearing to exert control. Kelso (1995, p. 8) explains that self-organization is defined by "spontaneous pattern formation" where the system organizes itself without any input from the "self, or other agent within the system doing the organizing."

self-regulation—In coaching this is a chain of events from a situation where the coach provides direct feedback to one where the coach asks questions and the athlete provides more and more input to the correction of errors.

Setchenov phenomenon—After exercising to exhaustion, directing attention to an external stimulus permits more work to be done (discovered by Setchenov (1903/1935).

somatic anxiety—Defined as "one's perception of the psychological affective elements of the anxiety experience; that is, indications of autonomic arousal and unpleasant feeling states such as nervousness and tension" (Morris, Davis, & Hutchings, 1981, p. 541). Somatic anxiety refers to the perception of one's physiological arousal symptoms, such as a rapid heart rate, shortness of breath, clammy hands, butterflies in the stomach, and tense muscles.

somatosensory cortex—Responsible for the sense of touch, pressure, and feeling—capacities that are extremely important in all forms of movement.

spotlight for the attention—The act of extracting and processing high-priority information in the visual field. Selected features from a stimulus pop out more than anything else. Attention at that location permits the identification of the object integrated with memory processes.

stereoscopic perception—The ability to detect depth by the difference in what the two eyes see.

summative feedback—A form of corrective feedback that is given only after a number of attempts are performed. In summative feedback, the coach tries to sum up what occurred in terms of major technical, tactical, or other cues.

synaptogenesis—Occurs when one cell excites another repeatedly, and a change takes place in one or both cells characterized by the growth of more dendrites, more synaptic connections, and a condition called arborization. A neuron that has been stimulated many times results in more synaptic connections or arborization, a longer axon, and more synaptic buds, while neurons that do not experience the same degree of stimulation are smaller and without the longer axon and dendrites.

tactical tasks—The gaze and attention system is used to read complex patterns of moving objects (e.g., players, balls, pucks) resulting in appropriate actions. Think of reading the offense or defense in a team sport such as basketball, baseball, or soccer, or trying to discern the open part of a net where you want to make a shot in field hockey, or reading a race course as in skiing, kayaking, or mountain climbing.

tactics—May be defined as the science of organizing and maneuvering forces in games, battles, or other endeavors to achieve a limited or immediate aim. Tactics also involves the art of deploying forces in order to compete or engage in battle. Most tactical situations require the planning of maneuvers as they will occur during actual contact with a competitor or an enemy.

targeting tasks—The function of the gaze and attention system is to locate a target in space and control the aiming of an object to the target area. Within targeting tasks, there are three subcategories of tasks: gaze control to fixed targets, to abstract targets, and to moving targets. In these tasks, an object is propelled away from the body in an aiming movement toward a target, usually with the hands or feet. Accuracy and consistency in performance are the ultimate goals.

task constraints—In Newell (1986, p. 352), include "a) the goal of the task; b) the rules specifying or constraining response dynamics; and c) implements or machines specifying or constraining response dynamics." In addition, "all goals relate to the outcome of the product or outcome of the action."

top-down processing—"The flow of information is from the 'higher' to 'lower' centers, conveying knowledge derived from previous experience rather than sensory stimulation" (Corbetta & Shulman, 2002, p. 201). Top-down processing is affected by our memories, our goals and expectations, and the amount of knowledge and experience we have in a given situation. Top-down processing often occurs rapidly and has qualities linked to awareness, insight, and the degree of experience the person has in a sport.

topographical mapping—The process whereby certain spatial relations among locations are preserved in the brain.

total response time—The sum of reaction time plus movement time.

transfer tests—These tests determine if a skill learned earlier can be used in new situations.

travel fixations—Are carried along by the feet and there is a continuous flow of information a the speed of locomotion.

triggered reaction—Has a latency of 80-120 ms and takes into account feedback that is received when we act against an object or location in the environment. Imagine trying to hit a baseball and having your foot slip, or skiing down a slope and hitting a patch of ice.

unpredictable object motion—When the flight of the object spins, slides, curves, or moves erratically.

variable practice—The athlete practices variations of a single class of skills in a setting that simulates the conditions found in play or competition. Variable practice drills are called smart variations when the drills simulate conditions similar to those found in competition. Variable practice is easy to remember if you think of coaching one class or pattern of skills.

ventral stream—The pathway that conducts signals from the occipital cortex to the temporal lobe. It is known as the "what stream" and is associated with the cognitive long-term processing of information and higher executive processes. The ventral stream is responsible for assigning meaning to events, and it guides the anticipation and planning of actions.

video feedback—Performers view their own movements in an effort to improve their performance.

vigilance network—Responsible for coordinating the posterior and anterior networks and preventing unwanted or distracting information from gaining access to the other networks during periods of sustained focus. The vigilance network is responsible for the sustained concentration seen in elite players, especially during pressure-filled games of long duration.

vision-in-action paradigm—A research method where the athlete's gaze is recorded as he or she performs in a manner that is very similar to that found in the sport; therefore, there is always a coupling of perception and action. The athlete performs a well-known sports task that, whenever possible, has published international standards of achievement (e.g., race times, shots made, goals saved). In this way athletes can be grouped into skill categories based on objective standards of achievement. The athlete is tested within an experimental environment that is very similar to that found in the sport. Finally, whenever possible, the athlete performs the task until an equal number of successful and unsuccessful trials are accomplished.

visual angle—Indicates the size of an image on the retina, and it is determined by extending lines from the edges of the object as viewed in space through the lens to the retina.

visual awareness—When a person is conscious of what is being viewed, for example, they know an apple is red versus being green.

visual field—It is the total amount of space that can be viewed by the retina when the eye is fixated straight ahead. It is also the total amount of light that stimulates your eye at any moment in time. It is therefore the region of the world that is seen by the eyes.

visual pivot—The centering of the gaze in a display and the use of peripheral vision to control and monitor the action.

visual reaction time—The time it takes from the presentation of a visual stimulus (e.g., light) until the first observable movement for a naive participant to respond to the stimulus (average 180-160 ms).

visual search—Defined as "the process by which one locates a target in a cluttered scene" (Zelinsky, Rao, Hayhoe, & Ballard, 1997). It has also been described as "the scan of an environment for particular features—actively looking for something when you are not sure where it will appear" (Sternberg, 2003, p. 83).

visual-search paradigm—A research paradigm where participants' eye movements or gaze are recorded as they view videotapes or photographs and search for aspects in the display in response to experimental conditions.

visual-spatial intelligence—"The ability to navigate across town, comprehend an animated display of the functioning human heart, view complex multivariate data on a company's website, or read an architectural blueprint and form a three-dimensional mental picture of a house are all tasks involving visuospatial thinking" (Shah & Miyake, 2005, p. i). It is central to sport performance and requires an ability to read complex patterns of movements, resulting in actions that lead to a goal being attained.

visuomotor coordination—The ability to use visual information to generate appropriate motor commands (McLeod, 1994). It is the process whereby visual (gaze) information is used to direct and control movements.

visuomotor workspace—This is the spatial environment within which objects and locations exist that command the performer's gaze and attention and upon which specific motor behaviors are enacted.

REFERENCES

Abernethy, B. (1986). Enhancing sports performance through clinical and experimental optometry. *Clinical and Experimental Optometry, 69,* 189-196.

Abernethy, B. (1991). Visual search strategies and decision-making in sport. *International Journal of Sport Psychology, 22,* 189-210.

Abernethy, B. (1996). Training the visual-perceptual skills of athletes: Insights from the study of motor expertise. *American Journal of Sports Medicine, 24* (6), 89-93.

Abernethy, B., & Woods, J. (2000). Do generalized programmes in sports really work? An experimental investigation. *Journal of Sport Sciences, 19,* 203-222.

Abrams, R.A., Meyer, D.E., & Kornblum, S. (1989). Speed and accuracy of saccadic eye movements: Characteristics of impulse variability in the oculomotor system. *Journal of Experimental Psychology, 15* (3), 529-543.

Abrams, R.A., Meyer, D.E., & Kornblum, S. (1990). Eye–hand coordination and oculomotor control in rapid aimed limb movements. *Journal of Experimental Psychology: Human Perception and Performance, 16* (2), 248-267.

Adolphe, R.M., Vickers, J.N., & LaPlante, G. (1997). The effects of training visual attention on gaze behaviour and accuracy: A pilot study. *International Journal of Sports Vision, 4* (1), 28-33.

Allard, F., & Starkes, J.L. (1980). Perception in sport: Volleyball. *Journal of Sport Psychology, 2,* 22-23.

Allard, F., & Starkes, J.L. (1991). Motor-skill experts in sports, dance, and other domains. In K.A. Ericsson & J. Smith (Eds.), *Toward a general theory of expertise: Prospects and limits* (pp. 126-152). Cambridge: Cambridge University Press.

Alpenfels, E., & Christina, R. (2005). The new way to putt. *Golf Magazine,* October, 95-99.

Altman, J., & Das, G.D. (1965). Autoradiographic and histological evidence of postnatal hippocampal neurogenesis in rats. *Journal of Comparative Neurology, 124,* 319-335.

Applegate, R.A. (1992). Set shot shooting performance and visual acuity in basketball. *Optometry & Vision Science, 69* (19), 765-768.

Assmussen, E., & Mazin, B. (1978a). Recuperation after muscular fatigue by "diverting activities." *European Journal of Applied Physiology, 38,* 1-8.

Assmussen, E., & Mazin, B. (1978b). A central nervous component in local muscular fatigue. *European Journal of Applied Physiology, 38,* 9-15.

Bahill, A.T., & LaRitz, T. (1984). Why can't batters keep their eyes on the ball? *American Scientist, 72,* 249-253.

Bard, C., & Fleury, M. (1976). Analysis of visual search activity during sport problem situations. *Journal of Human Movement Studies, 3,* 214-222.

Bard, C., & Fleury, M. (1981). Considering eye movements as predictor of attainment. In I.M. Cockerill & W.W. MacGillvary (Eds.), *Vision and sport* (pp. 28-41). Cheltenham: Stanley Thornes.

Bard, C., Fleury, M., Carriere, L., & Halle, M. (1980). Analysis of gymnastic judges' visual search. *Research Quarterly, 51* (2), 267-273.

Battig, W.F. (1956). Transfer from verbal pretraining to motor performance as a function of task complexity. *Journal of Experimental Psychology, 51,* 371-378.

Battig, W.F. (1966). Facilitation and interference. In E.A. Bilodeau (Ed). *Acquisition of skill* (pp. 215-240). New York: Academic Press.

Battig, W.F. (1972). Intratask interference as a source of facilitation in transfer and retention. In R.F. Thompson & J.F. Voss (Eds.), *Topics in learning and performance* (pp. 131-159). New York: Academic Press.

Battig, W.F. (1979). The flexibility of human memory. In L.S. Cermak & F.I.M. Craik (Eds.), *Level of processing in human memory* (pp. 22-44). Hillsdale, NJ: Erlbaum.

Baumeister, R. (1984). Choking under pressure: Self-consciousness and paradoxical effects of incentives on skillful performance. *Journal of Personality and Social Psychology, 46,* 610-620.

Bear, M.F., Connors, B.W., & Paradiso, M.A. (2007). *Neuroscience: Exploring the brain* (2nd ed.). Philadelphia: Lippincott, Williams & Wilkins.

Bernstein, N. (1967). *The co-ordination and regulation of movements.* Oxford: Pergamon Press.

Bleilock, S.L., & Carr, T.H. (2001). On the fragility of skilled performance: What governs choking under pressure. *Journal of Experimental Psychology: General, 130* (4), 701-725.

Bootsma, R.J. (1991). Predictive information and the control of action: What you see is what you get. *International Journal of Sport Psychology, 22,* 271-278.

Bootsma, R.J., & van Wieringen, P.C.W. (1988). Visual control of attacking forehand drive in table tennis. In O.G. Meijer & K. Roth (Eds.), *Complex movement behavior: The motor-action controversy* (pp. 189-199). Amsterdam: Elsevier Science Publishers.

Bootsma, R.J., & van Wieringen, P.C.W. (1990). Timing an attacking forehand drive in table tennis. *Journal of Experimental Psychology, 16* (1), 21-29.

Borg, G. (1971). The perception of physical performance. In R.J. Shepherd (Ed.), *Frontiers of fitness* (pp. 280-294). Springfield, IL: Charles C. Thomas.

Borg, G. (1982a). Psychological bases of perceived exertion. *Medicine and Science in Sports and Exercise, 14,* 377-381.

Borg, G. (1982b). Ratings of perceived exertion and heart rates during short-term cycle exercise and their use in a new cycling strength test. *International Journal of Sports Medicine, 3,* 153-158.

Brancazio, P.J. (1981). Physics of basketball. *American Journal of Physics, 49,* 356-365.

Breen, J. (1967). What makes a great hitter? *Journal of Health, Physical Education and Recreation, April,* 36-39.

Bridgeman, G., Hendry, D., & Start, L. (1975). Failure to detect displacement of visual world during saccadic eye movements. *Vision Research, 15,* 719-722.

Bridgeman, B., Kirch, M., & Sperling, A. (1981). Segregation of cognitive and motor aspects of visual information using induced motion. *Perception and Psychophysics, 29,* 336-342.

Brown, J., Cooper-Kuhn, C.M., Kempermann, G., van Praag, H., Winkler, J., Gage, F.H., et al. (2003). Enriched environment and physical activity stimulate hippocampal but not olfactory bulb neurogenesis. *European Journal of Neuroscience, 17,* 2042-2046.

Buckolz, E., & Vigars, B. (1987). Sprint start reaction time: On the advisability of sensory vs motor sets. *Canadian Journal of Sport Science, 12* (1), 51-53.

Buller, J. (2001). Integrated model of visual processing. *Brain Research Reviews, 36,* 96-107.

Calvin, William H. (1983). *The throwing Madonna: Essays on the brain.* New York: Bantam Books.

Calvo-Merino, B., Glaser, D.E., Grezes, D.E., Passingham, R.E., & Haggard, P. (2004). Action observation and acquired motor skills: An fMRI study with expert dancers. *Cerebral Cortex, 15,* 1243-1249.

Cao, L., Xiangyang, J., Zuzga, D., Liu, Y., Fong, D., Young, D., et al. (2004). VEGF links hippocampal activity with neurogenesis, learning and memory. *Nature Genetics, 36,* 827-835.

Carl, J., & Gellman, R. (1987). Human smooth pursuit: Stimulus-dependent responses. *Journal of Neurophysiology, 57,* 1446-1463.

Carlen, M., Classify, R.M., Breismar, H., Smith, G.A., Enquist, L.W., & Freisen, J. (2002). Functional integration of adult-born neurons. *Current Biology, 12,* 606-608.

Carlton, L.G. (1981a). Processing visual feedback information for movement control. *Journal of Experimental Psychology: Human Perception and Performance, 7,* 1019-1030.

Carlton, L.G. (1981b). Visual information: The control of aiming movements. *Journal of Experimental Psychology: Human Perception and Performance, 33A,* 87-93.

Carpenter, R.H.S. (1988). *Movements of the eyes* (2nd ed.). London: Pion.

Cave, T.R., & Bichot, N.P. (1999). Visuospatial attention: Beyond the spotlight metaphor. *Psychonomic Bulletin & Review, 6* (2), 204-223.

Chambers, K.L., & Vickers, J.N. (2006). The effect of bandwidth feedback and questioning on competitive swim performance. *The Sport Psychologist, 20* (2), 184-197.

Corbetta, M. (1998). Frontoparietal cortical networks for directing attention and the eye to visual locations: Identical, independent, or overlapping. *Proceedings of the National Academy of Sciences, 95,* 831-838.

Corbetta, M., Akbudak, E., Conturo, T.E., Snyder, A.Z., Ollinger, J.M., Drury, H.A., et al. (1998). A common network of functional areas for attention and eye movements. *Neuron, 21* (4), 761-773.

Corbetta, M., & Shulman, G.L. (2002). Control of goal-directed and stimulus driven attention in the brain. *Nature Reviews, 3,* 201-215.

Coren, S., Ward, L., & Enns, J.T. (2004). *Sensation and perception* (6th ed.). Hoboken, NJ: Wiley.

Crews, D.J., & Landers, D.M. (1993). Electroencephalographic measures of attentional patterns prior to the golf putt. *Medicine and Science in Sports and Exercise, 25,* 116-126.

Crick, F., & Koch, C. (1995). Are we aware of neural activity in primary visual cortex? *Nature, 375,* 121-123.

Cross, N., & Lyle, J. (Eds.). (1999). *The coaching process: Principles and practice for sport.* Woburn, MA: Reed.

Cutting, J.E. (1996). Wayfinding from multiple sources of local information in retinal flow. *Journal of Experimental Psychology, 22,* 1299-1313.

Dapretto, M., Davies, M.S., Pfeifer, J.H., Scott, A.A., Sigman, M., Bookheimer, S.Y., et al. (2006). Understanding emotions in others: Mirror neuron dysfunction in children with autism spectrum deficits. *Nature Neuroscience, 9* (1), 28-30.

Davids, K., Savelsbergh, G., Bennet, S., & van der Kamp, J. (Eds.) (2002). *Interceptive actions in sport: Information and movement.* London: Routledge.

Davidson, R.J., & Hughdahl, K. (Eds.). (1995). *Brain asymmetry.* Cambridge, MA: MIT Press.

Davidson, R.J., & Schwartz, G.E. (1976a). The psychobiology of gait transitions: Effects of load and grade. *Journal of Motor Behavior, 30,* 60-78.

Davidson, R.J., & Schwartz, G.E. (1976b). The psychobiology of relaxation and related states: A multiprocess theory. In D.I. Mostofsky (Ed.), *Behavior control and modification of physiological activity* (pp. 237-252). Englewood Cliffs, NJ: Prentice-Hall.

Dennet, D. (1987). Information theory. In R.L. Gregory (Ed.), *The Oxford companion to the mind* (pp. 160). Oxford: Oxford University Press.

Deubel, H., & Schneider, W.X. (1996). Saccade target selection and object recognition: Evidence of a common attentional mechanism. *Vision Research, 36* (12), 1827-1837.

Doane, S.M., Alderton, D., Sohn, Y., & Pelligrino, J. (1996). Acquisition and transfer of skilled performance: Are visual discrimination skills stimulus specific? *Journal of Experimental Psychology: Human Perception and Performance, 22* (5), 1218-1248.

Doane, S.M., Sohn, Y.W., & Schreiber, B. (1999). The role of processing cognitive strategies in the acquisition and transfer of a cognitive skill. *Journal of Experimental Psychology: Human Perception and Performance, 25* (5), 1390-1410.

Douge, B., & Hastie, P. (1993). Coach effectiveness. *Sport Science Review, 2* (2), 14-29.

Dozier, R.M., Hicks, M.W., Cornille, T.A., & Peterson, G.W. (1998). The effect of Tomm's therapeutic questioning style on therapeutic alliance: A clinical analog study. *Family Processes, 37* (2), 189-200.

Draganski, B., Gaser, C., Busch, V., Schuierer, T., Bogdahn, U., & May, A. (2004). Neuroplastiity: Changes in grey matter induced by training. *Nature, 427,* 311-312.

Driver, J. (2001). A selective review of selective attention research from the past century. *British Journal of Psychology, 92* (1), 53-79.

Druckman, D., & Bjork, R.A. (Eds.). (1991). *In the mind's eye: Enhancing human performance.* Washington, DC: National Academy Press.

Easterbrook, J.A. (1959). The effect of emotion on cue utilization and organization of behavior. Psychological Review, 66, 183-201

Elliott, B. (1992). A kinematic comparison of the male and female two-point and three-point jump shots in basketball. *Australian Journal of Science and Medicine in Sport, 24,* 111-118.

Elliott, B., & White, E. (1989). A kinematic and kinetic analysis of the female two point and three point jump shots in basketball. *Australian Journal of Science and Medicine in Sport, 21,* 7-11.

Emes, C., Vickers, J.N., & Livingston, L. (1994). Gaze control of children with high versus low motor proficiency. *Adapted Physical Activity* (pp. 147-154). Tokyo: Springer-Verlag.

Engel, A.K., & Singer, W. (2001). Temporal correlates and the neural correlates of sensory awareness. *Trends in Cognitive Science, 5,* 16-25.

Ericsson, K.A. (1996). The acquisition of expert performance: An introduction to some of the issues. In K.A. Ericsson (Ed.), *The road to excellence: The acquisition of expert performance in the arts and sciences, sports, and games* (pp. 1-50). Mahwah, NJ: Erlbaum.

Ericsson, K A. (2002). Attaining excellence through deliberate practice: Insights from a study of expert performance. In M. Ferrari (Ed.), The pursuit of excellence in education (pp. 21-55). Hillsdale, NJ: Erlbaum.

Ericsson, K.A. (2003). How the expert performance approach differs from traditional approaches to expertise in sport: In search of a shared theoretical framework for studying expert performance. In J.L. Starkes & K.A. Ericsson (Eds.), *Expert performance in sports: Advances in research on sport expertise* (pp. 371-402). Champaign, IL: Human Kinetics.

Ericsson, K.A., & Kintsch, W. (1995). Long-term working memory. *Psychological Review, 102,* 211-245.

Ericsson, K.A., Krampe, R., & Tesch-Romer, C. (1993). The role of deliberate practice in the acquisition of expert performance. *Psychological Review, 100* (3), 363-406.

Ericsson, K.A., & Simon, H.A. (1993). *Protocol analysis: Verbal reports as data* (rev. ed.). Cambridge, MA: MIT Press.

Eriksson, P.S., Perfilieva, E., Bjork-Eriksson, T., Alborn, A., Nordborg, C., Peterson, D., et al. (1998). Neurogenesis in the adult human hippocampus. *Nature Medicine, 4* (11), 1313-1317.

Eysenck, M.W. (1982). *Attention and arousal: Cognition and performance.* Berlin: Springer.

Eysenck, M.W. (1992). *Anxiety: The cognitive perspective.* Hove, UK: Erlbaum.

Eysenck, M.W. (1994). *The Blackwell dictionary of cognitive psychology.* Oxford: Blackwell.

Eysenck, M.W., & Carvello, M.G. (1992). Anxiety and performance: The processing efficiency theory. *Cognition and Emotion, 6,* 409-434.

Fabel, K., Tam, B., Kaufer, D., Baiker, A., Simmons, N., Kuo, C.J., et al. (2003). VEGF is necessary for exercise-induced adult hippocampal neurogenesis. *European Journal of Neuroscience, 18,* 2803-2812.

Farr, M.J. (1987). *The long-term retention of knowledge and skills: A cognitive and instructional perspective.* New York: Springer-Verlag.

Fields, D.R., & Stevens-Graham, B. (2002). New insights into neuron-cell glia communication. *Science, 298* (18), 556-562.

Fischer, B. (1987). The preparation of visually guided saccades. *Reviews of Physiology, Biochemistry, and Pharmacology, 106,* 2-35.

Fischer, B., & Weber, H. (1993). Express saccades and visual attention. *Behavioral and Brain Sciences, 16,* 553-610.

Fitts, P.M. (1954). The information capacity of the human motor system in controlling the amplitude of movement. *Journal of Experimental Psychology, 47,* 381-391.

Fitts, P.M., & Posner, M.I. (1967). *Human performance.* Belmont, CA: Brooks/Cole.

Fowler, G.A., & Sherk, H. (2003). Gaze during visually guided locomotion in cats. Behavioral *Brain Research, 139,* 83-96.

Franks, I.M., & Harvey, T. (1997). Cues for goalkeepers: High-tech methods used to measure penalty shot response. *Soccer Journal, 42,* 30-33.

Gagne, R., & Briggs, L.J. (1979). *Principles of instructional design* (2nd ed.). New York: Holt, Rinehart and Winston.

Gauthier, G.M., Nommay, D., & Vercher, J.L. (1990). The role of ocular muscle proprioception in visual localization of targets. *Science, 249,* 58-61.

Gauthier, G.M., Semmlow, J.L., Vercher, J.L., Pedrono, C., & Obrecht, G. (1991). Adaptation of eye and head movements to reduced peripheral vision. In R. Schmid & D. Zambarbieri (Eds.), *Oculomotor control and cognitive processes* (pp. 179-196). Amsterdam: Elsevier Science.

Gibson, E.J., & Pick, A. (2001). *Perceptual learning and development: An ecological approach.* New York: Oxford University Press.

Gibson, J.J. (1966). *The senses considered as perceptual systems.* Boston: Houghton Mifflin.

Gibson, J.J. (1979). *The ecological approach to visual perception.* Boston: Houghton Mifflin.

Gladwell, M. (2005). *Blink: The power of thinking without thinking.* New York: Little, Brown.

Goldstein, E.B. (2007). *Sensation and perception* (7th ed.). Belmont, CA. Thompson Wadsworth.

Goode, S., & Magill, R. (1986). Contextual interference effects in learning three badminton serves. *Research Quarterly for Exercise and Sport, 53,* 308-314.

Goodwin, J.E., & Meeuwsen, H.J. (1995). Using bandwidth feedback of results to alter relative frequencies during motor skill acquisition. *Research Quarterly for Exercise and Sport, 66* (2), 99-104.

Gopher, D. (1993). The skill of attention control: Acquisition and execution of attention strategies. In D. Meyer & S. Kornblum (Eds.), *Attention and performance XIV* (pp. 299-322). Cambridge, MA: MIT Press.

Gould, E., Beylin, A.V., Tanapat, P., Reeves, A., & Shors, T.J. (1999). Learning enhances adult neurogenesis in the adult hippocampal formation. *Nature Neuroscience, 2,* 260-265.

Gould, E., & Gross, G. (2002). Neurogenesis in adult mammals: Some progress and problems. *Journal of Neuroscience, 22,* 619-623.

Gould, E., McEwan, B.S., Tanapat, P., Galea, L.A.M., & Fuchs, E. (1997). Neurogenesis in the dentate gyrus of the adult tree shrew is regulated by psychosocial stress and NMDA receptor activation. *Journal of Neuroscience, 17,* 2492-2498.

Gregory, R.L. (1987). *The Oxford companion to the mind.* Oxford: Oxford University Press.

Gregory, R.L. (1997). *Eye and brain: The psychology of seeing* (5th ed.). Princeton, NJ: Princeton University Press.

Groslambert, A., Candau, R., Grappe, F., Dugue, B., & Rouillon, J.D. (2003). Effects of autogenic and imagery training on the shooting performance in biathlon. *Research Quarterly for Exercise and Sport, 74,* (3) 337-342.

Gross, C.G. (2000). Neurogenesis in the adult brain: Death of a dogma. *Nature Reviews, 1,* 67-73.

Guitton, D., & Volle, M. (1987). Gaze control in humans: Eye–head coordination during orienting movements to targets within and beyond the oculomotor range. *Journal of Neurophysiology, 58,* 427-459.

Hache, A. (2002). *The physics of hockey.* Baltimore, MD: Johns Hopkins University Press.

Hall, K., Domingues, D., & Cavazos, R. (1994). The effects of contextual interference on college level baseball players. *Perceptual and Motor Skills, 78,* 838.

Halpern, D.F. (1998). Teaching critical thinking for transfer across domains: Dispositions, skills, structure training, and metacognitive monitoring. American Psychologist, 53, 449-455.

Hardy, L. (1990). A catastrophe model of performance in sport. In J.G. Jones & L. Hardy (Eds.), *Stress and performance in sport* (pp. 81-106). New York: Wiley.

Hardy, L., & Fazey, J. (1987). The inverted-U hypothesis: A catastrophe for sports psychology and a statement of a new hypothesis. *Psychology and Motor Behaviour Abstracts, NASPSPA.* 29, Vancouver.

Hardy, L., & Parfitt, G. (1991). A catastrophe model of anxiety and performance. *British Journal of Psychology, 82,* 163-178.

Hardy, L., Parfitt, G., & Pates, J. (1994). Performance catastrophes in sport: A test of the hysteresis hypothesis. *Journal of Sport Sciences, 12,* 327-334.

Harle, S.K., & Vickers, J.N. (2001). Training quiet eye improves accuracy in the basketball free throw. *Sport Psychologist, 15,* 289-305.

Hastie, P.A. (1994). Selected teacher behaviors and student ALT-PE in secondary school physical education. *Journal of Teaching in Physical Education, 13* (3), 242-259.

Hatfield, B.D., & Hillman, C.H. (2001). The psychophysiology of sport: A mechanistic understanding of the psychology of superior performance. In R.N. Singer, H.A. Hausenblas, & C.M. Janelle (Eds.), *Handbook of sport psychology* (2nd ed.) (pp. 362-388). New York: Wiley.

Hatfield, B.D., Hillman, C.H., Apparies, R., & Vickers, J. (1999). Expert performance states: Psychophysiological perspectives in efficiency. [Abstract]. *Journal of Exercise and Sport Psychology, 21,* 55.

Hatfield, B.D., Landers, D.M., & Ray, W.J. (1987). Cardiovascular-CNS interactions during a self-paced, intentional attentive state: Elite marksmanship performance. *Psychophysiology, 24,* 542-549.

Haufler, A.J., Spalding, T., Santa Maria, D.L., & Hatfield, B.D. (2000). Neuro-cognitive activity during a self-paced visuospatial task: Comparative EEG profiles in marksmen and novice shooters. *Biological Psychology, 53,* 131-160.

Hay, J.G. (1985). *The biomechanics of sports techniques* (3rd ed.). Englewood Cliffs, NJ: Prentice Hall.

Hay, J.G. (1993). *The biomechanics of sports techniques* (4th ed.). Englewood Cliffs, NJ: Prentice Hall.

Haywood, K.M. (1984). Use of image-retina and eye-head movement visual systems during coincident anticipation performance. *Journal of Sports Sciences, 2,* 139-144.

Hebb, D.O. (1949). *Organization of behavior.* New York: Wiley.

Helsen, W.F., Elliot, D., Starkes, J.L., & Ricker, K.L. (1998). Temporal and spatial coupling of point of gaze and hand movements in aiming. *Journal of Motor Behaviour, 30,* 249-259.

Helsen, W., & Pauwels, J.M. (1992). A cognitive approach to visual search in sport. In D. Brogan, A. Gale, & K. Carr (Eds.), *Visual search 2* (pp. 379-388). London: Taylor & Francis.

Helsen, W., & Pauwels, J.M. (1993). The relationship between expertise and visual information processing in sport. In J.L. Starkes & F. Allard (Eds.), *Cognitive issues in motor expertise* (pp. 109-134). Amsterdam: Elsevier Science.

Helsen, W.F., Starkes, J.L., & Buekers, M.J. (1997). Effects of target eccentricity on temporal costs of point of gaze and the hand in aiming. *Motor Control, 1,* 161-177.

Helsen, W.F., Starkes, J.L., & Hodges, N.J. (1998). Team sports and the theory of deliberate practice. *Journal of Sport & Exercise Psychology, 20,* 12-34.

Henderson, J.M. (2003). Human gaze control during real-world scene perception. *Trends in Cognitive Sciences, 7* (11), 498-504.

Henderson, J.M., & Hollingsworth, A. (2003). Global transaccadic change blindness during scene perception. *Psychological Science, 14* (5), 493-497.

Henry, F.M. (1980). Use of simple reaction time in motor programming studies: A reply to Klapp, Wyatt and Lingo. *Journal of Motor Behavior, 12,* 163-168.

Henry, F.M., & Rogers, D.E. (1960). Increased response latency for complicated movements and a "memory drum" theory of neuromotor reaction. *Research Quarterly, 31,* 448-458.

Hernandez-Peon, R. (1964). Psychiatric implications of neurophysiological research. *Bulletin of the Menninger Clinic, 28,* 165-185.

Hick, W.E. (1952). On the rate of gain of information. *Quarterly Journal of Experimental Psychology, 4,* 11-26.

Hodges, N.J., Chua, R., & Franks, I.M. (2003). The role of video in facilitating perception and action of a novel coordination movement. *Journal of Motor Behavior, 35,* 247-260.

Hoffman, H.G. (2004). Virtual reality therapy. Scientific American, August, 58-65.

Hoffman, H.G., Patterson, D.R., & Carrougher, G. J. (2000). Use of virtual reality for adjunctive treatment of adult burn pain during physical therapy: A controlled study. *Clinical Journal of Pain, 16* (3), 244-250.

Hoffman, J.E. (1998). Visual attention and eye movements. In H. Pashler (Ed.), *Attention* (pp.119-153). East Sussex, UK: Psychology Press.

Hoffman, J.E., & Subramaniam, B. (1995). Saccadic eye movements and selective visual attention. *Perception and Psychophysics, 57,* 787-795.

Hollands, M.A., Patla, A.E., & Vickers, J.N. (2002). Look where you are going! Gaze behaviour associated with maintaining and changing direction. *Experimental Brain Research, 143,* 221-230.

Horn, R.R., Williams, A.M., Scott, M.A., & Hodges, N.J. (2005). The role of feedback and demonstrations in skill acquisition. *Journal of Motor Behavior, 37* (4), 265-279.

House, B.M., Chassie, M.B., & Spohn, B.B. (1990). Questioning: An essential ingredient in effective teaching. *Journal of Continuing Education in Nursing, 21* (5), 196-201.

Howe, M.J.A., Davidson, J.W., & Sloboda, J.A. (1998). Innate talents: Reality or myth? *Behavioural and Brain Sciences, 21,* 399-442.

Hubbard, A.W., & Seng, C.N. (1954). Visual movements of batters. *Research Quarterly, 25,* 42-57.

Hudson, J.L. (1985). Prediction of basketball skill using biomechanical variables. *Research Quarterly for Exercise and Sport, 56,* 115–121.

Iacoboni, M., & Dapretto, M. (2006). The mirror neuron system and the consequences of its dysfuntion. *Nature Reviews Neuroscience, 7,* 942-95.

Irwin, D. (1996). Integrating information across saccadic eye movements. *Current Directions in Psychological Science, 5,* 94-100.

Irwin, D., & Brockmole, J.R. (2004). Suppressing where but not what. The effects of saccades on norsal and ventral stream visual processing. *Psychological Science, 15,* (7), 467-473.

Itti, L., & Koch, C. (1999). A saliency-based search mechanism for overt and covert shifts of visual attention. *Vision Research, 40,* 1489-1506.

Itti, L., & Koch, C. (2001). Computational modeling of visual attention. *Nature Neuroscience Reviews, 2,* 194-203.

James, W. (1890/1981). *The principles of psychology.* Cambridge, MA: Harvard University Press.

Janelle, C.M. (2002). Anxiety, arousal and visual attention: A mechanistic account of performance variability. *Journal of Sports Sciences,* March, 237-251.

Janelle, C.M., Barba, D.A., Frehlich, L., Tennant, L.K., & Cauraugh, J.H. (1997). Maximizing performance feedback effectiveness through videotape replay and a self-controlled learning environment. *Research Quarterly for Exercise and Sport, 68* (4), 269-279.

Janelle, C.M., Hillman, C.H., Apparies, R.J., Murray, N.P., Meili, L., Fallon, E.A., et al. (2000). Expertise differences in cortical activation and gaze behavior during rifle shooting. *Journal of Sport and Exercise Psychology, 22* (2), 167-182.

Janelle, C.M., Singer, R.N., & Williams, A.M. (1999). External distraction and attentional narrowing: Visual search evidence. *Journal of Sport & Exercise Psychology, 21,* 70-91.

Jones, J.G. (1995). More than just a game: Research developments and issues in competitive anxiety in sport. *British Journal of Psychology, 86,* 449-478.

Jones, S.M., & Miles, T.R. (1978). Use of advanced cues in predicting the flight of a lawn tennis ball. *Journal of Human Movement Science, 4,* 231-235.

Kahneman, D. (1973). *Attention and effort.* Englewood Cliffs, NJ: Prentice Hall.

Kalat, J. (2004). *Biological psychology* (8th ed.). Belmont, CA: Thompson Wadsworth.

Kandel, E.R., Schwartz, J.H., & Jessell, T.M. (2000). *Principles of neural science* (4th ed.). New York: McGraw-Hill.

Kelso, J.A.S. (1982). *Human motor behavior.* Hillsdale, NJ: Erlbaum.

Kelso, J.A.S. (1995). *Dynamic patterns: The self organization of brain and behavior.* Boston: MIT Press.

Kempermann, G. (2002). Why new neurons? Possible functions for adult hippocampal neurogenesis. *Journal of Neuroscience, 22,* 635-638.

Kinomura, S., Larson, J., Gulyas, B., & Roland, P.E. (1996). Activation by attention of the human reticular formation and thalamic intranuclei, *Science, 271,* 512-515.

Kirby, R., & Roberts, J.A. (1985). *Introductory biomechanics.* Ithaca, NY: Mouvement Publications.

Klapp, S.T. (1977). Reaction time analysis of programming control. *Exercise and Sport Sciences Reviews, 5,* 231-253.

Klein, G. (1999). *Sources of power: How people make decisions.* Cambridge, MA: MIT Press.

Klein, G., & Hoffman, R. (1993). Seeing the invisible: The perceptual cognitive aspects of expertise. In M. Rabinowtz (Ed.), *Cognitive science foundations of instruction* (pp. 203-226). Mahawah, NJ: Lawrence Earlbaum Associates.

Knight, G.W., Guenzel, P.J., & Feil, P. (1997). Using questions to facilitate motor skill acquisition. *Journal of Dental Education, 61* (1), 56-65.

Knudson, D. (1993). Biomechanics of the basketball jump shot: Six key teaching points. *Journal of Physical Education, Recreation & Dance, 64,* 67-73.

Knudson, D.V., & Morrison, C.S. (1997). *Qualitative analysis of human movement.* Champaign, IL: Human Kinetics.

Kolb, B., & Whishaw, I. Q. (2001). *An introduction to brain and behavior.* New York: Worth Publishers.

Kolb, B., & Whishaw, I.Q. (2006). *An introduction to brain and behavior* (2nd ed.). New York: Worth Publishers.

Komi, P.V. (1992). *Strength and power in sport.* Oxford: Blackwell Scientific.

Kowler, E., Anderson, E., Dosher, B., & Blaser, E. (1995). The role of attention in the programming of saccades. *Vision Research, 35* (13), 1897-1916.

Krane, V. (1994). The mental readiness form as a measure of competitive state anxiety. *Sport Psychologist, 8,* 189-202.

Krebs, C., Huttmann, K., & Steinhauser, C. (2005). The forgotten brain emerges. *Scientific American Mind, 14* (5), 40-43.

Kuhn, T.S. (1970). *The structure of scientific revolutions.* Chicago: University of Chicago Press.

Kurz, M.J., & Stergiou, N. (2004). Applied dynamic systems theory for analysis of movement. In N. Stergiou (Ed.), *Innovative analysis of human movement: Analytical tools for human movement research* (pp. 93-119). Champaign, IL: Human Kinetics.

Kustov, A.A., & Robinson, D.L. (1996). Shared neural control of attentional shifts and eye movements. *Nature, 384* (7), 74-77.

Ladd, G.T., & Woodworth, R.S. (1911). *Elements of Physiological Psychology.* New York: Charles Scribner's Sons.

Land, M. (1998). The visual control of steering. In L.R. Harris & M. Jenkin (Eds.), *Vision and action* (pp. 163-180). Cambridge, UK: Cambridge University Press.

Land, M., & Lee, D.N. (1995). Which parts of the road guide steering? *Nature, 377,* 339-340.

Land, M.F., & McLeod, P. (2000). From eye movements to actions: How batsmen hit the ball. *Nature Neuroscience, 3,* 1340-1345.

Landers, D.M., Han, M., Salazar, W., Petruzzello, S.J., Kubitz, K.A., & Gannon, T.L. (1994). Effect of learning on electroencephalographic and electrocardiographic patterns on novice archers. *International Journal of Sport Psychology, 25,* 313-330.

Latash, M., & Turvey, M.T. (Eds.). (1996). *Dexterity and its development.* Mahwah, NJ: Erlbaum.

Lavery, J.J. (1962). The retention of simple motor skills as a function of type of knowledge of results. *Canadian Journal of Psychology, 16,* 300-311.

Lee, D.N. (1976). A theory of visual control of braking based on information about time to collision. *Perception, 5,* 437-459.

Lee, D.N. (1980). Visuomotor coordination in space-time. In G.E. Stelmach & J. Requin (Eds.), *Tutorials in motor behavior* (pp. 281-295). Amsterdam: North-Holland.

Lee, D.N., & Aronson, E. (1974). Visual proprioceptive control of standing in human infants. *Perception and Psychophysics, 15,* 527-532.

Lee, D.N., Lishman, J.R., & Thomson, J.A. (1982). Regulation of gait in long jumping. *Journal of Experimental Psychology: Human Perception and Performance, 8,* 448–459.

Lee, T.D. & Magill, R.A. (1983). The locus of contextual interference in motor-skill acquisition. *Journal of Experimental Psychology: Learning, Memory and Cognition, 9,* 730-746.

Lee, D.N., & Young, D.S. (1985). Visual timing of interceptive action. In D. Ingle, M. Jeannerod, & D.N. Lee (Eds.), *Brain mechanisms and spatial vision* (pp. 1-30). Dordrecht: Martinus Nijhoff.

Lee, D.N., Young, D.S., Reddish, P.E., Lough, S., & Clayton, T.M.H. (1983). Visual timing in hitting an accelerating ball. *Quarterly Journal of Experimental Psychology, 35A,* 333–346.

Lee, T.D., & Carnahan, H. (1990). Bandwidth knowledge of results and motor learning: More than just a relative frequency effect. *Quarterly Journal of Experimental Psychology, 42A,* 777-789.

Lee, T.D., Swinnen, S., & Serrien, D. (1994). Cognitive effort and motor learning. *Quest, 46,* 328-344.

Lee, T.D., White, M.A., & Carnahan, H. (1990). On the role of knowledge of results in motor learning: Exploring the guidance hypothesis. *Journal of Motor Behavior, 22* (2), 191-208.

Lewis, B.P., & Linder, D.E. (1997). Thinking about choking? Attentional processes and paradoxical performance. *Personality and Social Psychology Bulletin, 23* (9), 937-947.

Liebert, R.M., & Morris, L.W. (1967). Cognitive and emotional components of test anxiety: A distinction and some initial data. *Psychological Reports, 20,* 975-978.

Mack, A. (2003). Inattention blindness. *Current Directions in Psychological Science, 12* (5), 180-184.

Magill, R.A. (2004). *Motor learning: Concepts and applications* (7th ed.). Boston, MA: McGraw-Hill.

Martell, S., & Vickers, J.N. (2004). Gaze characteristics of elite and near-elite ice hockey players. *Human Movement Science, 22,* 689-712.

Martens, R., Burton, D., Vealey, R., Bump, L.A., & Smith, D.E. (1990). Competitive state anxiety 2. In R. Martens, R. Vealey, & D. Burton (Eds.), *Competitive anxiety in sport* (pp. 117-190). Champaign, IL: Human Kinetics.

Martens, R., Vealey, R., & Burton, D. (Eds). (1990). *Competitive anxiety in sport.* Champaign, IL: Human Kinetics.

Masters, J.P., Masters, R.S.W., & Eves, F.F. (2000). From novice to no know-how: A longitudinal study of implicit motor learning. *Journal of Sports Sciences, 18,* 111-122.

Masters, R.S.W. (1992). Knowledge, knerves and know-how: The role of explicit versus implicit knowledge in the breakdown of a complex motor skill under pressure. *British Journal of Psychology, 83,* 343-358.

Masters, R.S.W., & Maxwell, J.P. (2004). Implicit motor learning, reinvestment, and movement disruption: What you don't know won't hurt you. In A.M. Williams & N. J. Hodges (Eds.), *Skill acquisition in sport: Research, theory and practice* (pp. 207-228). London: Routledge.

McArdle, W.D., Katch, F., & Katch, V. (2001). *Exercise physiology: Energy, nutrition and human performance* (5th ed.). Philadelphia: Lea & Febiger.

McLeod, P. (1994). Perceptual motor co-ordination. In M.W. Eysenck (Ed.), *Blackwell dictionary of cognitive psychology* (pp. 262-264). Oxford: Blackwell.

McMorris, T., & Colenso, S. (1996). Anticipation of professional soccer goalkeepers when facing right- and left-footed penalty kicks. *Perceptual and Motor Skills, 82,* 931-934.

McMorris, T., Copeman, R., Corcoran, D., Saunders, G., & Potter, S. (1993). Anticipation of soccer goal-keepers facing penalty kicks. In T. Reilly, J. Clarys, & A. Stibbe (Eds.), *Science and football II* (pp.250-253). London: E&FN Spon.

McMorris, T., & Hauxwell, B. (1997). Improving antici-pation of soccer goalkeepers using video observation. In T. Reilly, J. Bangsbo, & M. Hughes (Eds.), *Science and football III* (pp. 250-253). London: E&FN Spon.

McNevin, N.H., Wulf, G., & Carlson, C. (2003). Effects of attentional focus, self-control, and dyad training on motor learning: Implications for physical rehabilita-tion. *Physical Therapy, 80* (4), 373-385.

McPherson, S.L. (1993). Knowledge representation and decision-making in sport. In J. Starkes & F. Allard (Eds.), *Cognitive issues in motor expertise* (pp. 159-188). Amsterdam: Elsevier.

McPherson, S.L., & Vickers, J.N. (2004). Cognitive con-trol in motor expertise. *International Journal of Sport and Exercise Psychology, 2,* 274-300.

Mestre, D.R., & Durand, S. (2001). Flow matters. ARVO annual meeting, Fort Lauderdale, Florida, 29 April-4 May 2001. *Investigative Ophthalmology and Visual Science, 42,* 4977.

Mestre, D.R., Mars, F., Durand, S., Vienne, F., & Espie, S. (2005). *Proceedings of the Third International Driving Symposium on Human Factors in Driver Assessment, Training and Vehicle Design.* Rockport, ME, June 27-30, 2005 pp. 304-310.

Metzler, M.W. (2000). *Instructional models for physical education.* Needham Heights, MA: Allyn & Bacon.

Michaels, C.F., & Carello, C. (1981). *Direct perception.* Englewood Cliffs, NJ: Prentice-Hall.

Miller, G.A. (1956). The magical number seven, plus or minus two: Some limits on our capacity to process information. *Psychological Review, 63,* 81-97.

Miller, S., & Bartlett, R.M. (1993). The effects of shoot-ing distance in the basketball jump shot. *Journal of Sports Sciences, 11,* 285-293.

Miller, S., & Bartlett, R.M. (1996). The relationship between basketball shooting kinematics, distance and playing position. *Journal of Sports Sciences, 14,* 243-253.

Millslagle, D.G. (1988). Visual perception, recognition, recall and mode of visual search control in basketball involving novice and inexperienced basketball play-ers. *Journal of Sport Behaviour, 11,* 32-44.

Milner, A.D., & Goodale, M. A. (1995). *Visual brain in action.* Oxford: Oxford University.

Mirescu, C., Peters, J.D., & Gould, E. (2004). Early life experience alters response to adult neurogenesis to stress. *Nature Neuroscience, 7* (8), 841-846.

Montagne, G., Laurent, A., & Ripoll, H. (1993). Visual information pick-up in ball-catching. *Human Move-ment Science, 12,* 273-297.

Montello, D. (2005). Navigation. In P. Shah & A. Miyake (Eds.), *The Cambridge handbook of visual spatial think-ing* (pp. 257-294). New York: Cambridge University Press.

Morris, L.W., Davis, M.A., & Hutchings, C. (1981). Cognitive and emotional components of anxiety: Literature review and revised worry emotional scale. *Journal of Educational Psychology, 73,* 541-555.

Morya, E., Ranvaud, R., & Pinheiro, W.M. (2003). Dynamics of visual feedback in a laboratory simula-tion of a penalty kick. *Journal of Sports Sciences, 21,* 87-95.

Murphy, B.J., Kowler, E., Steinman, R.M. (1975). Slow oculomotor control in the presence of moving back-grounds. *Vision Research, 15,* 1263-1268.

Neisser, U. (1967). *Cognitive psychology.* New York: Appleton-Century Crofts.

Neisser, U. (1976). *Cognition and reality.* San Francisco: Freeman.

Neisser, U. (1979). The control of information pickup in selective looking. In A.D. Pick (Ed.), *Perception and its development: A tribute to Eleanor Gibson* (pp. 201-219). Hillsdale, NJ: Erlbaum.

Neisser, U. (1983). The rise and fall of the sensory register. *Behavioral and Brain Sciences, 6,* 35.

Newell, K.M. (1985). Coordination, control and skill. In D. Goodman, R.B. Wilberg, & I.M. Franks (Eds.), *Differing perspectives in motor learning, memory and control* (pp. 516-536). Amsterdam: Elsevier.

Newell, K.M. (1986). Constraints on the development of coordination. In M. Wade & H.T.A. Whiting (Eds.), *Motor development in children: Aspects of coordination and control* (pp. 341-360). Maastricht, Netherlands: Nijhoff.

Newell, K.M., & McDonald, P.V. (1992). Searching for solutions to the coordination function: Learning as exploratory behavior. In G.E. Stelmach & J. Requin (Eds.), *Tutorials in motor behavior II* (pp. 517-532). Amsterdam: Elsevier.

Newell, K.M., & McDonald, P.V. (1994). Learning to coordinate redundant biomechanical degrees of freedom. In S. Swinnen, H. Heuer, J. Massion, & P. Casaer (Eds.), *Interlimb coordination: Neural, dynamical, and cognitive constraints* (517-531). New York: Academic Press.

Newell, K.M., & Vaillancourt, D.E. (2001). Dimensional change in motor learning. *Human Movement Science, 20* (4-5), 695-715

Noble, B.J., Borg, G., Jacobs, I., Ceci, R., & Kaiser, P. (1983). A category-ratio perceived exertion scale: Relationship to blood and muscle lactates and heart rate. *Medicine Science Sports and Exercise, 15*, 523-528.

Noton, D., & Stark, L. (1971). Eye movements and visual perception. *Scientific American, 224*, 34-43.

Noton, D., & Stark, L. (1971). Scanpaths in saccadic eye movements during pattern perception. *Science*, 308-311.

Nottebohm, F. (1985). Neural replacement in adulthood. *Annual Review New York Academy of Science, 457*, 143-161.

Optican, L.M. (1985). Adaptative properties of the saccadic system. In A. Berthoz & M. Melvine-Jones (Eds.), *Adaptative mechanisms in gaze control: Facts and theories* (pp. 71-79). New York: Elsevier Science.

Ota, D., & Vickers, J.N. (1999). The effects of variable practice on the retention and transfer of two volleyball skills in male club-level athletes. *International Journal of Volleyball Research, 1* (1), 18-24.

Otero, J., & Graesser, A.C. (2001). PREG: Elements of a model of question asking. *Cognition & Instruction, 19* (2), 143-175.

Oudejans, R.R.D., Koedijker, J.M., Bleijendaal, I., & Bakker, F.C. (2005). The education of attention in aiming at a far target: Training visual control in basketball jump shooting. *International Journal of Sport Psychology, 3*, 197-221.

Oudejans, R.R.D., van de Langenberg, R.W., & Hutter, R.I. (2002). Aiming at a far target under different viewing conditions: Visual control in basketball jump shooting. *Human Movement Science, 21*, 457-480.

Panchuk, D., & Vickers, J.N. (2005). Gaze behaviors of goaltenders under spatial–temporal constraints. *Journal of Sport and Exercise Psychology, 27*, 119.

Panchuk, D., & Vickers, J. N. (2006). Gaze behaviors of goaltenders under spatial–temporal constraints. *Human Movement Science, 25* (6), 733-752.

Patla, A., & Vickers, J.N. (1997). When and where do we look as we approach and step over an obstacle in the travel path? *NeuroReport, 8* (17), 3661-3665.

Pearsall, J., & Trumble, B. (1996). *The Oxford English Dictionary*. Oxford: Oxford University Press.

Pellison, D., Prablanc, C., Goodale, M. A., & Jeannerod, M. (1986). Visual control of reaching movements without vision of the limb. II. Evidence of fast unconscious processes correcting the trajectory of the hand to the final position of a double-step stimulus. *Experimental Brain Research, 62*, 303-311.

Pelz, D. (1994). A study of golfers' abilities to read greens. In A.J. Cochran & M.R. Farally (Eds.), *Science and golf II: Proceedings of the World Congress of Golf* (pp. 181-185). London: E&F Spon.

Pelz, D. (2000). *Dave Pelz's putting bible*. New York: Doubleday.

Penrose, T., & Blanksby, B. (1976). Two methods of basketball jump shooting techniques by two groups of different ability. *Australian Journal of Health, Physical Education and Recreation, 71*, 14-23.

Pola, J., & Wyatt, H.J. (1991). Smooth pursuit: Response characteristics, stimuli and mechanisms. In R.H.S. Carpenter (Ed.), *Eye movements* (pp.138-156). Boca Raton, FL: CRC Press.

Pollen, D.A. (1999). On the neural correlates of visual perception. *Cerebral Cortex, 9*, 4-19.

Poskiparta, M., Kettunen, T., & Liimatainen, L. (1998). Reflective questions in health counselling. *Qualitative Health Research, 8* (5), 682-693.

Posner, M.I. (1980). Orienting of attention. *Quarterly Journal of Experimental Psychology, 32*, 3-25.

Posner, M.I., & Raichle, M.E. (1994). *Images of mind*. New York, NY: Scientific American Library.

Raab, M., Masters, R.S.W., & Maxwell, J.P. (2005). Improving the 'how' and 'what' decisions of elite table tennis players. *Human Movement Science, 24*, 326-344.

Ramachandran, V.S. (2000). Mirror neurons and imitation learning as the driving force behind "the great leap forward" in human evolution. *Edge, 69*, 3-10.

Ramage, B., Gotch, M., Ronsky, J., Vickers, J., Morton, B., Panchuk, D., et al. (2006). Ankle joint power during lunge in elite ballet dancers, controls, and ACL-deficient subjects. (Poster session). *Canadian Society of Biomechanics*.

Rensink, R.A. (2002). Change detection. *Annual Review of Psychology, 53*, 245-277.

Riemersma, S.B.J. (1981). Visual control during straight road driving. *Acta Psychologica, 48*, 215-225.

Ripoll, H. (1991). The understanding-acting process in sport: The relationship between semantic and sensorimotor visual function. *International Journal of Sport Psychology, 22*, 221-243.

Ripoll, H., Bard, C., & Paillard, J. (1986). Stabilization of head and eye movements on target as a factor in successful basketball shooting. *Human Movement Science, 5*, 47-58.

Ripoll, H., Bard, C., Paillard, J., & Grosgeorge, B. (1982). Caracteristiques de la centration de l'oeil et de la tete sur la cible et son role dans l'execution du tir en basketball. In T. Orlick, J.T. Partington, & J.H. Salmela (Eds.), *New paths to sport learning* (pp. 33-36). Ottawa: Perceptives in Sport.

Ripoll, H., & Fleurance, P. (1988). What does keeping one's eye on the ball mean? *Ergonomics, 31*, 1647-1654.

Ripoll, H., Papin, J.P., Guezennec, J.Y., Verdy, J.P. & Philip, M. (1985). Analysis of visual scanning patterns of pistol shooters. *Journal of Sports Sciences, 3* (2), 93-101.

Rizzolatti, G., & Craighero, L. (2004). The mirror-neuron system. *Annual Review of Neuroscience, 27*, 169-192.

Rizzolatti, G., Fadagia, L., Gallese, V., & Figassi, L. (1996). Premotor cortex and the recognition of mirror actions. *Cognitive Brain Research, 3*, 131-141.

Rizzolatti, G., Fogassi, L. & Vittorio, G. (2006). Mirrors in the mind. *Scientific American, 295* (5), 54-61.

Rodrigues, S.T., Vickers, J.N., & Williams, A.M. (2002). Head, eye and arm coordination in table tennis: An exploratory study. *Journal of Sport Sciences, 20* (3), 171-186.

Rossetti, Y. (1998). Implicit short-lived motor representations of space in brain damaged and healthy participants. *Consciousness and Cognition. 7*, 520-558.

Roth, K. (1989). *Taktik im Sportspiel [Tactics in games].* Schorndorf, Germany: Hofmann.

Rothstein, A., & Arnold, R. (1976). Application of research on videotape feedback and bowling. *Motor Skills: Theory into Practice, 1*, 36-61.

Rotstein, A., Jablonowsky, S., Bar-Sela, S., Malamud, G., Tenenbaum, G & Inbar, O. (1999). The effect of diverting activity on fatigue during isokinetic exercise using large muscle groups. *Journal of Strength and Conditioning Research, 13* (1), 72-75.

Sachdeva, A.K. (1996). Use of effective questioning to enhance the cognitive abilities of students. *Journal of Cancer Education, 11* (1), 17-24.

Salmela, J.H., & Fiorito, P. (1979). Visual cues in ice hockey goaltending. *Canadian Journal of Applied Sport Science, 4* (1), 56-59.

Sanders, G.S., Baron, R.S., & Moore, D.L. (1978). Distraction and social facilitation effects. *Journal of Experimental Social Psychology, 14*, 291-303.

Sanes, J.N., & Donoghue, J.P. (2000). Plasticity and motor cortex. *Annual Reviews of Neuroscience, 23*, 395-415.

Savelsbergh, G.J.P., & Rosengren, K.S. (2001). The separation of action and perception and the issue of affordances. *Ecological Psychology, 13*, 167-172.

Savelsbergh, G.J.P., van der Kamp, J., Williams, A.M., & Ward, P. (2005) Anticipation and visual search behaviour in expert soccer goalkeepers: A within-group comparison. *Ergonomics, 48*, 11-14, 1686-1697.

Savelsbergh, G.J.P., Whiting, H.T.A., & Bootsma, R.J. (1991). Grasping tau. *Journal of Experimental Psychology, 17* (2), 315-322.

Savelsbergh, G.J.P., Williams, A.M., van der Kamp, J., & Ward, P. (2002). Visual search, anticipation and expertise in soccer goalkeepers. *Journal of Sports Sciences, 20*, 279-287.

Schell, R.M. (1998). Organizational behavior management: Applications with professional staff. *Journal of Organizational Behavior Management, 18*, 157-171.

Schmid, R., & Zambarbieri, D. (1991). Strategies of eye–head coordination. In R. Schmid & D. Zambarbieri (Eds.), *Oculomotor control and cognitive processes* (pp. 229-246). Amsterdam: Elsevier Science.

Schmidt, R.A. (1985). The search for invariance in skilled movement behaviour. *Research Quarterly, 56* (2), 188-200.

Schmidt, R.A. (1991). *Motor learning and performance: From principles to practice.* Champaign, IL: Human Kinetics.

Schmidt, R.A., & Bjork, R. (1992). New conceptualizations of practice: Common principles in three paradigms suggest new concepts for training. *Psychological Science, 3*, 207-217.

Schmidt, R.A., & Lee, T.D. (1999). *Motor control and learning: A behavioral emphasis* (3rd ed.). Champaign, IL: Human Kinetics.

Schmidt, R.A., & Lee, T.D. (2005). *Motor control and learning: A behavioral emphasis* (4th ed.). Champaign, IL: Human Kinetics.

Schmidt, R.A., & Wrisberg, C.A. (2004). *Motor learning and performance* (3rd ed.). Champaign, IL: Human Kinetics.

Seidentop, D. (1976). *Developing teaching skills in physical education.* Mountain View, CA: Mayfield.

Selder, D.J., & Del Rolan, N. (1979). Knowledge of performance, skill level and performance on the balance beam. *Canadian Journal of Applied Sport Sciences, 4*, 226-229.

Setchenov, I.M. (1903/1935). Zur frage nach der einwirkung sensitiver reize auf die muskelarbeit des menchen. In *Selected works* (pp. 246-240). Moscow.

Shah, P., & Miyake, A. (2005). *The Cambridge handbook of visual spatial thinking.* New York: Cambridge University Press.

Shank, M.D., & Haywood, K.M. (1987). Eye movements while viewing a baseball pitch. *Perceptual and Motor Skills, 64*, 1191-1197.

Sharp, R.H., & Whiting, H.T.A. (1974). Exposure and occluded duration effects in a ball catching skill. *Journal of Human Movement Studies, 6* (3), 139-147.

Sharp, R.H., & Whiting, H.T.A. (1975). Information processing and eye movement behaviour in ball catching skill. *Journal of Motor Behavior, 1,* 124-131.

Shea, J., & Morgan, R. (1979). Contextual interference effects on the acquisition, retention, and transfer of a motor skill. *Journal of Experimental Psychology, 5,* 179-187.

Shepherd, M., Findlay, J.M., & Hockey, R.J. (1986). The relationship between eye movements and spatial attention. *Quarterly Journal of Experimental Psychology, 38A,* 475-491.

Sherwood, D.E. (1988). Effect of bandwidth knowledge of results on movement consistency. *Perceptual and Motor Skills, 66,* 535-542.

Sidaway, B., & Hand, J. (1993). Relative frequency of modeling effects on the acquisition and retention of a motor skill. *Research Quarterly for Exercise and Sport, 64* (1), 122-126.

Simons, D.J., & Levin, D. (1998). Failure to detect changes to people during a real-world interaction. *Psychonomic Bulletin & Review, 5,* 644-649.

Singer, R.N., Cauraugh, J.H., Chen, D., Steinberg, G.M., & Frehlich, S.G. (1996). Visual search, anticipation, and reactive comparisons between skilled and beginning tennis players. *Applied Sport Psychology, 8,* 18-35.

Skinner, B.F. (1953). *Science and human behavior.* New York: Free Press.

Smeeton, N., Ward, P., & Williams, A.M. (2004). Transfer of perceptual skill in sport. *Journal of Sports Sciences, 19* (2), 3-9.

Smeeton, N.J., Williams, A.M., Hodges, N.J., & Ward, P. (2005). The relative effectiveness of explicit instruction, guided-discovery and discovery learning techniques in enhancing perceptual skill in sport. *Journal of Experimental Psychology: Applied, 11* (2), 98-110.

Soderkvist, I., & Wedin, P.A. (1993). Determining the movement of the skeleton using well-configured markers. *Journal of Biomechanics, 26,* 1473-1477.

Solso, R. (1995). *Cognitive psychology* (4th ed.). Boston: Allyn & Bacon.

Starkes, J.L. (1987). Skill in field hockey: The nature of cognitive advantage. *Journal of Sport Psychology, 9,* 146-160.

Starkes, J.L., & Deakin, J. (1984). Perception in sport: A cognitive approach to skilled performance. In W.F. Straub & J.M. Williams (Eds.), *Cognitive sport psychology* (pp.115-128). Lansing, NY: Sport Science Associates.

Starkes, J.L., & Ericsson, K.A. (Eds.). (2003). *Expert performance in sports: Advances in research on sport expertise.* Champaign, IL: Human Kinetics.

Sternberg, R. (2003). *Cognitive psychology* (3rd ed.). Belmont, CA: Thompson & Wadsworth Barnes.

Summers, J.J. (2004). A historical perspective on skill acquisition. In A.M. Williams & N.J. Hodges (Eds.), *Skill acquisition in sport: Research, theory and practice* (pp. 1-26). London: Routledge.

Swinnen, S., Schmidt, R.A., Nicholson, D.E., & Shapiro, D.C. (1990). Information feedback for skill acquisition: Instantaneous knowledge of results degrades performance. *Journal of Experimental Psychology, 16,* 706-716.

Tenenbaum, G. (2003). Expert athletes: An integrated approach to decision making. In J.L. Starkes & K.A. Ericsson (Eds.), *Expert performance in sports: Advances in research on sport expertise* (pp. 191-218). Champaign, IL: Human Kinetics.

Thomas, P.F. (2000). On the art of questioning. *Horizon, 27* (1).

Thorndike, E.L. (1911). *Animal intelligence.* New York: Macmillan.

Titel, K., & Wutscherk, H. (1992). Anatomical and anthropometric fundamentals of endurance. In R. Shepard & P.O. Astrand (Eds.), *Endurance in sport* (pp. 35-46). Oxford: Blackwell Scientific.

Tong, F. (2003). Primary visual cortex and visual awareness. *Cognitive Neuroscience, 4,* 219-229.

Tononi, G., & Edelman, G.M. (1998). Consciousness and complexity. *Science, 282,* 1846-1851.

Treisman, A. (1986a). Properties, parts and objects. In K.R. Boff, L. Kaufman, & J.P. Thomas (Eds.), *Handbook of perception and human performance* (pp. 1-70). New York: Wiley.

Treisman, A. (1986b). Features and objects in visual processing. *Scientific American, 255,* 106-115.

Treisman, A. (1988). Features and objects: The fourteenth Bartlett memorial lecture. *Quarterly Journal of Experimental Psychology, 40A,* 201-237.

Treisman, A. (1993). The perception of features and objects. In A. Baddeley & L. Weiskrantz (Eds.), *Attention: Selection, awareness and control* (pp. 5-35). Oxford: Clarendon Press University.

Treisman, A. (1998). Feature binding, attention and object perception. *Philosophical Transactions of the Royal Society, 353* (1373), 1295-1306.

Treisman, A. (1999). Solutions to the binding problem. *Neuron, 24,* 105-110.

Treisman, A., Cavanagh, P., Fischer, B., Ramachandran, V., & von der Heydt, R. (1990). From perception to attention: Striate cortex and beyond. In L. Spillman

& J. Werner (Eds.), *Visual perception: The neurophysiological foundations* (pp. 273-316). Boston: Academic Press.

Treisman, A., & Gelade, G. (1980). A feature-integration theory of attention. *Cognitive Psychology, 12,* 97-136.

Treisman, A., & Gormican, S. (1988). Feature analysis in early vision. *Psychologcal Review, 95,* 15-30.

Turvey, M.T. (1977a). Preliminaries to a theory of action with reference to vision. In R. Shaw & J. Bransford (Eds.), *Perceiving, acting, and knowing: Toward an ecological psychology* (pp. 211-265). Hillsdale, NJ: Erlbaum.

Turvey, M.T. (1977b). Contrasting orientations to a theory of visual information processing. *Psychological Review, 84,* 67-88.

Turvey, M.T., Fitch, H.L., & Tuller, B. (1982). The Bernstein perspective: I. The problem of degrees of freedom and context-conditioned variability. In J.A. Kelso (Ed.), *Human motor behavior: An introduction* (pp. 239-252). Hillsdale, NJ: Lawrence Erlbaum & Associates.

Tversky, B. (2005). Functional significance of visuospatial representations. In P. Shah & A. Miyake (Eds.), *The Cambridge handbook of visual spatial thinking* (pp. 1-34). New York: Cambridge University Press.

Tyldesley, D.A., Bootsma, R.J., & Bomhoff, G.T. (1982). Skill level and eye movement patterns in a sport orientated reaction time task. In H. Rieder, H. Mechling, & K. Reischle (Eds.), *Proceedings of an international symposium on motor behaviour: Contribution to learning in sport* (pp. 290-296). Cologne: Hofmann.

Valet, M., Sprenger, T., Boecker, H., Willoch, F., Rummeny, E., Conttrad, B., et al. (2004). *Pain, 109,* 399-498.

van der Kamp, J. (2006). A field simulation study of the effectiveness of penalty kick strategies in soccer: Late alterations of kick direction increase errors and reduce accuracy. *Journal of Sports Sciences, 24* (5), 467-477.

van Praag, H., Kempermann, G., & Gage, F.H. (1999). Running increases cell proliferation and neurogenesis in the adult mouse dentate gyrus. *Nature Neuroscience, 2,* 266-270.

van Praag, H., Kempermann, G., & Gage, F. (2000). Neural consequences of environmental enrichment. *Nature Reviews, 1,* 191-198.

van Praag, H., Schinder, A.F., Christie, B.R., Toni, N., Palmer, T.D., & Gage, F. (2002). Functional neurogenesis in the adult hippocampus. *Nature, 415,* 1030-1034.

Vereijken, B., van Emmerik, R.E.A., Whiting, H.T.A., & Newell, K. (1992). Free(z)ing degrees of freedom in skill acquisition. *Journal of Motor Behavior, 24,* 133-142.

Vickers, J.N. (1988). Knowledge structures of elite–novice gymnasts. *Journal of Human Movement Science 7,* 4-72.

Vickers, J.N. (1990). *Instructional design for teaching physical activity: A knowledge structures approach.* Champaign, IL: Human Kinetics.

Vickers, J.N. (1991a). Eye movements of low and high handicapped golfers in putting (hits vs. misses). [Abstract]. *North American Society for Psychology of Sport and Physical Activity.* Ansilomar 123.

Vickers, J.N. (1991b). Look and launch. *Golf Magazine,* October, 74.

Vickers, J.N. (1992). Gaze control in putting. *Perception, 21,* 117-132.

Vickers, J.N. (1994a). Psychological research in sport pedagogy: Exploring the reversal effect. *Sport Science Review, 3* (1), 28-40.

Vickers, J.N. (1994b). The reversal effect. In A. Jewett, L. Bain, & C. Ennis (Eds.), *The curriculum process in physical education* (pp. 348-353). Madison, WI: Brown & Benchmark.

Vickers, J.N. (1996a). Visual control when aiming at a far target. *Journal of Experimental Psychology: Human Perception and Performance, 22,* 342-354.

Vickers, J.N. (1996b). Control of visual attention during the basketball free throw. *American Journal of Sports Medicine, 3* (Suppl. 1), 93-97.

Vickers, J.N. (1996c). Location of fixation, landing position of the ball and accuracy during the free throw. *International Journal of Sports Vision, 3* (1), 54-60.

Vickers, J.N. (2000a). *Decision training: A new approach in coaching.* Vancouver: Coaching Association of British Columbia.

Vickers, J.N. (2000b). Quiet eye in sport. *Dragon Fly: A Magazine for Young Investigators.* Arlington, VA: National Science Teachers Association, 2, 6-8.

Vickers, J.N. (2003). Decision training: An innovative approach to coaching. *Canadian Journal for Women Coaches Online.* Retrieved October 22, 2006, from www.coach.ca/WOMEN/e/journal/.

Vickers, J.N. (2004). The quiet eye: It's the difference between a good putter and a poor one. *Golf Digest,* January, 96-101.

Vickers, J.N. (2006). Gaze of Olympic speed skaters while skating at full speed on a regulation oval: Perception-action coupling in a dynamic performance environment. *Cognitive Processing,* (Suppl.1):S102-105.

Vickers, J.N. (in progress). Gaze of shooters during the ice hockey shoot-out.

Vickers, J.N., & Adolphe, R.A. (1997). Gaze behaviour during a ball tracking and aiming skill. *International Journal of Sports Vision, 4* (1), 18-27.

Vickers, J.N., Bales, J., Allison, T., Jensen, M., Cluff, M., & Bowman, L. (1996a). *Decision training in free style skiing.* Calgary: National Coaching Institute.

Vickers, J.N., Bales, J., Davidson, M., Curry, J., Johnson, M. & Rennie, T. (1996b). *Decision training in ice hockey.* Calgary: National Coaching Institute.

Vickers, J.N., Bales, J., Pike, R., Dolan, C., Lemieux, C., & Ryan, G. (1996c). *Decision training in volleyball.* Calgary: National Coaching Institute.

Vickers, J.N., & Crews, D. (2002). Short term memory characteristics of golfers: Concurrent measures of gaze and EEG. Presentation to the World Congress of Science in Golf. St. Andrews, Scotland, July.

Vickers, J.N., & Crews, D. (in progress). Decay of the distance: Short-term memory characteristics of golfers during the concurrent measurement of gaze and EEG.

Vickers, J.N., Livingston, L., Umeris, S., & Holden, D. (1999). Decision training: The effects of complex instruction, variable practice and reduced delayed feedback on the acquisition and transfer of a complex motor skill. *Journal of Sport Sciences, 17,* 357-367.

Vickers, J.N., Morton, B. & Panchuk, D. (in progress). Quiet eye training in golf.

Vickers, J.N., Panchuk, D., Morton, B., & Martell, S. (in progress a). Gaze control during the basketball free throw and jump shot.

Vickers, J.N., Panchuk, D., Morton, B., & Martell, S. (in progress b). The effects of screen training in the basketball jump shot.

Vickers, J.N., & Patla, A.E. (1999). Object and travel gaze fixation during successful and unsuccessful stepping stone task. *Gait & Posture, 9* (1), S3.

Vickers, J.N., Reeves, M., Chambers, K.L., & Martell, S. (2004). Decision training: Cognitive strategies for enhancing motor performance. In A.M. Williams and N.J. Hodges (Eds.), *Skill acquisition in sport: Research, theory and practice* (pp. 103-120). New York: Routledge.

Vickers, J.N., Rodrigues, S.T., & Brown, L.N. (2002). Gaze pursuit and arm control of adolescent males diagnosed with attention deficit hyperactivity disorder (ADHD) as compared to normal controls: Evidence of dissociation in processing short and long-duration visual information. *Journal of Sport Sciences, 20* (3), 201-216.

Vickers, J.N., Rodrigues, S.T., & Edworthy, G. (2000). Quiet eye and accuracy in the dart throw. *International Journal of Sports Vision, 6,* 30-36.

Vickers, J.N., Ronsky, J., Ramage, B., Panchuk, D., Morton, B., Gotch, M., Ferber, R., et al. (2006). Gaze control and COP during quiet stance and lunge of ballet dancers, normal controls & ACL-deficient. *Cognitive Processing.* (Suppl.1):S176.

Vickers, J.N., & Sinclair, G. (1984). The physical education teaching laboratory: An on-campus theory to practice interface. *Journal of Physical Education, Recreation and Dance,* October, 16-18.

Vickers, J.N., & Williams, A.M. (in press). Performing under pressure: The interactive effects of physiological arousal, cognitive anxiety and gaze control in elite biathlon shooters. *Journal of Motor Behavior.*

Vickers, J.N., Williams, A.M. Rodrigues, S.T., Hillis, F., & Coyne, G. (1999). Eye movements of elite biathlon shooters during rested and fatigued states. [Abstract]. *Journal of Exercise and Sport Psychology, 21,* 116.

Vinger, P. (1996). The eye and sports medicine. In P. Vinger, J.G. Classe, & T. Woods (Eds.), *The eye and sports medicine manual* (pp. 1-108). Harrisburg, PA: International Academy of Sports Vision.

Volkmann, F., Riggs, L., & Moore, R. (1981). Eyeblinks and visual suppression. *Science, 207,* 900-902.

Ward, P., Williams, A.M., and Bennett, S. (2002) Visual search and biological motion perception in tennis. *Research Quarterly for Exercise and Sport, 73* (1), 107-112.

Warren, W.H. & Shaw, R.E. (1985). Events and encounters as units of analysis for ecological psychology. In W.H. Warren & R.E. Shaw (Eds.), *Persistence and Change: Proceedings of the First International Conference on Event Perception* (pp. 1-27). Hillsdale, NJ: Lawrence Erlbaum Associates Publishers.

Warren, W.H., Young, D.S., & Lee, D.N. (1986). Visual control of step length during running over irregular terrain. *Journal of Experimental Psychology: Human Perception and Performance, 12* (3), 259-266.

Watson, J. B. (1924/1998). *Behaviorism.* London: Transaction Publications.

Weber, E. (1914). Eine physiologische Methode die Leistungsfahigkeit exmudeter menschlicher Muskeln zu erhohen. Ergographische Untersuchungen. Archiv fur Physiologie, 385-420.

Weeks, D., Hall, A.K., & Anderson, L.P. (1996). A comparison of imitation strategies in observational learning of action patterns. *Journal of Motor Behavior, 28,* 348-358.

Weeks, D.L., & Kordus, R.N. (1998). Relative frequency of knowledge of performance and motor skill learning. *Research Quarterly for Exercise and Sport, 69* (3), 224-230.

Werner, S., & Theis, B. (2002). Is "change blindness" attenuated by domain-specific expertise? An expert-novices comparison of change detection in football images. *Visual Cognition, 7* (1-3), 163-173.

Whaley, M.H., Woodall, T., Kaminsky, L., & Emmett, J. (1997). Reliability of perceived exertion during graded exercise testing in apparently healthy adults. *Journal of Cardiopulmonary Rehabilitation, 17,* 37-42.

Wheeler, M.E., & Treisman, A. (2002). Binding in short term-memory. *Journal of Experimental Psychology, 131* (1), 48-64.

Wilkinson, E J., & Sherk, H.A. (2005). The use of visual information for planning accurate steps in a cluttered environment. *Behavioral Brain Research, 164,* 270-274.

Williams, A.M. (2002) Visual search behaviour in sport. *Journal of Sports Sciences, 20,* 169-170.

Williams, A.M., & Burwitz, L. (1993). Advanced cue utilization in soccer. In T. Reilly, J. Clarys, & A. Stibbe (Eds.), *Science and football II* (pp. 239-243). London: E&FN Spon.

Williams, A.M., & Davids, K. (1995). Declarative knowledge in sport: A by-product of experience or a characteristic of expertise. *Journal of Sport and Exercise Psychology, 17* (3), 259-275.

Williams, A.M., & Davids, K. (1998). Visual search strategy, selective attention and expertise in soccer. *Research Quarterly for Exercise and Sport, 69* (2), 111-128.

Williams, A.M., Davids, K., Burwitz, L., & Williams, J.G. (1994). Visual search strategies of experienced and inexperienced soccer players. *Research Quarterly for Sport and Exercise, 65,* 127-135.

Williams, A.M., Davids, K., & Williams, J.G. (1999). *Visual perception and action in sports.* London: E&FN Spon.

Williams, A.M., & Elliott, D. (1999). Anxiety and visual search strategy in karate. *Journal of Sport and Exercise Psychology, 21* (4), 362-375.

Williams, A.M., & Ericsson, K.A. (2005). Some considerations when applying the expert performance approach in sport. *Human Movement Science, 24,* 283-307.

Williams, A.M., & Grant, A. (1999). Training perceptual skill in sport. *International Journal of Sports Psychology, 30,* 194-220.

Williams, A.M., & Hodges, N.J. (2005). Practice, instruction and skill acquisition: Challenging tradition. *Journal of Sports Sciences, 23* (6), 637-650.

Williams, A.M., Janelle, C.K., & Davids, K. (2004). Constraints on the search for visual information in sport. *International Journal of Sports Psychology, 2* (3), 301-318.

Williams, A.M., Singer, R.A., & Frehlich, S. (2002). Quiet eye duration, expertise, and task complexity in a near and far aiming task. *Journal of Motor Behavior, 34,* 197-207.

Williams, A.M., Vickers, J.N., & Rodrigues, S.T. (2002). The effects of anxiety on visual search, movement kinematics, and performance in table tennis: A test of Eysenck and Calvo's processing efficiency theory. *Journal of Sport and Exercise Science, 24* (4), 438-456.

Williams, A.M., & Ward, P. (2003). Perceptual expertise: Development in sport. In J.L. Starkes, & K.A. Ericsson (Eds.), *Expert performance in sport* (pp. 219-251). Champaign, IL: Human Kinetics.

Williams, A.M., Ward, P., & Chapman, C. (2003). Training perceptual skill in field hockey: Is there transfer from the laboratory to the field? *Research Quarterly for Exercise and Sport, 74* (1), 98-104.

Williams, A.M., Ward, P., Knowles, J.M., & Smeeton, N. (2002). Perceptual skill in real-world tasks: Training, instruction, and transfer. *Journal of Experimental Psychology: Applied, 8* (4), 259-270.

Wine, J. (1971). Test anxiety and direction of attention. *Psychological Bulletin, 76,* 92-104.

Wink, D.M. (1993). Using questioning as a teaching strategy. *Nurse Educator, 18* (5), 11-15.

Winstein, C.J., & Schmidt, R.A. (1990). Reduced frequency of knowledge of results enhances motor skill learning. *Journal of Experimental Psychology: Learning, Memory, and Cognition, 16,* 677-691.

Wiren, G. (1991). *The PGA manual of golf.* New York: MacMillan.

Wissel, H. (1994). *Basketball: Steps to success.* Champaign, IL: Human Kinetics.

Wong-Riley, M.T.T., Hevner, R.F., Cutlan, R., Earnest, M., Egan, R., Frost J., et al. (1993). Cytochrome oxidase in the human visual cortex: Distribution in the developing and the adult brain. *Visual Neuroscience, 10,* 41-58.

Wooden, J.R. (1988). *Practical modern basketball.* New York: Wiley.

Woods, T. (2001). *How I play golf.* New York: Warner Books.

Wrisberg, C., & Liu, Z. (1991). The effect of contextual variety on practice, retention and transfer of an applied skill. *Research Quarterly for Exercise and Sport, 62* (4), 406-412.

Wulf, G., McConnel, N., Gartner, M., & Schwarz, A. (2002). Enhancing the learning of sport skills through external-focus feedback. *Journal of Motor Behaviour, 34* (2), 171-182.

Wulf, G., McNevin, N.H., Fuchs, T., Ritter, F., & Toole, T. (2000). Attentional focus in complex skill learning. *Research Quarterly for Exercise & Health, 71* (3), 229-239.

Wulf, G., McNevin, N., & Shea, C.H. (2001). The automaticity of complex motor skill learning as a function of attentional focus. *Quarterly Journal of Experimental Psychology, 54* (4), 1143-1154.

Wulf, G., Mercer, J., McNevin, N., & Gaudagnoli, M.A. (2004). Reciprocal influences of attentional focus on postural and suprapostural task performance. *Journal of Motor Behavior, 36* (2), 189-199.

Wulf, G., Prinz, W., & Hob, M. (1998). Instructions for motor learning: Differential effects of internal versus external focus of attention. *Journal of Motor Behavior, 30* (2), 169-180.

Wulf, G., Shea, C., & Park, J.H. (2001). Attention and motor performance: Preferences for and advantages of an external focus. *Research Quarterly for Exercise & Health, 72* (4), 335-344.

Zangemeister, W.H., & Stark, L. (1982). Gaze latency: Variable interaction of head and eye latency. *Experimental Neurology, 75,* 389-406.

Zelinsky, G.J., Rao, R.P.N., Hayhoe, M.M., & Ballard, D.H. (1997). Eye movements reveal the spatial temporal dynamics of visual search. *Psychological Science, 8* (6), 448-453.

ADDITIONAL QUIET-EYE AND DECISION-TRAINING RESOURCES

Quiet-Eye and Decision-Training Certification Courses

Are you interested in learning more about the quiet eye and decision training? Certification courses are available in both quiet-eye training and decision training at http://conted.ucalgary.ca/business/professionaldesignations/decision/index.html.

Quiet Eye Solutions

Quiet Eye Solutions is a program that synchronizes the gaze data collected by a mobile eye tracker with a video of the athlete's movements as taken by an external camera. A simple interface plays both videos perfectly in time, thus permitting the simultaneous coding and analysis of the individual's gaze and movements. Output is an Excel data file that can be read by most statistical and graphical programs. This data file includes the location, onset, duration, and offset of the gaze (including the quiet eye) coupled with the phases of the movement or events being performed. Quiet Eye Solutions is also a great quiet-eye training tool, as it permits the frame-by-frame viewing of vision-in-action data, as explained in this book. For information about this program, go to www.quieteyesolutions.com. In addition, this Web site presents many of the vision-in-action and decision-training videos presented in this book.

INDEX

Note: The italicized *f* and *t* following page numbers refer to figures and tables, respectively.

ABOUT THE AUTHOR

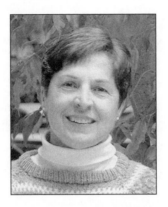

Joan N. Vickers, PhD, is a researcher who has been conducting research in gaze control and motor behavior in sport since 1980. From her research, she originated the vision-in-action method, discovered the quiet eye, and developed decision training. Vickers' work has been featured on CNN, with Alan Alda on PBS, and in *Golf Digest.* She is currently a kinesiology professor at the University of Calgary where she also provides decision training as a professional certification.

Dr. Vickers previously wrote *Instructional Design for Teaching Physical Activity,* is a reviewer for many journals, and is a member of the North American Society for Psychology of Sport and Physical Activity (NASPSPA) and other professional organizations. An internationally known speaker, she has introduced and taught decision training throughout Canada, and many sport organizations in Canada have adopted the approach.

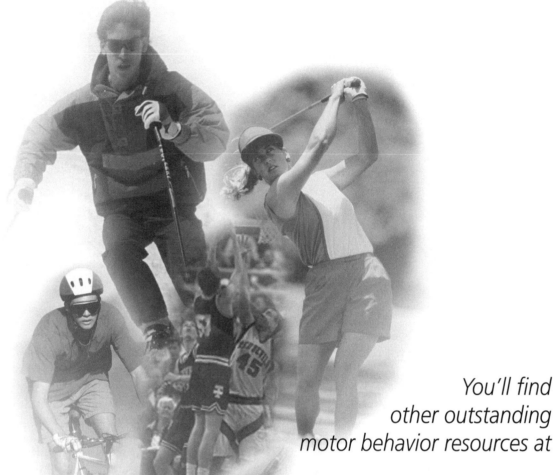

You'll find
other outstanding
motor behavior resources at

www.HumanKinetics.com

In the U.S. call

1-800-747-4457

Australia..08 8372 0999
Canada 1-800-465-7301
Europe..+44 (0) 113 255 5665
New Zealand...0800 222 062

HUMAN KINETICS
The Information Leader in Physical Activity & Health
P.O. Box 5076 • Champaign, IL 61825-5076 USA